MRI
of the Liver
A Practical Guide

MRI

of the Liver

A Practical Guide

Philip J. A. Robinson
University of Leeds
St. James's University Hospital
Leeds, U.K.

Janice Ward
St. James's University Hospital
Leeds, U.K.

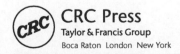

CRC Press
Taylor & Francis Group
Boca Raton London New York

CRC Press is an imprint of the
Taylor & Francis Group, an **informa** business

CRC Press
Taylor & Francis Group
6000 Broken Sound Parkway NW, Suite 300
Boca Raton, FL 33487-2742

First issued in paperback 2019

© 2001 by Taylor & Francis Group, LLC
CRC Press is an imprint of Taylor & Francis Group, an Informa business

No claim to original U.S. Government works

ISBN-13: 978-0-8247-2871-7 (hbk)
ISBN-13: 978-0-367-39075-4 (pbk)

This book contains information obtained from authentic and highly regarded sources. While all reasonable efforts have been made to publish reliable data and information, neither the author[s] nor the publisher can accept any legal responsibility or liability for any errors or omissions that may be made. The publishers wish to make clear that any views or opinions expressed in this book by individual editors, authors or contributors are personal to them and do not necessarily reflect the views/opinions of the publishers. The information or guidance contained in this book is intended for use by medical, scientific or health-care professionals and is provided strictly as a supplement to the medical or other professional's own judgement, their knowledge of the patient's medical history, relevant manufacturer's instructions and the appropriate best practice guidelines. Because of the rapid advances in medical science, any information or advice on dosages, procedures or diagnoses should be independently verified. The reader is strongly urged to consult the relevant national drug formulary and the drug companies' and device or material manufacturers' printed instructions, and their websites, before administering or utilizing any of the drugs, devices or materials mentioned in this book. This book does not indicate whether a particular treatment is appropriate or suitable for a particular individual. Ultimately it is the sole responsibility of the medical professional to make his or her own professional judgements, so as to advise and treat patients appropriately. The authors and publishers have also attempted to trace the copyright holders of all material reproduced in this publication and apologize to copyright holders if permission to publish in this form has not been obtained. If any copyright material has not been acknowledged please write and let us know so we may rectify in any future reprint.

For permission to photocopy or use material electronically from this work, please access www.copyright.com (http://www.copyright.com/) or contact the Copyright Clearance Center, Inc. (CCC), 222 Rosewood Drive, Danvers, MA 01923, 978-750-8400. CCC is a not-for-profit organization that provides licenses and registration for a variety of users. For organizations that have been granted a photocopy license by the CCC, a separate system of payment has been arranged.

Trademark Notice: Product or corporate names may be trademarks or registered trademarks, and are used only for identification and explanation without intent to infringe.

A CIP record for this book is available from the British Library.

Library of Congress Cataloging-in-Publication Data available on application

**Visit the Taylor & Francis Web site at
http://www.taylorandfrancis.com**

**and the CRC Press Web site at
http://www.crcpress.com**

Preface

MRI of the liver has come of age. After a prolonged gradual period of development, MRI is now sufficiently accessible to radiologists with an interest in hepatobiliary imaging, and MRI techniques are sufficiently stable for this practical guide to be of value. We have been privileged to obtain extensive experience of liver MRI over the last 15 years, so committing to paper the knowledge, ideas, and opinions that we have accumulated during that time has been a natural consequence of our work.

This book is aimed at clinical professionals—from any discipline—who wish to develop or to supplement an interest in the clinical applications of MRI in patients with liver disease. After the first four chapters, which relate to the clinical indications, techniques, contrast agents, and anatomic aspects of liver MRI, we have taken a broadly systematic approach to the recognition and interpretation of different liver disorders.

For us it is axiomatic that by the time a patient is referred for MRI of the liver, he or she will already have undergone first line investigations which typically include sonography and liver function tests. Each of the Chapters 5–13 are based upon the outcome of preliminary liver screening results—for example, cysts and cyst-like lesions are dealt with in Chapter 5, solid focal lesions in the non-cirrhotic liver in Chapter 6 and so on.

One of our major aims in producing this book has been to offer the reader a large number of illustrative examples of different pathologies. We have deliberately included multiple examples of some pathologies in order to indicate the potential range of appearances, including atypical as well as typical cases. Essential technical aspects of image acquisition are included in each of the "clinical" chapters, but the reader is urged to refer to Chapters 2 and 3 for a more detailed discussion of the choice of acquisition sequences and the use of contrast agents. Wherever possible we have also included a discussion of the differential diagnosis of conditions that may appear similar, and illustrative examples have been provided. This has inevitably led to some overlap between the contents of different chapters, but it has also allowed us to reduce the frequency of cross-referencing between chapters.

Well over 99% of the images illustrated here are from our own department, so we have to admit that this book presents a personal and possibly idiosyncratic view of our subject. However, presenting personal experience does allow us to be more detailed and more specific in our recommendations for technique and interpretation, and we hope this aspect will improve the practical value of this guide to the less experienced reader. For the same reasons we have not provided exhaustive references to support all the points made in the text, but instead offer a limited selected bibliography.

Finally, this book is aimed at clinical professionals who share our view that the role of the investigating diagnostician is not just to interpret a set of images put in front of her or him, but to establish what is wrong with the patient. As mentioned above, when a patient presents for liver MRI the results of the first line investigations should have crystallized the clinical question, and a careful review of the history and results of initial investigations is often helpful in guiding the interpretation of the MRI findings and assessing their significance. Particularly in patients who have already undergone treatment, it is often critical to establish the details—has the patient had previous liver surgery? if so, exactly what procedure was carried out and what is the expected residual anatomy? has the patient been treated with chemotherapy? has the patient had thermal ablation of liver lesions, and if so, how long ago? The more you know when you start, the easier it is to interpret the result of further imaging.

There is a second reason for carrying out a thorough assessment of each patient before undertaking liver MRI—that is to ensure the correct technical approach. We need to establish what exactly we are trying to discover, in order to ensure the appropriate choice of contrast agents and to select the relevant acquisition sequences. In our view, liver MRI is not a "one size fits all" technique—each patient must be assessed individually. This is not to say that there is an infinite range of technical approaches—most patients can be successfully investigated by selecting from a short menu of protocols, each comprising a set of sequences with one or more contrast agents. Obtaining good results with liver MRI are only achieved with careful attention to practical details, and a thorough study of the clinical context.

This volume could not have been created without the help and support of our staff and colleagues at St. James's University Hospital. We have enjoyed enthusiastic and productive collaboration with colleagues in hepatology, liver surgery, and pathology. We have had the continuing support of an enthusiastic group of radiographers and radiographic assistants in the MR section. We are grateful to our radiologic colleagues for their co-operation and support, particularly Dr. M.B. Sheridan and Dr. H. Woodley. Our regular collaborator Dr. J. Ashley Guthrie has generously allowed us to use a large number of his cases. Dr. Daniel Wilson has given us sustained scientific support and much helpful discussion. We would like to thank Mrs. S. Callaghan for secretarial assistance and we are particularly indebted to Mrs. S. Boyes who has spent many hours retrieving images and preparing them for publication, in addition to her help with references and typing.

Philip J. A. Robinson
Janice Ward

Contents

Part B: MRI for Characterizing Focal Lesions in the Non-Cirrhotic Liver

Part D: MRI in Metastatic Disease of the Liver

Part E: Liver MRI for Biliary Obstruction

CHAPTER 1

An Introduction to the Role of MRI in Liver Disease

A FRAME OF REFERENCE FOR APPROACHING IMAGING IN LIVER DISEASE

In order to clarify the role of different imaging techniques in investigation of liver disease, we need first to answer two questions:

1. What are the attributes of the disease or condition we suspect?
2. What are the attributes of the imaging techniques available to us?

Choosing an effective imaging approach to diagnosis then becomes a matter of matching up the expected abnormalities with the techniques most likely to detect them. If the conditions we suspect to be present are manifest by minor anatomical changes (e.g., early diagnosis of malignant tumors), we need to select imaging techniques which will best demonstrate the detailed anatomy of the area in question. Conversely, if the disorders that we suspect are manifest by physiologic changes (e.g., abnormal liver function or altered blood flow), we need to consider which imaging methods will allow us to demonstrate both the abnormality itself, and the underlying cause of the disease (e.g., elucidating the cause of portal hypertension).

RECENT DEVELOPMENTS IN MR AND OTHER IMAGING TECHNIQUES

In contrast to MR applications in the musculoskeletal and central nervous systems, the development and acceptance into widespread use of MRI for liver disease has been relatively slow. One reason is that the liver is a large organ requiring a large field of view so that the spatial resolution available is less than with the smaller fields used for brain and joint imaging. A more significant problem in the development of liver MR has been motion artifact. Although this major handicap can now be overcome using breath-hold sequences, respiratory, and cardiac gating, and various motion suppression techniques, the acquisition of good quality images requires an unflagging attention to details of technique. However, probably the major reason for the relatively slow incorporation of MRI into diagnostic imaging of the liver is the relatively high level of accuracy available with sonography and computed tomography (CT), both more widely available and less costly.

During the last two decades, technical developments have dramatically improved the quality of liver MRI. These include increases in field strength, more powerful gradients, and more sensitive receiver coils, all of which contribute to substantially improved spatial resolution in the images. Faster switching of gradient amplifiers, together with fundamental changes in pulse sequence design, have improved temporal resolution to allow acquisition of high resolution images of the entire liver volume within a single breath-hold. The improved temporal resolution also allows a more detailed analysis of perfusion characteristics using conventional extracellular fluid contrast agents, and the creation of new tissue-specific contrast media has given us the opportunity to correlate abnormal anatomy with abnormal physiology in the liver parenchyma.

During the same period, CT has progressed from single slice incremental acquisitions to helical multislice volume imaging, producing improvements in both spatial resolution and temporal resolution. Concurrent developments in sonography focused on techniques aimed at improving tissue characterization, including pulsed, and power Doppler imaging, harmonic imaging, and phase inversion imaging. The new generation of sonographic contrast agents now offer considerable improvements in the specificity of sonographic discrimination of focal liver lesions.

CURRENT CHOICES FOR IMAGING THE LIVER

In terms of 3-dimensional spatial resolution, when imaging an organ as large as the liver in ideal conditions there is little to choose between sonography, CT, and MRI. The major differences are in intrinsic contrast resolution and in temporal resolution. The advantage of improved temporal resolution is that it gives us the opportunity to visualize rapid physiological changes—in the liver this means flow in blood vessels and tissue perfusion. Although rapid sequential imaging of a single slice is available with both CT and MR ("CT fluoroscopy" and "MR Fluoroscopy"), these approaches have not received much attention for characterizing liver lesions. It is with sonography using the second generation contrast agents that the rapid flow changes in focal liver lesions have been most effectively charted. However, at the time of writing it is not yet clear how specific these characteristics will be in discriminating between various types of benign liver lesions and malignant tumors.

The advantages of MRI over sonography and CT depend on its superior contrast resolution which arises from several sources.

Firstly, whereas sonography illustrates tissue interfaces and CT records x-ray attenuation, MRI can demonstrate several different tissue characteristics, so that acquisition sequences can be chosen to enhance or isolate the features which are most likely to discriminate individual pathologies.

Secondly, MRI is unique in offering the possibility of modifying the signal characteristics of tissues in vivo—for example by frequency-selective fat suppression or water excitation techniques.

Thirdly, while the contrast agents used in CT and sonography have an intravascular/extracellular distribution similar to that of conventional MRI gadolinium agents, intracellular contrast agents are also available for use with liver MRI, giving an additional dimension to the characterization of the two main cell populations of the liver—hepatocytes and Kupffer cells.

DEFINING THE APPROPRIATE CLINICAL APPLICATIONS OF LIVER MRI

It is inappropriate to define strict or exclusive roles for each imaging technique in investigating liver disease, since local practice in each center will be influenced by the access to each type of imaging device, the availability of technical and radiological expertise, the clinical case-mix, and the established referral practices. The following outline is based on current practices at a large university hospital which is a referral center for oncology and for liver transplantation.

Sonography is the first choice imaging technique for patients presenting with upper abdominal pain, clinical jaundice or abnormal liver function tests. Sonography is also the first line procedure for investigating post-operative complications and suspected vascular abnormalities in the upper abdomen. The majority of image-guided interventions are most conveniently performed using sonography. Finally, sonography combined with alpha-fetoprotein measurement forms a regular screening procedure for patients with cirrhosis who are at risk of developing hepatocellular carcinoma.

Computed Tomography is the mainstay of imaging for staging known malignancies, and for the surveillance of cancer patients during and after treatment. CT is usually preferred for investigating patients presenting with a surgical acute abdomen, and with abdominal trauma. CT is also used as a second test when the results of sonography are unexpected, equivocal, or technically unsatisfactory.

Hepatobiliary scintigraphy is mainly used to demonstrate abnormalities of the flow of bile (leaks, fistulae, dyskinetic gallbladder, unilobar obstruction) and occasionally to investigate regional or segmental liver function.

What does this leave for MRI?
Applications of MRI largely fall into two categories:

1. **Problem Cases**—Patients with unsolved questions remaining after initial imaging, particularly:

   Is there a liver lesion?
   (a) A lesion is suspected but not definite on sonography and/or CT
   (b) Sonography and/or CT are normal, but tumor markers are raised

What is the nature of the lesion?

A focal abnormality was found on sonography and/or CT but it was not possible to characterize the lesion.

Examples include patients in whom an incidental liver lesion has been found during an examination performed for an unrelated indication, patients who are at risk of metastatic disease, and who are found to have one or more liver abnormalities of uncertain character, also patients with cirrhosis in whom sonography shows a dominant or changing nodule. In the great majority of cases MRI will eliminate the necessity for biopsy.

2. **Surgical Cases**—Patients who are candidates for liver resection, for transplantation or for non-surgical local therapies (ablation or chemoembolization) of tumors.

The last decade has seen a dramatic increase in the use of surgical resection and various ablation techniques for the treatment of malignant liver tumors. In selecting patients for treatment, we need to use the most sensitive technique available for detecting small metastases, and differentiating them from small benign liver lesions. Pre-operative mapping to show the relationships of tumors to the main vascular structures, and the anatomy of the portal circulation in cirrhotic patients who are candidates for liver transplantation, is also conveniently incorporated into the MR examination.

The results of liver MRI—Is it worthwhile?

(a) Like other workers in the field, we have found liver MRI to be more sensitive than multislice CT in detecting small metastases, particularly from colorectal cancer (1–13).

(b) Like other workers in the field, we have found liver MRI to be more specific in characterizing various benign pathologies presenting as focal abnormalities within the liver (6,7,10,12–17).

(c) Like other workers in the field, we have found MRI to be the most effective technique for the early detection and characterization of hepatocellular cancer in cirrhotic patients (18–24).

However, it must be emphasised that MRI of the liver is not a "plug, play, and walk away" technique. Obtaining good results requires consideration of the clinical question in each individual patient, appropriate choice of techniques, and contrast agents, and meticulous attention to detail in the acquisition and interpretation of the images.

Technical developments in MRI continue apace, and it is inevitable that the snapshot provided above will change in coming years. The introduction of parallel imaging and the use of 3T field strength are examples of the new technology which will no doubt impact on hepatobiliary applications of MRI in the near future. We can look forward to further improvements.

REFERENCES

1. Hagspiel KD, Neidl KF, Eichenberger AC, Weder W, Marincek B. Detection of liver metastases: comparison of superparamagnetic iron oxide-enhanced and unenhanced MR imaging at 1.5T with dynamic CT, intraoperative US, and percutaneous US. Radiology 1995; 196:471–478.
2. Huppertz A, Haraida S, Kraus A, et al. Enhancement of focal liver lesions at gadoxetic acid-enhanced MR imaging: correlation with histopathologic findings and spiral CT-initial observations. Radiology 2005; 243:468–478.
3. Kondo H, Kanematsu M, Hoshi H, et al. Preoperative detection of malignant tumors: comparison of combined methods of MR imaging with combined methods of CT. Am J Roentgenol 2000; 174:947–954.
4. Lencioni R, Della Pina C, Bruix J, et al. Clinical management of hepatic malignancies: ferucarbotran-enhanced magnetic resonance imaging versus contrast-enhanced spiral computed tomography. Dig Dis Sci 2005; 50:533–537.
5. Muller RD, Vogel K, Neumann K, et al. SPIO-MR imaging versus double-phase spiral CT in detecting malignant lesions of the liver. Acta Radiol 1999; 40:628–635.
6. Poeckler-Schoeniger C, Koepke J, Gueckel F, et al. MRI with superparamagnetic iron oxide: efficacy in the detection and characterization of focal hepatic lesions. Magn Reson Imaging 1999; 17:383–392.

7. Reimer P, Jähnke N, Fiebich M, et al. Hepatic lesion detection and characterization: value of non-enahnced MR imaging, superparamagnetic iron oxide-enhanced MR imaging and spiral CT-ROC analysis. Radiology 2000; 217:152–158.

8. Semelka RC, Cance WG, Marcos HB, Mauro MA. Liver metastases: comparison of current MR techniques and spiral CT during arterial portography for detection in 20 surgically staged cases. Radiology 1999; 213:86–91.

9. Seneterre E, Taourel P, Bouvier Y, et al. Detection of hepatic metastases: ferumoxides-enhanced MR imaging versus unenhanced MR imaging and CT during arterial portography. Radiology 1996; 200:785–792.

10. Takahama K, Amano Y, Hayashi H, et al. Detection and characterization of focal liver lesions using superparamagnetic iron oxide-enhanced magnetic resonance imaging: comparison between ferum-oxides-enhanced T1-weighted imaging and delayed-phase gadolinium-enhanced T1-weighted imaging. Abdom Imaging 2003; 28:525–530.

11. Ward J, Guthrie JA, Wilson D, et al. Colorectal hepatic metastases: detection with SPIO-enhanced breath-hold MR imaging—comparison of optimized sequences. Radiology 2003; 228:709–718.

12. Ward J, Naik KS, Guthrie JA, et al. Hepatic lesion detection: comparison of MR imaging after the administration of superparamagnetic iron oxide with dual-phase CT by using alternative-free response receiver operating characteristic analysis. Radiology 1999; 210:459–466.

13. Ward J, Robinson PJ, Guthrie JA, et al. Liver metastases in candidates for hepatic resection: comparison of helical CT and gadolinium- and SPIO-enhanced MR imaging. Radiology 2005; 237:170–180.

14. Hawighorst H, Schoenberg S, Knopp MV, et al. Hepatic lesions: morphologic and functional characterization with multiphase breath-hold 3D gadolinium-enhanced MR angiography—initial results. Radiology 1999; 210:89–96.

15. Ito K, Mitchell DG. Imaging diagnosis of cirrhosis and chronic hepatitis. Intervirology 2004; 47:134–143.

16. Low RN. MR imaging of the liver using gadolinium chelates. In: MR Imaging of the liver 1: techniques and contrast agents. Magn Reson Imaging Clin N Am 2001:717–743.

17. Ward J, Robinson PJ. Combined use of MR contrast agents for evaluating liver disease. Magn Reson Imaging Clin N Am 2001; 9:767–802.

18. Burrel M, Llovet JM, Ayuso C, et al. Barcelona clinic liver cancer group. MRI angiography is superior to helical CT for detection of HCC prior to liver transplantation: an explant correlation. Hepatology 2003; 38:1034–1042.

19. Ichikawa T. MRI in the evaluation of hepatocellular nodules: role of pulse sequences and contrast agents. Intervirology 2004; 47:252–270.

20. Kwak HS, Lee JM, Kim CS. Preoperative detection of hepatocellular carcinoma: comparison of combined contrast-enhanced MR imaging and combined CT during arterial portography and CT hepatic arteriography. Eur Radiol 2004; 14:447–457.

21. Oi H, Murakami T, Kim T, et al. Dynamic MR imaging and early-phase helical CT for detecting small intrahepatic metastases of hepatocellular carcinoma. Am J Roentgenol 1996; 166:369–374.

22. Rode A, Bancel B, Douek P, et al. Small nodule detection in cirrhotic livers: evaluation with US, spiral CT, and MR and correlation with pathologic examination of explanted liver. J Comput Assist Tomogr 2001; 25:327–336.

23. Ward J, Guthrie JA, Scott DJ, et al. Hepatocellular carcinoma in the cirrhotic liver: double-contrast MR imaging for diagnosis. Radiology 2000; 216:154–162.

24. Yamamoto H, Yamashita Y, Yoshimatsu S, et al. Hepatocellular carcinoma in cirrhotic livers: detection with unenhanced and iron oxide-enhanced MR imaging. Radiology 1995; 195:106–112.

CHAPTER 2

Techniques for MRI of the Liver

T he success of liver MR is primarily dependent on technique and the optimization of pulse sequences. We aim to achieve high lesion-to-liver contrast, avoid motion artifact, and use MR contrast agents appropriately. Fast breathhold sequences with both T1 and T2 weighting are now routine, and motion induced artifacts which hampered the success of abdominal imaging for so long are no longer a significant problem. Fast spin echo (FSE) techniques facilitate high quality breathhold T2w imaging while faster gradient echo (GRE) sequences allow rapid T1w imaging with higher resolution matrixes and thinner effective slice thickness (Fig. 1).

GRADIENTS, SAMPLING FREQUENCY, BANDWITH, AND ECHO TIME (TE)

Imaging speed and spatial resolution are influenced by gradient performance. Both gradient strength and the time taken to achieve maximum gradient amplitude (rise time) are important. Recent developments in gradient coil design and technology have resulted in the routine use of gradients with a maximum strength of 30–40 mT/m, approximately three times the strength of those previously used (standard gradient strength typically 10–15 mT/m). Gradient rise times have also been substantially reduced to approximately 200 µsec (traditionally approximately 600 µsec).

Increasing the speed of scanning is generally achieved at the expense of signal to noise ratio (SNR) but this is largely compensated by the use of body phased array coils. Refinements in gradient technology have enabled rapid imaging without compromising SNR. With 2D imaging, high performance gradients can allow a shorter TE (enabling more slices for a given TR) at a fixed bandwidth, or a narrower bandwidth giving better SNR for the same TE. With 3D imaging they enable shorter TRs which allow more slices or better resolution for a given acquisition time. Receiver bandwidth is an important determinant of SNR. The bandwidth represents the range of frequencies contained within the MR signal and determines the rate at which an echo is sampled. TE is determined by the duration of the dephasing lobe of the readout gradient and the length of acquisition, with maximum signal amplitude of the echo occurring when the amount of rephasing equals dephasing. With a low bandwidth sequence the echo is sampled at a lower sampling frequency for longer. This results in high SNR but the center of the echo occurs later, TE is longer and fewer slices are available for a given TR. TE may be shortened by increasing the gradient amplitude and sampling at a higher frequency for less time (high bandwidth sequence) but then because more frequencies are being sampled there is more noise in the resultant image (Fig. 2). Although the sampling rate is fixed for a particular bandwidth, high performance gradients enable more rapid sampling at lower bandwidths because the dephasing gradient is applied at higher amplitude for less time, thus shortening the duration of image acquisition and TE. Also, because gradient rise time is much faster, the time to maximum signal amplitude occurs sooner, which further reduces TE while maintaining SNR. Further shortening of the TE at the same bandwidth may be achieved with the use of asymmetric echoes. By reducing either the duration or amplitude of the dephasing gradient the echo occurs towards the start of data acquisition instead of the center (Fig. 3). Although TE is shorter there is an overall decrease in SNR because only part of the echo is sampled; the degree of asymmetry determines how much of K space is filled, and the remainder is encoded with zero filling. Although low bandwidths are recommended for use with GRE sequences, they are generally not suitable for use with FSE sequences. As bandwidth decreases, echo spacing increases and this adversely effects image quality. With longer echo spacing, blurring, susceptibility, and edge-related artifacts are more pronounced, so with most FSE sequences the shortest possible echo spacing commensurate with adequate SNR is automatically implemented. Given the typically elliptical shape of the body outline, a rectangular field of view (FOV) may also be used to shorten acquisition times. With this technique the square raw data matrix is sampled unequally with fewer data points sampled in the phase encoding direction. If the increment between each phase-encoding step is doubled, FOV is halved. Since both the FOV and the number of phase-encoding steps is halved, pixel size in the phase encoding direction and therefore spatial resolution is unchanged. A 75% FOV is suitable for most patients but varies depending on patient shape. The technique incurs a small reduction in SNR because only part of K space is sampled.

PARALLEL ACQUISITION TECHNIQUES

Parallel imaging techniques further reduce scan time or allow higher resolution images to be obtained in the same time as conventional images (Fig. 4). With parallel imaging, spatial information from the different receiver channels of a multi-coil array is used to replace a proportion of the lines of K space and speed up acquisition time. Although the whole of K space is measured in a conventional fashion, the spacing in between the lines of K space is increased, so fewer echoes are measured and scan times are reduced without compromising spatial resolution. With conventional scanning fold-over may occur when the spacing between the lines of K space is increased to reduce FOV (Fig. 5). Parallel imaging eliminates wrap artifact either by using the coil sensitivities to "unfold" the image (e.g., SENSE) or by using the coil sensitivities to generate the missing lines of K space (e.g., SMASH/GRAPPA) to increase the FOV and eliminate fold-over. All the above parallel imaging techniques require some estimation of the individual coil sensitivities. These sensitivity maps are acquired either prior to, or during parallel image acquisition by acquiring a small number of calibration K space lines during the actual scan. The scan time in general, is reduced in proportion to the number of coil elements within the multi-coil array. Good image quality is currently achievable with scan time reductions of $\times 2$ to $\times 4$, but further reduction of scan time requires specialized hardware. The decrease in acquisition time is at the expense of SNR, which is reduced by approximately the square root of the scan time reduction factor.

REDUCING BREATHING ARTIFACT

Assuming an acceptable level of tissue contrast, the suppression of motion artifact is probably the most important determinant of diagnostic efficacy. Respiratory gating techniques are widely used to compensate for motion artifact but with mixed success. Gating techniques adequately suppress motion in patients who have a regular breathing pattern but artifacts remain severe when breathing is erratic (Fig. 6). Also, image acquisition always occurs at the same point of the respiratory cycle, typically end-expiration, so significant time penalties are incurred. The most effective way to eliminate motion is to use rapid imaging in conjunction with breathholding. Several studies have shown that breathhold versions of traditionally used sequences provide superior image quality and lesion detection at least as good as non-breathhold versions. Most patients are able to achieve repeated 20-second breathholds following a brief rehearsal using hyperventilation techniques. Wherever possible we image during suspended end-expiration to improve reproducibility and we instruct the patients to breath in and out twice before the "breath in, breath out, and hold" command. In some patients we have also found that coaching them to bear down in a Valsalva-type manoeuvre is beneficial. If patients find suspended inspiration easier to maintain they are instructed to perform comparable respiratory excursions for each breathhold to avoid mis-registration. Oxygen administration also improves the success rate with patients whose breathholding capacity is limited.

Recently introduced navigator pulses allow images free of motion artifacts to be acquired during free breathing. With this technique a small-boxed region of interest is placed over the diaphragm and a low-resolution GRE sequence is repeatedly implemented. The sequence employs a low flip angle to minimize saturation and the sharp change in the signal intensity of the lungs and liver along the axis of the box is used to determine the position of the diaphragm. An acceptance window is calculated from the preliminary pre-scan data after which the gated acquisition begins. The navigator detects the position of the diaphragm prior to each subsequent slice acquisition and imaging is only initiated when the diaphragm falls within the acceptance window. For this reason it is important to encourage patients to maintain a regular breathing pattern throughout the procedure. The effectiveness of the navigator is reduced if breathing is shallow or if the position of the diaphragm falls outside the acceptance window. Navigator techniques are faster and more robust than conventional gating methods. Typically the navigator adds only around 30 msec to each slice acquisition and respiratory belts are not needed. Navigator pulses also eliminate mis-registration and allow the correct anatomical alignment of sequential slices when multiple single slices are obtained during a single acquisition (Fig. 7). They also allow high-resolution non-breathhold images to be acquired over several minutes without motion artifact (Fig. 8).

REDUCING GHOSTING AND FLOW ARTIFACTS

Motion-induced ghost artifacts have the same configuration as the moving structure they arise from, and they always occur in the phase-encoding direction. In most patients breathholding effectively eliminates artifacts from structures such as the gallbladder or anterior abdominal wall, but pre-saturation or gradient motion rephasing (GMR) techniques are necessary to eliminate ghosting from vascular structures (Fig. 9). Flow artifacts may arise from any vessel but those from the aorta are usually more pronounced. They are readily identified because they occur at regular intervals along the phase encoding axis. The distance between the ghosts increases with increasing TR and they are more pronounced at longer TEs because more time is available for motion to occur. When the phase- and frequency-encoding directions are exchanged, the orientation of the artifact will also change (Fig. 10). With GMR, additional gradient lobes added to the standard dephasing and rephasing lobes of the slice select and readout gradients before the echo is sampled, compensate in advance for motion-induced phase shifts that occur between excitation and echo sampling. Because more time is needed to utilise the additional gradient lobes, GMR techniques—although effective—are only feasible with sequences using relatively longer TE. Use of a higher bandwidth will reduce the minimum TE feasible with GMR but at the expense of SNR. Regardless of TE, pre-saturation pulses positioned above and below the region of interest are also effective (Fig. 11). Their implementation will, however, reduce the number of slices available for a given scan time with 2D imaging or increase the TR for 3D imaging.

SUSCEPTIBILITY

Susceptibility artifacts are caused by a local distortion of the magnetic field due to the close proximity of objects or substances (mainly metallic foreign bodies and air) which are susceptible to the induction of magnetization. The severity of susceptibility artifacts is pulse sequence dependent. The 180° refocusing pulse of spin echo sequences reduces susceptibility by correcting dephasing and this is particularly effective on FSE sequences with a long echo train, due to the incorporation of multiple 180° refocusing pulses. Because of this, FSE sequences are relatively insensitive to this type of artifact. Susceptibility is also less pronounced at shorter TEs because there is less time for dephasing to occur (Fig. 12). GRE sequences are particularly sensitive to susceptibility artifact because they have no 180° refocusing pulse, but the artifact is minimized when very short TE is used.

CHEMICAL SHIFT

There are two types of chemical shift artifact, described as first order (caused by misregistration) and second order (caused by phase cancellation).

First-Order Chemical Shift

Fat protons resonate at a slightly lower frequency than water protons (with a difference of approximately 3.5 parts per million at 1.5T). In tissues where fat and water protons are adjacent, frequency encoding errors occur because the signal from the fat protons has a slightly lower frequency than that from the water protons. Since the spatial location of the MR signal in the frequency-encode direction is determined from the signal frequency, the fat protons are registered at a slightly different position to that of the water protons, and so are misregistered in the direction of the weaker end of the readout gradient. This results in an image in which the signals from fat have a different location to those of water, producing artifactual high and low signal bands at anatomic sites where watery and fatty tissues (e.g., kidney and perinephric fat) are in contact (Fig. 13). The degree of chemical shift misregistration increases with greater field strength and reduced sampling bandwidth. The artifact may be considerably smaller with a high bandwidth technique but this is achieved at the expense of SNR. However, chemical shift is effectively eliminated with all types of fat suppression.

Second-Order Chemical Shift

Because of their slightly different resonant frequencies, fat and water protons can be in- or out-of-phase with each other at different echo times on GRE images. At 1.5T, fat and water are in phase at TEs of 4.4 msecs and 8.8 msecs etc., and out of phase at 2.2 msecs, 6.6 msecs etc. With spin echo imaging the signals from fat and water are always in phase. When fat and water protons co-exist within a voxel their opposed phases cancel each other, producing a loss of signal. This is manifest as an edge artifact at the fat/water interface on opposed-phase (OP) GRE images (Fig. 14). The artifact is not a feature of spin-echo sequences or in-phase GRE images and again it is effectively eliminated with fat suppression. With very large or exophytic tumors, the fat/water cancellation artifact on opposed-phase T1w images is often helpful in determining the organ of origin and involvement of adjacent structures (Fig. 15). While the presence of an intact edge artifact between a mass and adjacent organs reliably excludes invasion, a disrupted artifact is suggestive of involvement (Fig. 15).

FAT SUPPRESSION

Fat suppression strategies are strongly recommended for abdominal imaging. They eliminate ghosting artifact from the high signal of fat on T2w FSE (Fig. 16) images and increase image contrast which accentuates gadolinium enhancement. For 2D imaging the authors routinely use a fat suppression technique which selectively excites water protons using a binomial pulse sequence. Compared with the standard frequency-selective method of fat suppression, this approach is more efficient and less sensitive to radiofrequency inhomogeneities. Consequently, more slices can be obtained for a given acquisition time and fat suppression is more homogeneous. A simple 1:1 binomial pulse sequence uses two short RF pulses of equal amplitude. The first pulse tips all spins by 45° after which a gap (2.2 msec at 1.5T) is left for fat and water protons to become out-of-phase with each other. The second RF pulse then tips the water protons over by another 45° into the transverse plane but because the fat protons are pointing in the opposite direction they are tipped back 45° towards the z-axis so only the water component generates signal (Fig. 17). Although the 2.2 msec gap and the use of two RF pulses results in a longer excitation time than a simple non-selective pulse sequence, the standard spectral fat-suppression method has an even longer excitation time since the duration of the fat-sat pulse is approximately 10 msec.

T2-WEIGHTED IMAGING

FSE sequences have replaced CSE for T2w imaging because they allow better resolution for a given acquisition time, or can use a shorter acquisition time to allow breathhold imaging. With FSE, multiple 180° refocusing pulses generate a train of echoes after each 90° excitation pulse. Compared with conventional SE, FSE sequences achieve a reduction in scan time which is proportional to echo train length (the number of phase-encoding lines acquired per TR). Contrast in FSE is manipulated by the ordering of K space. Although each echo is acquired with a different TE, the central lines of K space (i.e., the lowest ordered phase encoded steps), which determine image contrast are acquired at the time of the "effective" TE (TEeff). Theoretically TEeff may be assigned to any echo in the echo train although the degree of user flexibility varies between vendors. The low order phase encoding signals are obtained when the phase encoding gradient has the smallest amplitude so there is only minimal dephasing of the echo and signal is maximized. Traditionally, T2w images have been regarded as the most useful for depicting pathology, but liver-to-lesion contrast decreases as echo train length increases, and this has resulted in a rather poor detection rate for solid lesions on T2w FSE images (Fig. 18). The lower liver/lesion contrast with FSE is multi-factorial. Firstly, normal liver has a comparatively short T2 relaxation time of approximately 40 msec, probably due to hepatic iron stores and other paramagnetic substances which induce signal loss due to diffusion in adjacent water molecules. Metastases, hemangiomas and simple cysts have T2 relaxation times of approximately 80 msec, 160 msec and 240 msec respectively. Although cysts and hemangiomas are well seen on FSE, the inherent contrast between metastases and normal liver is relatively poor. Moreover FSE sequences are fairly insensitive to susceptibility so the signal intensity of the normal liver is slightly higher than with conventional SE. Secondly, FSE is influenced by magnetization transfer (MT) which causes solid tissues to lose signal intensity (tumor tissue is particularly affected) so lesion/liver contrast is further reduced. Fluid is unaffected by MT, so benign lesions are well shown on FSE (Fig. 19). Although MT occurs to some extent in all multislice techniques, the 180° off-resonance pulses in FSE significantly increase MT compared with conventional SE sequences. Restricted protons bound to macromolecules resonate over a much larger frequency range than free water. An RF pulse applied (on resonance) to a particular imaging section will act as an off-resonance pulse to other imaging sections in a multi-section acquisition and saturate the restricted pool. The saturation is transferred to adjacent mobile water protons and a net loss of signal occurs. Solid lesions have a large number of restricted protons and show large magnetization transfer effects compared to normal liver (Fig. 20). In general as echo train length increases (i.e., with more 180° refocusing pulses) MT effects increase, and lesion/liver contrast decreases even further. Gradient echo sequences are less affected by MT. MT effects and therefore lesion/liver contrast may be improved by reducing echo train length, but the longer acquisition time then necessitates respiratory gating to minimize motion artifacts. FSE sequences are also subject to blurring from tissues with short T2. Late echoes subject to pronounced T2 decay have a lower signal amplitude than echoes acquired at the start of data acquisition. For this reason it is important to minimize echo spacing as much as possible. Also the increased signal intensity of fat on FSE (due to a phenomenon known as J-coupling) increases motion artifact, so fat suppression is strongly recommended with FSE (Fig. 16). Effective echo times of 80–100 msec will maximize image contrast for lesion detection.

GREATER T2 WEIGHTING

More heavily T2w images are necessary to distinguish non-solid benign and malignant hepatic lesions. To avoid overlap between the signal intensity characteristics of solid lesions (particularly hypervascular metastases) and hemangiomas on standard T2w FSE images, TE must be increased to approximately 180 msec. At even longer echo times, hemangiomas—which have a T2 relaxation time of approximately 160 msec—start to lose their signal and mimic metastases (Fig. 21). Breathhold FSE sequences are suitable for characterizing lesions because the strong MT effects which effect only solid tumors accentuate the difference in the signal intensity between benign and malignant lesions.

SINGLE SHOT FSE SEQUENCES

With single shot FSE (SSFSE) techniques multiple echoes which fill the whole of K space are acquired after a single excitation pulse. Consequently scan times are extremely short with measurement times for a single image of approximately one-second. Since the excitation pulse is not repeated, SSFSE sequences do not have a true repetition time i.e., TR is "infinite". The denoted TR here is the acquisition time of a single slice and this is directly influenced by the number of phase encoding lines. Single shot FSE (SSFSE) sequences with partial Fourier techniques (e.g., half Fourier acquisition single shot fast spin echo [HASTE]) are particularly effective in distinguishing benign and malignant lesions. With the HASTE technique just over half of K space is encoded with a single echo train and the remainder filled with half Fourier transformation. Images are obtained in less than a second with virtually no motion artifact even during free breathing so HASTE is particularly useful in uncooperative patients. This is a single slice technique so MT effects are less significant, but because the duration of the echo train (approximately 400 msecs) is considerably longer than the T2 relaxation time of solid liver lesions (approximately 80 msecs), there is relatively little signal from short T2 tissues by the end of image acquisition. Conversely, tissues with a longer T2 exhibit a much higher signal and are well seen. Also, while blurring of short T2 tissues maybe particularly pronounced on HASTE, tissues with a longer T2 are generally well-defined. This results in improved sharpness and conspicuity of cysts and small fluid collections (Fig. 22). Edge definition is enhanced by using a high acquisition matrix, and also improves when the effective TE approaches the end of the echo train (long effective TE sequence) so that the high spatial frequencies which determine edge definition are collected at the earlier echoes. At our institution we use HASTE images at a TE of approximately 100 msecs to characterize focal liver lesions because motion artifacts are consistently negligible regardless of patient co-operation and non-solid benign lesions have a crisp well-defined edge (Fig. 23). However, HASTE is limited by a low SNR compared with standard FSE sequences, such that small low-contrast lesions are not well shown. Heavily T2w SSFSE (full Fourier) with TE of ≥500 msecs, and HASTE (half-Fourier) sequences are used to image the fluid filled biliary tree for MR cholangiopancreatography. Thick-slab SSFSE with a slab thickness of 30–80 mm and thin-slice multi-slice HASTE images have a complementary role. Thick-slab images are obtained with an extremely long TE to provide complete suppression of background tissue and an overview of bile duct anatomy, while thin-slice HASTE images with a slice thickness of 2–4 mm are obtained at a more moderate TE of approximately 100 msec to improve the visualization of fine structures since small caliber structures may be obscured with longer TE (Fig. 24).

STIR SEQUENCES

FSE-short tau inversion recovery (STIR) imaging is a valuable alternative to FSE for lesion detection. Breathhold FSE STIR has been shown to be superior to CSE and non-breathhold STIR for the detection of hepatic tumors. With STIR the inversion time is chosen to null the signal from fat and image contrast is provided by the additive effects of T1 and T2. Compared with a standard chemical shift saturation pulse, fat suppression on STIR is generally more homogeneous; at 1.5T an inversion time of approximately 150 msecs is optimum. Standard STIR is characterized by a fairly short TE (approximately 30 msecs) to maximize both the SNR and the number of slices obtained with a given TR. With FSE STIR, longer TEs are feasible without incurring time penalties, so allowing a greater T2 contribution in the images, which should improve the conspicuity of abnormalities. The combination of fat suppression and combined T1 and T2 effects with FSE STIR results in greater soft tissue contrast and increased lesion conspicuity (Fig. 25). However, because this is a breathhold sequence with a long echo train, MT effects are still a limitation and relatively fewer slices per breathhold are possible due to the initial 180° inversion pulse. One should also be aware that the signal of other substances such as melanin or proteinacious fluid which have T1 relaxation times similar to fat may also be suppressed on STIR. Breathhold STIR may also be used to characterize lesions. As with other types of heavily T2-weighted imaging, non-solid benign lesions are typically homogeneous and markedly hyperintense with crisply defined borders.

HYBRID SEQUENCES

Turbo gradient spin echo (TGSE) or gradient-recalled spin echo (GRASE) sequences combine echo planar (EPI) and FSE techniques. All echoes are gradient refocused with EPI whereas with FSE they are refocused spin echoes. With TGSE techniques, gradient echoes are generated before and after each spin echo. Image contrast results from the spin echo component of the sequence while the gradient echoes contribute only to resolution. Compared with FSE, TGSE is more efficient, MT effects are less and the high signal intensity of fat is less pronounced. However, image quality is variable due to degradation by motion and susceptibility artifacts. The EPI component (the number of gradient echoes) of the sequence is extremely sensitive to phase errors and variations in magnetic field homogeneity and at the longer EPI factors required for breathhold imaging artifacts maybe severe (Fig. 26). When TGSE is implemented with a shorter EPI factor, artifacts are reduced and lesion to liver contrast is improved compared with FSE (Fig. 27). However longer acquisition times prohibit breathholding and efficient respiratory gating is required to minimize motion artifact.

TRUE FISP/BALANCED FFE SEQUENCES

True fast imaging with steady state precession (True FISP, Siemens) or balanced fast field echo (FFE, Philips) sequences have the highest signal of all steady state sequences. The technique employs balanced gradients in all three axes at the time of radiofrequency excitation which compensate for motion-induced phase shifts. Although the contrast here is a function of T1 divided by T2, high contrast images which are essentially T2-weighted are generated. As with any steady-state free precession technique, both transverse and longitudinal magnetization contribute to the signal. True FISP is useful in patients who are unable to breathhold because each slice is acquired in approximately one second. It provides an excellent and quick anatomical survey, and is particularly useful for demonstrating vessels and lymphadenopathy (Fig. 28). Limitations include a sensitivity to magnetic field inhomogeneities which may result in fairly severe artifact, and low liver/tumor contrast (Fig. 29). True FISP is an out-of-phase GRE sequence so it is fairly sensitive to fatty infiltration. If severe, this produces an abnormally low liver signal on True FISP images, and occasionally an edge artifact at the interface between the liver parenchyma and the intra-hepatic vessels (Fig. 30). In milder cases of fat deposition, no signal change will be discernible on True FISP images since the signal intensity of normal liver is already low.

T2-WEIGHTED GRE

Contrast-to-noise ratio in the liver is generally poor on long TE GRE images. However, because T2*-weighted images are sensitive to susceptibility they are useful for depicting iron deposition in siderotic nodules, haemochromatosis, and the breakdown products of resolving hematomas (Fig. 31). They are also recommended for detecting focal lesions following the injection of superparamagnetic iron oxide particles (SPIO) but parameters must be optimized to minimize noise, to maximize the signal from solid lesions, and to minimize motion-related artifact which may be greater at longer TEs (Fig. 32). A detailed description of this pulse sequence can be found in chapter 3.

T1-WEIGHTED IMAGING

Contrary to early experience we now find that many lesions are better seen on T1w than on T2w images (Fig. 33). Gradient echo sequences are routinely used for T1w imaging because gradient refocusing of echoes is simpler and more efficient than radio frequency refocusing. Shorter TEs and more slices for a given TR are achieved with gradient echo sequences than with otherwise comparable SE sequences. With multi-section spoiled GRE sequences (e.g., FLASH, Siemens; SPGR, IGE; FFE, Philips) the entire liver is imaged in a single breathhold with high SNR and minimum inter-slice spacing. For 2D imaging TRs of 100–200 msec facilitate acquisition times short enough for breathholding with maximum SNR. TE should be kept as short as possible to maximize the number of available slices and minimize T2 influence, and a flip angle of 70–90° is chosen to provide optimum T1 contrast (Fig. 34).

CHEMICAL SHIFT IMAGING

Providing fat and water co-exist within a voxel, opposed-phase T1w GRE images are very sensitive to the fat content of tissues. This is particularly useful in liver imaging where the combination of in-phase (IP) and opposed-phase (OP) GRE images (chemical shift imaging) provides a reliable diagnosis of focal or diffuse fatty infiltration. The normal liver has the same signal intensity on IP and OP GRE images and it is always greater than the signal intensity of the spleen. Fatty and non-fatty liver have the same signal on IP images but on OP images the fatty liver shows a reduced signal intensity which may be equal to or less than that of the spleen (Fig. 35). We obtain IP and OP images in all patients undergoing liver MR because they are sensitive to quite small degrees of fatty infiltration. Chemical shift imaging also aids lesion characterization by demonstrating fat within tumors (see chapter. 7). In patients with a fatty liver, lesions may be isointense with the lower signal of fatty liver on OP images but lesion-to-liver contrast is greater on IP images (Fig. 36). Chemical shift imaging is also able to distinguish signal loss due to fatty liver from signal loss caused by excess iron deposition and to confirm the presence of surgical clips which may otherwise be wrongly interpreted as pathology (Fig. 37). Signal loss due to metal is caused by susceptibility effects which become more pronounced with increasing TE. In general in-phase TE is longer than opposed-phase TE so signal loss due to iron excess or clips is more pronounced on IP T1.

IP and OP images may be acquired together as part of a multi-echo technique in which two echoes per excitation pulse are acquired simultaneously. This approach avoids misregistration and facilitates the exact replication of anatomical structures at each TE. However, SNR may be reduced because the acquisition of two echoes in a breathhold necessitates the use of a higher bandwidth compared with a single echo sequence (see also chapter 7).

DYNAMIC GADOLINIUM-ENHANCED IMAGING

Effective imaging with extracellular space gadolinium-based contrast agents requires rapid sequential acquisitions at various critical time points after bolus injection. A T1-weighted GRE sequence with the shortest possible TE should be used to maximize the number of slices in order to obtain sufficient anatomic coverage in a breathhold. 2D spoiled GRE sequences have been widely used and have an established record of success but they are limited by relatively thick sections and inter-section gaps. Coverage of the entire liver in acquisition times short enough for breathholding comes at the expense of reduced spatial resolution and partial volume averaging which may limit the diagnosis of sub-cm lesions. The introduction of fast 3D T1w GRE sequences has overcome many of the problems associated with 2D sequences. 3D imaging methods give a higher SNR and thinner effective slice thickness than 2D methods, with no inter-slice gap or crosstalk. Combined with interpolation algorithms to facilitate high resolution matrices and the repeated application of fat suppression pulses, current 3D GRE sequences facilitate high resolution dynamic Gd-enhanced imaging with improved contrast resolution and superior depiction of small tumors. Flexible parameters allow scan times to be adjusted to accommodate the breathholding capacity of individual patients. Additionally parameters may be manipulated to produce isotropic voxels for optimal 3D reconstruction (Fig. 38). Isotropic resolution is achieved at the expense of anatomic coverage but this is largely overcome by parallel imaging techniques. In most patients a parallel imaging factor of two enables breathhold isotropic imaging of the whole liver in approximately 20 seconds. 3D T1w GRE sequences are obtained with minimum TR and TE to maximize the number of image sections for a given time. With short TEs, magnetic susceptibility artifacts are less apparent because there is less time for signal loss to occur. Minimum TEs also result in opposed-phase images which have a signal cancellation artifact at fat/water interfaces that may reduce the conspicuity of small abnormalities, particularly near the liver surface. The fat suppression pulse is an essential addition to this technique because it eliminates the fat/water cancellation artifact and accentuates gadolinium enhancement. A flip angle of approximately 15° minimizes the saturation of stationary tissues for the simultaneous display of liver parenchyma and hepatic vessels (Fig. 39) while a flip angle of 25° or more is used for dedicated MR angiography (Fig. 40). A more detailed description of 3D T1w GRE sequences for dynamic Gd-enhanced imaging is provided in chapter 3. Rapid 3D T1w GRE sequences may be used for any application requiring gadolinium enhancement. They are particularly helpful in distressed patients who are unable to stay still for higher resolution imaging with longer scan times (Fig. 41).

IMAGING THE NON-COMPLIANT PATIENT

Magnetization-prepared GRE sequences generate T1w images in less than a second with a reasonable SNR and minimum motion artifact even during free breathing. This approach is extremely valuable in patients who have difficulty breathholding but is not generally recommended for routine liver imaging because SNR is reduced and image contrast is less reliable than with multi-slice spoiled GRE techniques. Also, since this is a single slice technique, timing image acquisition to coincide with arrival of the gadolinium bolus in the tissue of interest is more difficult because timing will vary from slice to slice. The preparation and acquisition of each individual slice takes approximately one second and is completed before the next slice is acquired, so a stack of sequential slices is selected to encompass the whole liver. Typically 128 lines of K space are measured per slice. Magnetization-prepared GRE sequences comprise an initial 180° inversion pulse followed by a delay [the inversion time (TI)] and a standard spoiled GRE sequence which employs a small flip angle and a short TR and TE. Image contrast is determined by the preparatory phase and depends primarily on the effective TI, which is the time from application of the 180° pulse to acquisition of the central phase encoding lines. As with all inversion recovery sequences, different inversion times can be selected to suppress the signal from specific tissues and vary T1 contrast. A non-slice selective inversion pulse produces consistent image contrast across all slices providing the TR is long enough to allow sufficient recovery of the longitudinal magnetization between each inversion pulse (Fig. 42).

In patients who are unable to perform repeated breathholds, we obtain sequential True FISP and HASTE images during free breathing with navigator pulses applied to the HASTE sequence to eliminate mis-registration. A stack of magnetization-prepared GRE T1w images are then obtained before and at the arterial, portal and equilibrium phases after a bolus injection of gadolinium (Fig. 43). More delayed T1w images are obtained in selective cases. We use a low-resolution version of the same sequence for test bolusing with gadolinium. For more details of the test bolus technique see chapter 3.

ILLUSTRATIVE FIGURES

Gradients, sampling, frequency, bandwidth, and echo time (TE)—Figures 1–3
Parallel acquisition techniques—Figures 4, 5
Reduced breathing artifact—Figures 6–8
Reduced ghosting and flow artifacts—Figures 9–11
Susceptibility—Figure 12
Chemical shift—Figures 13–15
Fat suppression—Figures 16, 17
T2-weighted imaging—Figures 18–20
Greater T2 weighting—Figure 21
Single shot FSE sequences—Figures 22–24
STIR sequences—Figure 25
Hybrid sequences—Figures 26, 27
True FISP/balanced FFE sequences—Figures 28–30
T2-weighted GRE—Figures 31, 32
T1-weighted imaging—Figures 33, 34
Chemical shift imaging—Figures 35–37
Dynamic gadolinium-enhanced imaging—Figures 38–41
Imaging the non-compliant patient—Figures 42, 43

REFERENCES

1. Mitchell DG. MRI Principles. Philadelphia: W.B. Saunders, 1999.
2. Elster AD. Questions and answers in Magnetic Resonance Imaging. St. Louis, Missouri: Mosby, 1994.
3. Morrin MM, Rofsky NM. Techniques for liver MR imaging. Magn Reson Imaging Clin N Am 2001; 9:675–696.
4. Lee VS, Lavelle MT, Krinksy GA, Rofsy NM. Volumetric MR imaging of the liver and applications. Magn Reson Imaging Clin N Am 2001; 9:697–716.
5. Regan F. Clinical applications of half-fourier (HASTE) MR sequences in abdominal imaging. Magn Reson Imaging Clin N Am 1999; 7:275–288.
6. Barish MA, Jara H. Motion artifact control in body MR imaging. Magn Reson Imaing Clin N Am 1999; 7:289–302.
7. Blaimer M, Breuer F, Mueller M, Heidmann RM, Griswold MA, Jakob PM. SMASH, SENSE, PILS, GRAPPA: how to choose the optimal method. Top Magn Reson Imaging 2004; 15:223–236.
8. Margolis DJ, Bammer R, Chow LC. Parallel imaging of the abdomen. Top Magn Reson Imaging 2004; 15:197–206.

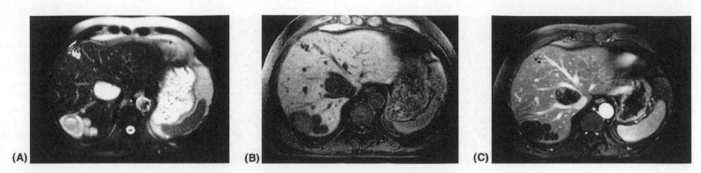

Figure 1. *Image quality*:   Breathhold T1w and T2w images in a patient with multiple metastases illustrating the typical image quality of current MR pulse sequences. Sub-second HASTE (**A**) and 3D T1w GRE (VIBE) images before (**B**) and after (**C**) gadolinium showed multiple lesions of varying size with high lesion/liver contrast and negligible motion artifact.

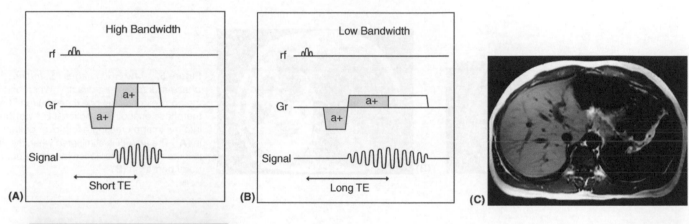

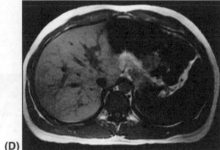

Figure 2. *Influence of receiver bandwidth on signal to noise*:   The readout gradient may be applied at a higher or lower sampling frequency (high or low bandwidth sequences). With a high bandwidth, the readout gradient (shown above the line) has twice the area (a+) of the dephasing gradient (shown below the line) and the peak of the echo occurs when the amount of rephasing equals dephasing (i.e., when the areas a+ are equal). With a lower bandwidth, there is less noise in the image because fewer frequencies are sampled but it takes longer to sample the echo, so echo time is increased (**B**). In this example, as sampling bandwidth is increased from 200 Hz/pixel on (**C**) to 380 Hz/pixel on (**D**) SNR decreases due to more noise in the higher bandwidth image.

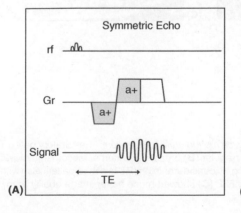

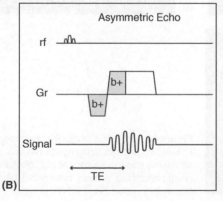

Figure 3. *Asymmetric echo sampling used to shorten TE*:   When the echo is sampled asymmetrically (**B**), only part of the echo is sampled. Compared with symmetric sampling of the whole echo (**A**), the peak of the echo occurs earlier and so TE is shorter.

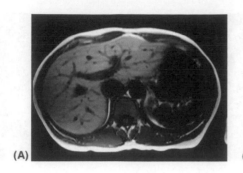

(A)

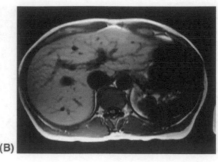

(B)

Figure 4. *Parallel imaging can reduce scan times without compromising image quality:* Typical image quality of an in-phase 2D T1w GRE image obtained without parallel imaging is illustrated in (**A**). The same sequence repeated with identical parameters but with a parallel imaging factor of two (**B**) showed only a slight reduction in SNR compared with (**A**). Scan time was reduced from 20 msecs in (**A**) to 13 secs in (**B**).

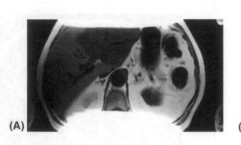

(A)

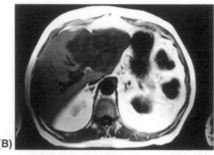

(B)

Figure 5. *T1w GRE images illustrating phase-axis fold-over artifact:* When part of the body extends beyond the acquired FOV in the phase encoding direction it is "wrapped" into the image creating a fold-over artifact as in (**A**). The artifact is eliminated when the FOV is increased to encompass the whole of the body part as in (**B**).

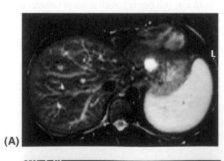

(A)

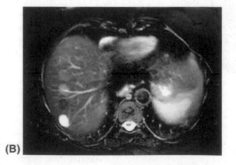

(B)

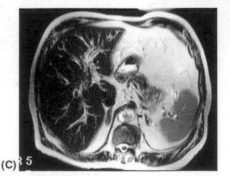

(C)

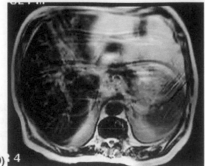

(D)

Figure 6. *The effect of respiratory gating on motion artifact reduction:* Respiratory gated T2w FSE in two patients with regular (**A**) and irregular (**B**) breathing patterns. Motion artifact was effectively suppressed on (**A**) but "ghosting" is considerable on (**B**). In a third patient also with an erratic breathing pattern, breathhold T2w FSE (**C**) showed much better image quality than respiratory gated T2w FSE (**D**) images.

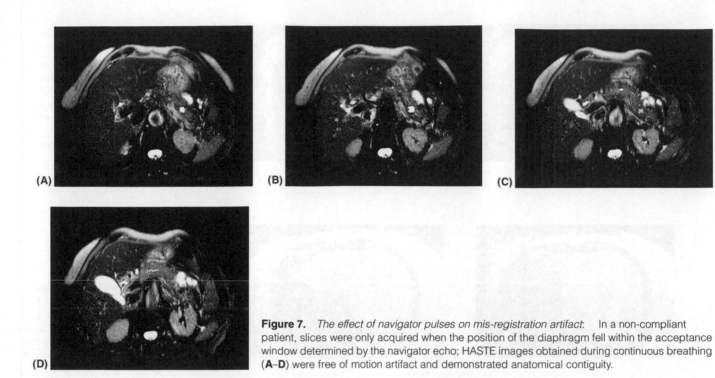

Figure 7. *The effect of navigator pulses on mis-registration artifact:* In a non-compliant patient, slices were only acquired when the position of the diaphragm fell within the acceptance window determined by the navigator echo; HASTE images obtained during continuous breathing (**A–D**) were free of motion artifact and demonstrated anatomical contiguity.

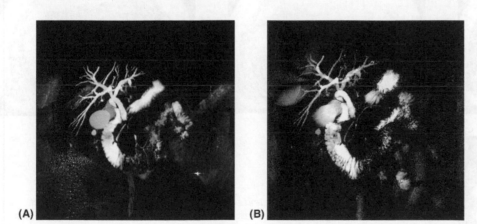

Figure 8. *Effective motion artifact suppression with navigator pulses:* MIP image derived from a heavily T2w 3D sequence acquired during free breathing over several minutes with navigator pulses (**A**) is free of motion artifact. This high resolution MIP image shows excellent depiction of the entire biliary tree with improved resolution of the finer anatomic structures compared with the corresponding single thick-slab breathhold SSFSE MRCP image (**B**).

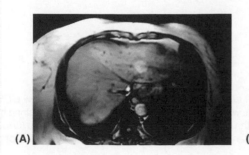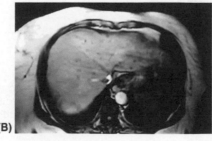

Figure 9. *Effect of GMR on aortic ghosting artifact:* T2w GRE images obtained without GMR (**A**) and with GMR (**B**) demonstrate a substantial artifact reduction on (**B**) compared with (**A**).

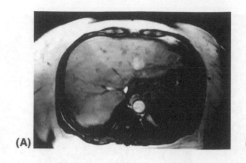
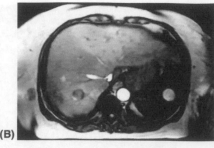

(A) **(B)**

Figure 10. *Effect of exchanging the phase encoding and frequency encoding directions on the orientation of aortic ghost artifact:* T2w GRE images demonstrate a change in the location of the aortic ghost artifact from the usual antero-posterior phase encoding direction on (**A**) to the right-to-left phase encoding direction on (**B**).

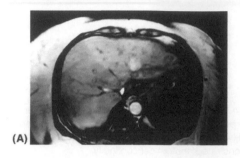
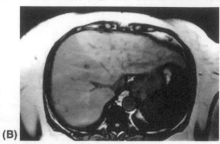

(A) **(B)**

Figure 11. *Effect of pre-saturation pulses on vascular ghost artifacts:* On the T2w GRE image without pre-saturation (**A**), there is pronounced ghost artifact from the aorta. The artifact has been effectively reduced on the identical image with pre-saturation bands (**B**).

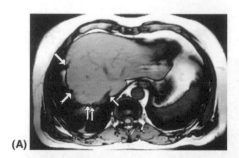
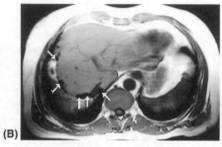
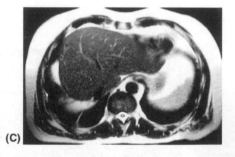

(A) **(B)** **(C)**

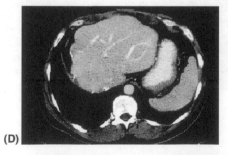

(D)

Figure 12. *Effect of pulse sequence and echo time on severity of susceptibility artifact:* The signal void (arrows) due to surgical clips at the right hepatectomy resection margin is less severe on OPT1w (TE 2.4 msec) (**A**) than on IPT1w imaging (TE 4.7 msec) (**B**). The artifact appears larger and more pronounced on (**B**) due to greater dephasing at the longer TE. The artifact is imperceptible on HASTE (**C**) due to the multiple 180° refocusing pulses, which minimize susceptibility. Surgical clips were confirmed on the corresponding CT image (**D**).

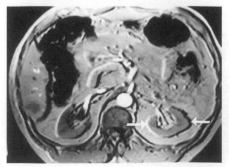

Figure 13. *First-order chemical shift mis-registration artifact on low bandwidth T2w GRE image:* Relative to the signal from fat, water from the kidney is incorrectly mapped along the frequency encoding direction toward the right. This is illustrated by a black signal void (arrow) at the lateral margin of the left kidney and a high signal band (arrow) on the medial aspect.

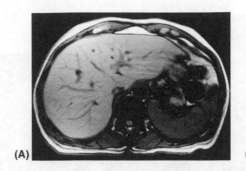
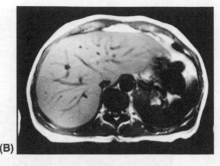

(A) **(B)**

Figure 14. *Fat/water cancellation artifact on OPT1w GRE:* Dark lines around the periphery of organs at the fat/water interface are apparent on the OPT1w image (**A**), but the artifact was not present on the corresponding IPT1w image (**B**).

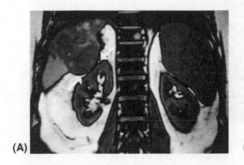
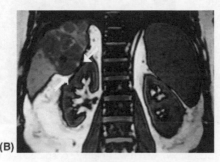

(A) **(B)**

Figure 15. *Fat/water cancellation artifact on OPT1w GRE helps to determine the extent of tumor invasion:* The edge artifact between the kidney and the tumor (arrows) was intact, but was absent between the tumor and the liver. Primary liver lesion, not invading the kidney, was confirmed at surgery.

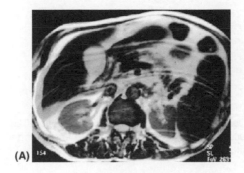
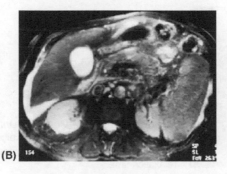

(A) **(B)**

Figure 16. *Importance of fat suppression to eliminate ghosting artifact from the high signal of fat on T2w FSE:* Identical breathhold T2w FSE images acquired without (**A**) and with fat suppression (**B**); pronounced ghosting of the anterior abdominal wall is apparent on (**A**) due to the increased signal of fat on FSE. Fat suppression diminishes fat signal intensity and eliminates the artifact (**B**).

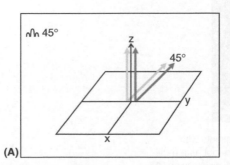
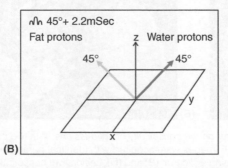
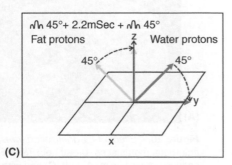

(A) **(B)** **(C)**

Figure 17. *Fat suppression using a 1:1 binomial water excitation pulse sequence:* After the first 45° pulse which tips the equilibrium magnetization toward the transverse plane, (**A**) a delay of 2.2 msec allows the fat and water protons to precess out of phase with each other and point in opposite directions. (**B**) When a second 45° pulse is applied, (**C**) the fat protons (light grey) are tipped back into the z-axis; only the water protons (dark grey) are tipped into the transverse plane so signal intensity in the resulting image is mostly from water.

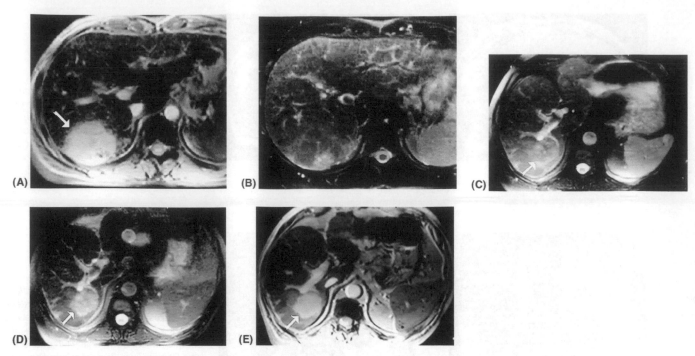

Figure 18.   *Reduced liver/lesion contrast on breathhold T2w FSE in two patients with advanced cirrhosis and hepatocellular carcinoma*:   A 6 cm HCC (arrow), which was highly conspicuous on SPIO-enhanced T2w GRE (**A**), was barely visible on the corresponding unenhanced T2w FSE image (**B**). In a second patient a poorly seen HCC (arrow) on unenhanced T2w FSE (**C**) was more conspicuous on the corresponding T2w FSE images after SPIO (**D**) and seen even more clearly on post-SPIO T2w GRE imaging (**E**).

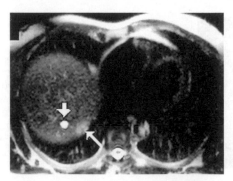

Figure 19.   *Benign versus malignant lesion conspicuity on T2w FSE*:   Breathhold T2w FSE images showed a highly conspicuous high signal intensity cyst (short arrow), and a metastasis (long arrow), which was less conspicuous due to MT effects and its shorter T2 relaxation time.

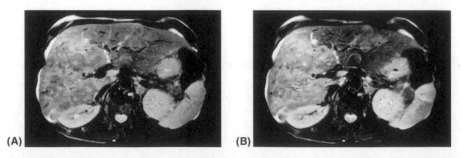

Figure 20.   *Effect of magnetization transfer on the conspicuity of solid lesions*:   In two patients with colorectal metastases, breathhold T2w FSE images were acquired with identical parameters but as a multi-section acquisition in (**A**) and (**C**) and with single slices in (**B**) and (D). Lesion/liver conspicuity was less on (**A**) than (**B**) because of MT effects. Tissue contrast is diminished in multi-slice acquisitions due to partial saturation of macromolecules within the acquisition volume by radiofrequency pulses applied to a single image section within the volume. The central necrotic components of the posterior metastasis in both (**C**) and (**D**) (arrow) were unaffected by MT and had a high signal intensity relative to the background liver on both images. The solid component of the lesion was highly conspicuous on the single slice acquisition but difficult to see on the multislice acquisition. (*Continued*)

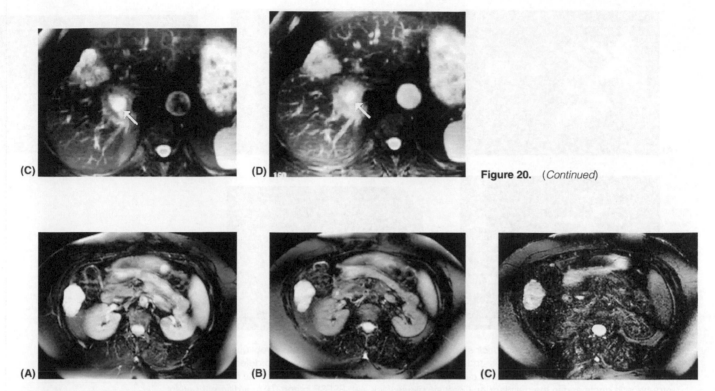

(C)   (D)   **Figure 20.** (*Continued*)

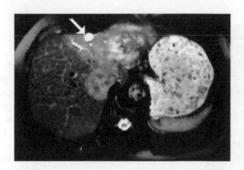

(A)   (B)   (C)

Figure 21. *Effect of increasing TE on the signal intensity of hemangiomas*:   Breathhold T2w FSE images were obtained at TEs of 90 (**A**), 180 (**B**), and 320 msec (**C**). The hemangioma had a signal intensity similar to CSF on (**A**) and (**B**), but at the longest TE (**C**), the lesion had less signal intensity than CSF due to its shorter T2 relaxation time.

Figure 22. *Effectiveness of HASTE in depicting small cysts*:   Simple cysts are well-defined and have a very high signal intensity on HASTE images. In a patient with co-existent cysts and metastases, a small cyst was highly hyperintense and sharply defined (arrow) while the metastasis was less well-defined and relatively inconspicuous due to a shorter relaxation time and blurring of short T2 tissues.

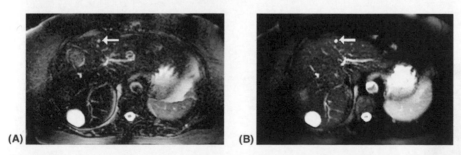

(A)   (B)

Figure 23. *HASTE verses heavily T2w breathhold FSE for depicting small cysts*:   On heavily T2w FSE images (TE 180 msec) (**A**), although the large right lobe cyst had a very high signal intensity and was well-defined, the small cyst in the left lobe (arrow) was ill-defined and difficult to characterize. Ghosting artifacts from the aorta and large cyst were pronounced despite patient compliance. On HASTE imaging (**B**) the small cyst was conspicuous, sharply defined and more reliably characterized. Motion artifacts were also negligible on HASTE images.

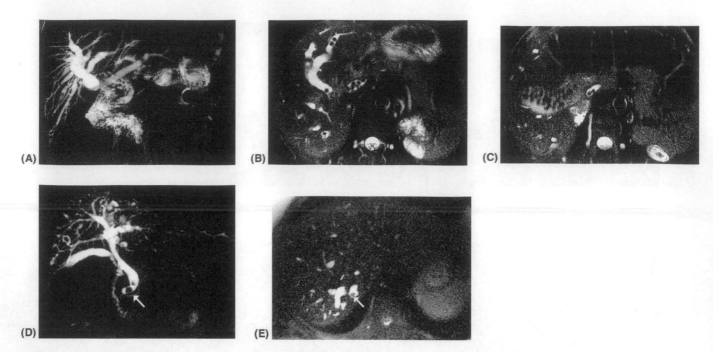

Figure 24. *Complementary role of thick slab MRC and thin-slice HASTE:* Coronal/oblique thick slab SSFSE imaging (**A**) showed a tortuous and dilated biliary tree and questionable filling defects in the CBD. Axial thin-slice HASTE images (**B** and **C**) clearly showed multiple, dependent filling defects in the CBD and intra-hepatic ducts and in the gallbladder. Coronal/oblique thick slab SSFSE image (**D**) in a different patient with Caroli's disease showed an apparently solitary filling defect in the distal CBD (arrow). Axial thin-slice HASTE image (**E**) showed additional stones in the right-sided intra-hepatic ducts (arrow).

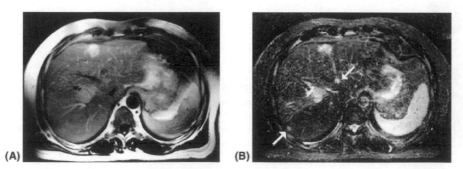

Figure 25. *Improved conspicuity with STIR compared with T2w FSE:* Two metastases were visible on breathhold T2 FSE images (**A**). Both lesions were more conspicuous on breathhold STIR imaging (**B**) due to the additive effects of T1 and T2 contrast. Two additional, previously unsuspected sub-cm metastases were also well shown on (**B**) (arrows).

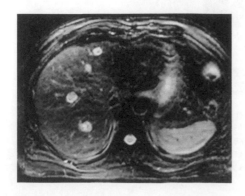

Figure 26. *Artifact associated with long EPI factor on breathhold TGSE:* There was high lesion/liver contrast on the breathhold TGSE images, but they were degraded by phase artifact (ghosting) due to the long gradient echo train (EPI factor).

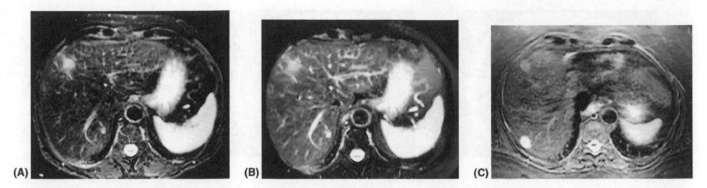

Figure 27. *Lesion/liver contrast on non-breathhold TGSE compared with T2w FSE*:   In a patient with a regular breathing pattern, motion artifacts were effectively eliminated with respiratory gating, and lesion/liver contrast was better on non-breathhold TGSE (**A**) than on non-breathhold FSE images (**B**). In a second patient with more erratic breathing, respiratory gating was ineffective and non-breathhold TGSE images (**C**) were severely degraded by motion.

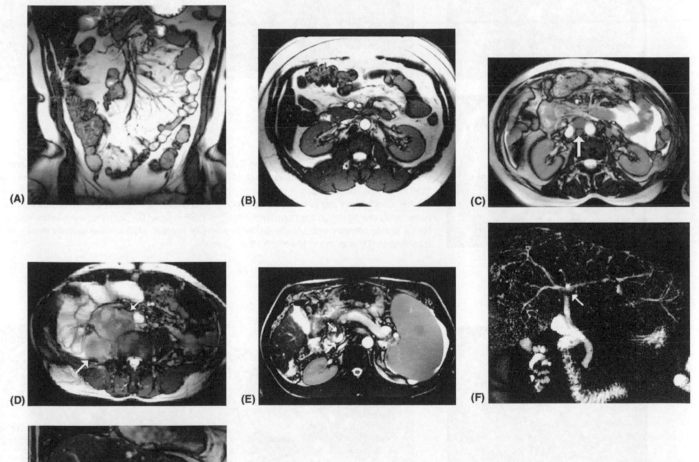

Figure 28. *Role of True FISP imaging*:   Single breathhold coronal (**A**) and axial (**B**) True FISP images illustrate the value of True FISP in obtaining a rapid anatomical survey of the abdomen with high contrast and negligible motion artifact. Axial True FISP images in two other patients (**C** and **D**) showed conspicuous nodal disease (arrows). Axial True FISP image in a fourth patient with non-occluding thrombus of the portal vein showed high contrast between the low signal intensity thrombus (arrow) and the high signal of flowing blood (arrow) (**E**). A coronal/oblique thick-slab MRCP image (**F**) in a fifth patient showed a typical hepatic artery compression artifact at the bile duct bifurcation (arrow) mimicking a filling defect. The corresponding coronal/oblique True FISP image (**G**) demonstrated the hepatic artery (arrow) and confirmed its position adjacent to the signal void.

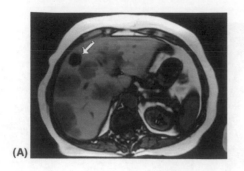

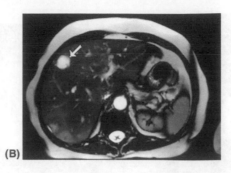

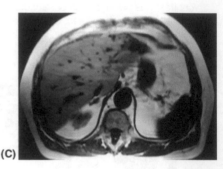

Figure 29. *Low liver/tumor contrast on True FISP in a patient with co-existent benign and malignant lesions*:   Multiple metastases which were well seen on OPT1w images (**A**) were barely visible on the corresponding True FISP image (**B**) and only detectable because of their mass effect. Conversely, a benign lesion with a high fluid content (arrow) was highly conspicuous on True FISP.

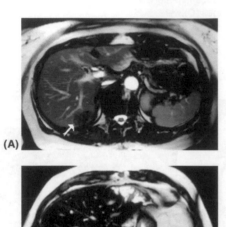

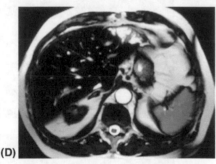

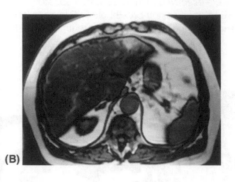

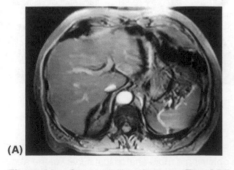

Figure 30. *Signal intensity change on True FISP due to fatty infiltration*:   True FISP image in a patient with a fat-containing adenoma (arrow) (**A**) illustrated a lower signal intensity in the lesion than in normal liver tissue. In a second patient with fairly severe fatty change as illustrated by a marked drop of liver signal on OPT1w (**B**) compared with IPT1 images (**C**), the whole liver had an abnormally low signal on the corresponding True FISP image (**D**). Note that the normal liver in (**A**) had a signal intensity close to the signal intensity of spleen, whereas the signal intensity of the fatty liver in (**D**) was much lower than the spleen.

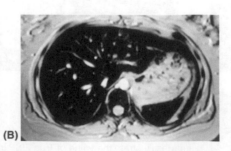

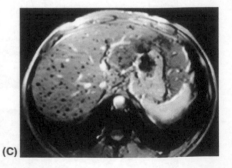

Figure 31. *Susceptibility effects on T2w GRE*:   The normal liver has a signal intensity only slightly lower than adipose tissue on unenhanced T2w GRE images (**A**) and contrast is poor. In a patient with excess iron deposition in the liver and spleen due to transfusional siderosis, there was a marked reduction in the signal intensity of the liver and spleen on unenhanced T2w GRE images (**B**). In a different patient, siderotic nodules were clearly seen as punctate areas of very low signal on T2W GRE (TE 14 msec) images (**C**). They were much less conspicuous on the corresponding in-phase T1W GRE (TE 4.7 msec) image (**D**) and undetectable on the opposed-phase T1w GRE (TE 2.4 msec) image (**E**). Susceptibility effects diminish as TE is reduced. (*Continued*)

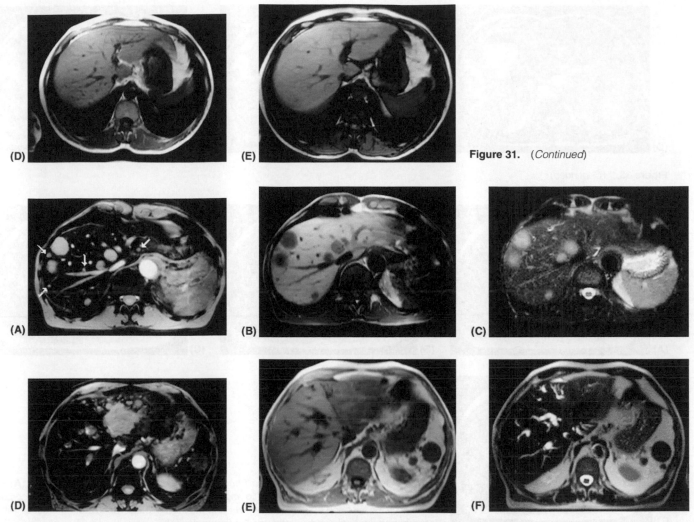

Figure 31. (Continued)

Figure 32. *Optimized SPIO-enhanced T2w GRE imaging*: T2w GRE image obtained with optimized parameters after SPIO (**A**) illustrates high lesion-to-liver contrast and negligible artifact. Note the improved conspicuity of sub-cm lesions (arrows) compared with corresponding unenhanced IPT1w GRE (**B**) and HASTE (**C**) images. In a second patient with a large colorectal metastasis and numerous satellite lesions the individual tumor deposits were more clearly defined on SPIO-enhanced T2w GRE (**D**) than on unenhanced IPT1 GRE (**E**) and HASTE (**F**) images.

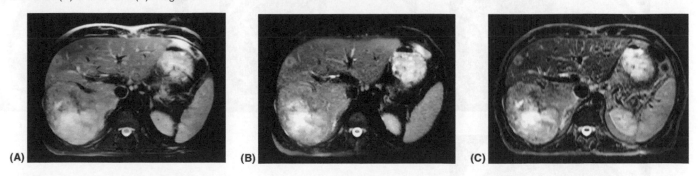

Figure 33. *Comparison of lesion/liver contrast on current breathhold, non-contrast T1w and T2w sequences*: T2w FSE (**A**), HASTE (**B**), STIR (**C**), True FISP (**D**), OPT1w GRE (**E**), and IPT1w GRE (**F**) images were obtained in a patient with multiple colorectal metastases. Image quality was good and motion artifacts were negligible on all images. Lesion/liver contrast was poor on (**A**) probably due to MT effects. Compared with (**A**), lesion/liver contrast was better on (**B**) probably due to less MT, and better on (**C**) because of the additive effects of T1 and T2 contrast. Only the central necrotic portion of the larger lesion was visible on (**D**). Compared with the four T2w sequences, lesion/liver contrast was considerably better on both T1w sequences (**E** and **F**), due to greater SNR and lack of MT effects. (*Continued*)

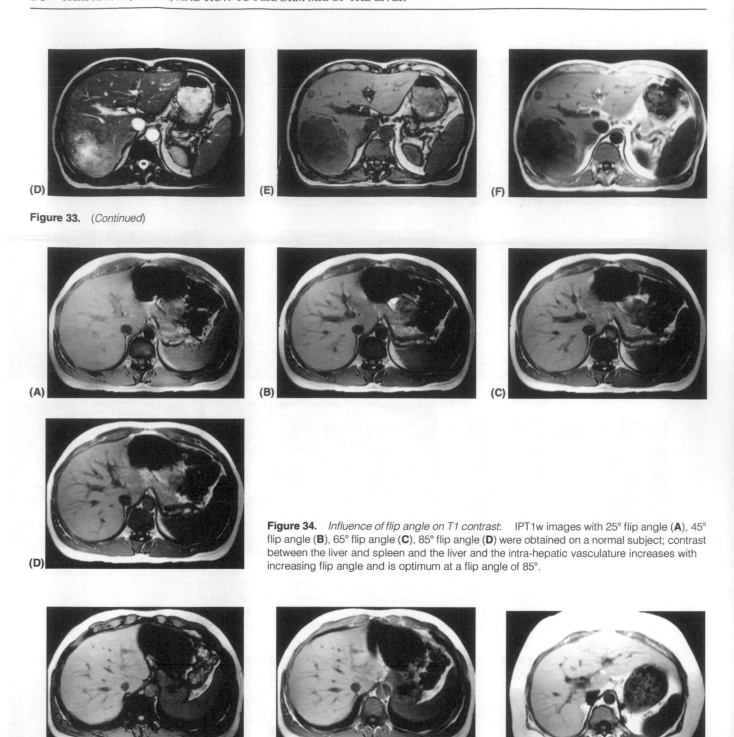

Figure 33.   (*Continued*)

Figure 34.   *Influence of flip angle on T1 contrast:*   IPT1w images with 25° flip angle (**A**), 45° flip angle (**B**), 65° flip angle (**C**), 85° flip angle (**D**) were obtained on a normal subject; contrast between the liver and spleen and the liver and the intra-hepatic vasculature increases with increasing flip angle and is optimum at a flip angle of 85°.

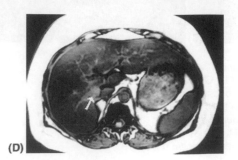

Figure 35.   *Fatty infiltration of the liver identified by T1w GRE in-phase (TE 4.7 msec) and opposed-phase (TE 2.4 msec) (imaging):*   the normal liver has the same signal on IPT1w (**A**) and OPT1w images (**B**) and liver signal is brighter than the spleen in both. In a different patient with diffuse fatty infiltration, the liver had a normal signal on IPT1w (**C**) but a much lower signal on OPT1w images (**D**) and on (**D**) the liver signal was lower than the signal intensity of the spleen. An area of focal fatty sparing (arrow) had a higher signal than the liver and spleen on (**D**) and was homogeneously isointense with the adjacent liver on (**C**).

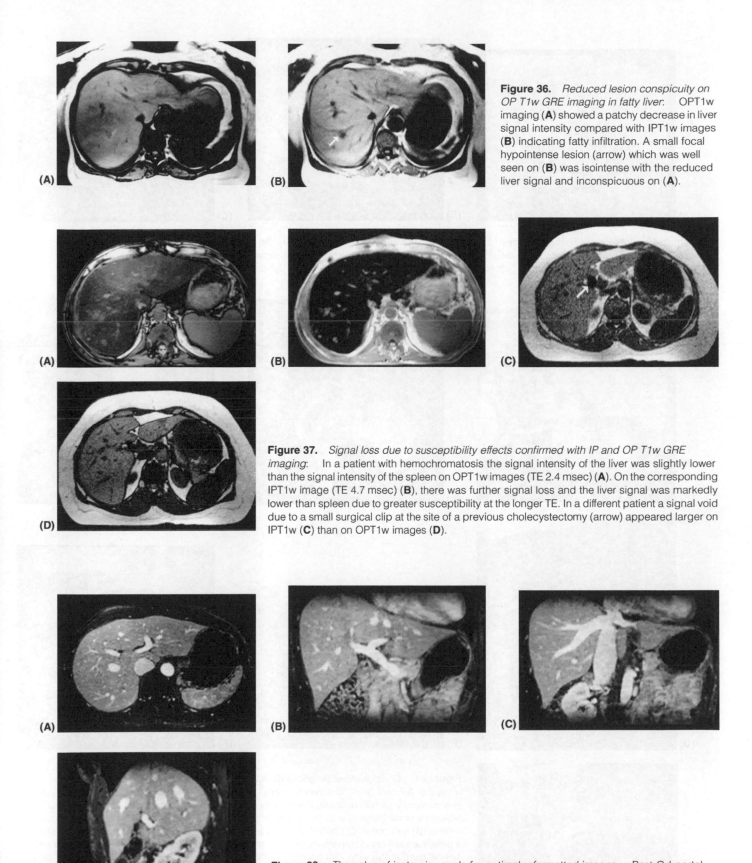

Figure 36.   *Reduced lesion conspicuity on OP T1w GRE imaging in fatty liver:*   OPT1w imaging (**A**) showed a patchy decrease in liver signal intensity compared with IPT1w images (**B**) indicating fatty infiltration. A small focal hypointense lesion (arrow) which was well seen on (**B**) was isointense with the reduced liver signal and inconspicuous on (**A**).

Figure 37.   *Signal loss due to susceptibility effects confirmed with IP and OP T1w GRE imaging:*   In a patient with hemochromatosis the signal intensity of the liver was slightly lower than the signal intensity of the spleen on OPT1w images (TE 2.4 msec) (**A**). On the corresponding IPT1w image (TE 4.7 msec) (**B**), there was further signal loss and the liver signal was markedly lower than spleen due to greater susceptibility at the longer TE. In a different patient a signal void due to a small surgical clip at the site of a previous cholecystectomy (arrow) appeared larger on IPT1w (**C**) than on OPT1w images (**D**).

Figure 38.   *The value of isotropic voxels for optimal reformatted images:*   Post-Gd portal phase axial 3D T1w GRE source images were obtained with near isotropic voxels (**A**). Reformatted images in coronal (**B**) coronal/oblique (**C**) and sagittal (**D**) planes, derived from the same source data as (**A**), have comparable image quality.

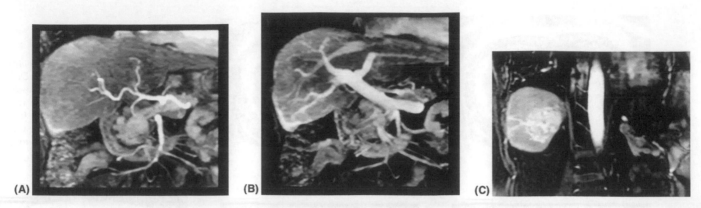

Figure 39. *Vascular MIP images derived from a 3D T1w GRE acquisition obtained with a flip angle of 15° for optimal parenchymal evaluation:* Post-Gd arterial (**A**) and portal (**B**) phase MIP images show normal arterial and portal vasculature. Arterial phase coronal/oblique source image (**C**) clearly shows a hypervascular tumor.

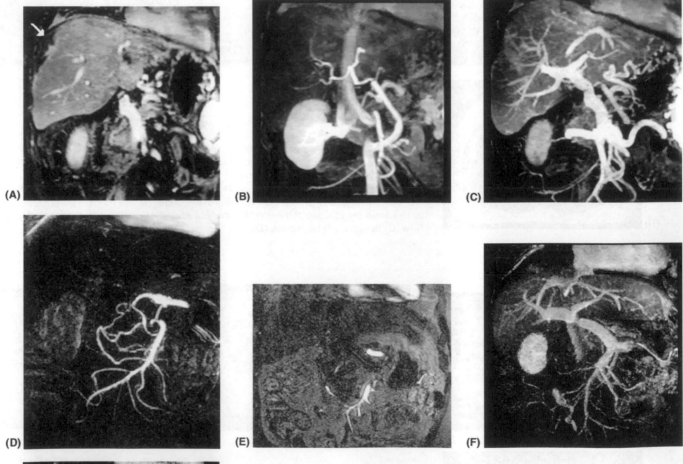

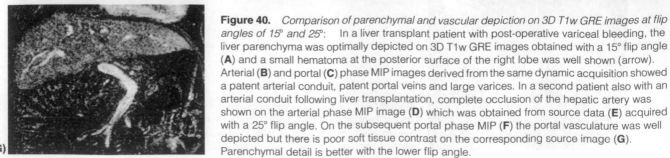

Figure 40. *Comparison of parenchymal and vascular depiction on 3D T1w GRE images at flip angles of 15° and 25°:* In a liver transplant patient with post-operative variceal bleeding, the liver parenchyma was optimally depicted on 3D T1w GRE images obtained with a 15° flip angle (**A**) and a small hematoma at the posterior surface of the right lobe was well shown (arrow). Arterial (**B**) and portal (**C**) phase MIP images derived from the same dynamic acquisition showed a patent arterial conduit, patent portal veins and large varices. In a second patient also with an arterial conduit following liver transplantation, complete occlusion of the hepatic artery was shown on the arterial phase MIP image (**D**) which was obtained from source data (**E**) acquired with a 25° flip angle. On the subsequent portal phase MIP (**F**) the portal vasculature was well depicted but there is poor soft tissue contrast on the corresponding source image (**G**). Parenchymal detail is better with the lower flip angle.

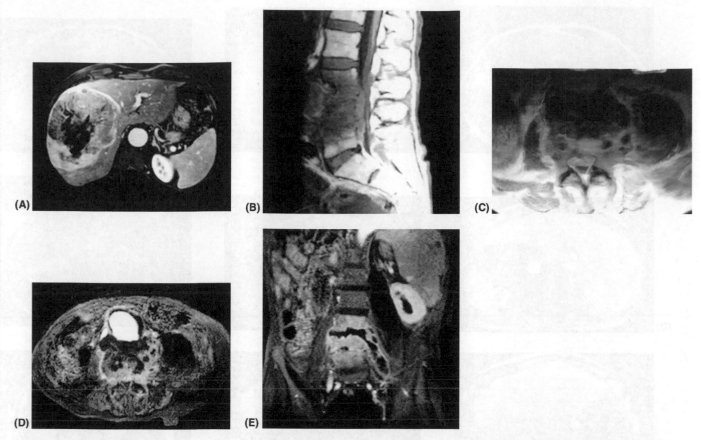

Figure 41. *Role of Gd-enhanced rapid 3D T1w GRE imaging for non-hepatic applications*: In a patient with severe lower back pain following an extended right hepatectomy for a large HCC (**A**), routine spinal imaging showed an extensive abnormality at L3/4 (**B** and **C**) but the images were badly degraded by movement artifact due to the acquisition time of several minutes. Subsequent rapid 3D T1w GRE images obtained in axial (**D**) and coronal (**E**) planes after bolus injection of gadolinium, each with an acquisition time of 20 seconds, provided excellent demonstration of the abnormality with negligible motion artifact. These post-contrast images showed a large psoas abscess communicating with the L3/4 disc space, and extending anteriorly to erode the posterior wall of a large infra-renal aortic aneurysm.

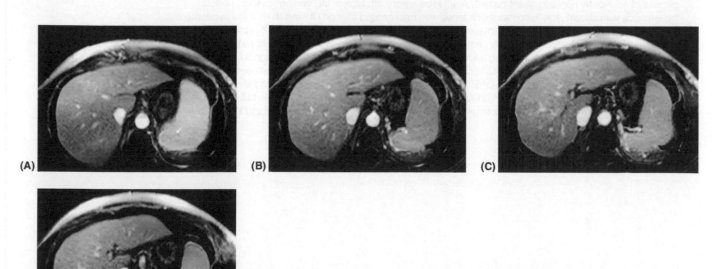

Figure 42. *Image contrast on magnetization-prepared GRE T1w images using a non-selective inversion pulse*: There is minimal contrast change between sequential images (**A–D**) at a TR of 1200 msec due to adequate recovery of the longitudinal magnetization between each inversion pulse. Since each slice is acquired in just over one second, the images which were obtained during free breathing were free of motion artifact.

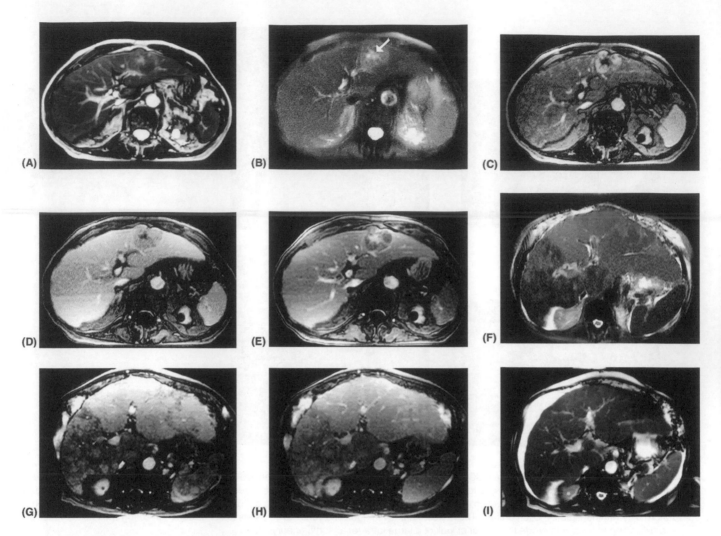

Figure 43. *Non-breathhold imaging in compromised patients*: True FISP (**A**), HASTE (**B**) and magnetization-prepared post-Gd T1w GRE images were obtained at arterial (**C**), portal (**D**), and delayed (**E**) phases in an elderly non-compliant patient. A left lobe lesion with typical MR findings of focal nodular hyperplasia was shown. The lesion was isointense with background liver on (**A**) and (**B**) but the hyperintense scar was visible (arrow). The lesion displayed marked enhancement on (**C**), which faded rapidly on (**D**), and there was delayed enhancement of the central scar on (**E**). In a second encephalopathic patient with end-stage liver disease, HASTE (**F**) imaging showed an enlarged left lobe with increased signal intensity consistent with edema. An infiltrative HCC occupying most of the small right lobe was well seen on immediate post-Gd magnetization-prepared T1w GRE images (**G**). Liver/lesion contrast was less in the subsequent portal phase (**H**). The corresponding True FISP image (**I**) showed a large volume of ascites but no abnormality in the liver parenchyma. High quality motion-free images were obtained during free breathing in both patients.

CHAPTER 3

Contrast Agents for Liver MRI

D espite the inherently high contrast resolution of MR the use of contrast agents has great diagnostic value for liver imaging. In many cases lesions become much more conspicuous, benign, and malignant masses are more reliably distinguished, and contrast enhancement characteristics often allow a specific diagnosis of pathology. Moreover, since the replacement of non-breathhold T2w sequences with breathhold T2w sequences—which are less sensitive for detecting solid lesions—the role of contrast enhancement has become even more important.

Several different contrast agents are available for liver MR (Table 1). Dynamic gadolinium (Gd)-enhanced techniques have been widely used in liver MR for several years and more recently liver-specific agents have been developed to increase and prolong the contrast between normal and abnormal tissues and further aid lesion detection. These agents target either the hepatocytes or Kupffer cells to allow an assessment of pathology at cellular level so they also have particular value for characterizing hepatocellular lesions.

NON-SPECIFIC EXTRA-CELLULAR (ECF) GADOLINIUM AGENTS

Gd is a paramagnetic metal ion, which shortens T1 relaxation time, producing positive enhancement on T1w images. Following initial distribution within the intravascular compartment the ECF Gd agents rapidly disperse throughout the extracellular space after which they are eliminated by renal excretion. Liver-to-lesion contrast peaks in the first minute after injection and then declines fairly quickly, so maximum lesion detection relies on dynamic imaging with rapid sequential acquisitions during the first 90 seconds after injection. Because the various perfusion and extraction characteristics of different tissues can be observed at different phases of enhancement, a specific pathologic diagnosis is often possible (Fig. 1).

Contrast Dosage and Administration

ECF Gd is administered as a rapid bolus at a dose of approximately 0.1 mmol/kg and the first acquisition is timed to coincide with arrival of the contrast in the tissue or vessel of interest during acquisition of the central lines of k-space, which determines tissue contrast within the image. Best results are obtained when the contrast is administered by a power injector at a rate of 2–4 ml per second followed by a 20–30 ml saline flush.

Choice of Acquisition Sequence Parameters

To enable sequential imaging of the entire liver during suspended respiration (~ 20 secs), a T1w gradient echo sequence with the shortest possible TE should be used to maximize the number of slices for a given TR. 3D sequences are preferred because they result in a higher signal-to-noise and thinner effective slice thickness than do 2D methods, with no inter-slice gap or crosstalk. We recommend a 3D T1w GRE sequence which comfortably allows thin-section coverage of the whole liver in a single breathhold. This technique known as VIBE, (Volume Interpolated Breathhold Examination) was first developed for abdominal imaging

Table 1   Contrast Agents for Liver MRI

Agents	Target	Effect
Extracellular Gd chelates (gadopentetate, etc.)	Intravascular and extracellular fluid	Positive T1 enhancement
Extra/intracellular T1 agents (gadobenate, gadoxetic acid)	Intravascular and extracellular fluid, then hepatocytes, biliary tract	Positive T1 enhancement
Intracellular T1 agents (mangafodipir)	Hepatocytes, then biliary tract	Positive T1 enhancement
Superparamagnetic iron oxide agents (ferucarbotran, ferumoxides)	Intravascular fluid initially, then reticuloendothelial cells of liver and spleen	Positive T1, then negative T1 and T2* enhancement

on a Siemens system by Rofsky and colleagues in 1998 but other manufacturers now offer comparable sequences (e.g., Philips WAVE, GE FAME). The use of a short repetition time (TR) and echo time (TE) facilitates a higher resolution matrix and the intermittent application of a chemically-selective fat saturation pulse before each partition loop achieves homogeneous fat suppression with minimal time penalty. The parameters we use are as follows: TR 3.8 msec, TE 1.55 msec, flip angle (FA) 15° and bandwidth (BW) 490 Hz/pixel. Acquisition of k-space is linear. We use a slightly asymmetric echo in the read out direction (kx), to reduce TE and TR although at the expense of some signal-to-noise. With symmetric echoes, the peak of the echo and the acquisition of the central lines of k-space occur at the center (echo position 50%) of echo sampling. With asymmetric sampling the central parts of k-space are acquired earlier at an echo position of 38%; approximately 80% of k-space is filled and the remainder encoded by zero-filling. The matrix in the readout direction is 256. We do not use partial Fourier in the in-plane phase encoding direction (ky) and acquire approximately 125 phase encoding points. We use a rectangular (typically 75%) field of view (FOV) of 280–400 mm depending on patient size to yield a pixel size of about 1.6 mm in the frequency encoded direction and 2.4 mm in the phase-encoding direction. Partial Fourier reconstruction is applied in the slice-select direction (kz) with 48–53 data points interpolated to achieve 72–80 partitions. A slab thickness of 180–240 mm provides full coverage of the liver with an interpolated slice thickness of 2.5–3.0 mm. The small FA of 15° minimizes saturation to maximize the signal from stationary tissues for simultaneous display of liver parenchyma and hepatic vessels (Fig. 2). Fat suppression is particularly helpful because it increases the dynamic range within the image and accentuates Gd enhancement (Fig. 3).

Tailoring the Acquisition for Individual Patients

Compared with 2DFT techniques at a comparable voxel size, 3DFT techniques theoretically generate images with higher signal-to-noise ratio, so even when parameters are compromised the image quality of 3D imaging is usually superior to that of conventional 2D imaging. VIBE is a very flexible sequence and can be easily adapted to achieve full liver coverage in acquisition times as short as 12 seconds. In patients with a reduced breathholding capacity we increase the effective slice thickness to 4 mm thereby reducing the slab thickness needed to encompass the liver and we reduce the number of data points in the phase encoding direction. Conversely if less anatomic coverage is required, the use of a targeted coronal/oblique slab permits higher resolution images with an effective slice thickness of 1–1.5 mm also in a breathhold period (Fig. 4). Furthermore, artifacts from surgical clips, stents, and coils are minimal because short TE sequences are relatively insensitive to susceptibility.

It should be recognized that a TE of approximately 2 msec produces opposed-phase images which in the presence of fatty infiltration results in reduced liver signal and rarely this may be decreased still further following Gd due to paradoxical enhancement. We no longer use dedicated MRA sequences to image the hepatic vasculature, since the VIBE sequence produces MIP reconstructions of comparable quality with excellent soft tissue contrast (Fig. 5).

Timing the Dynamic Acquisition Phases

At least three phases of enhancement (arterial, portal, and equilibrium) are necessary. Of these, the arterial-dominant phase—which is identified by marked enhancement of the hepatic arteries, pancreas, and spleen with early filling of the main portal vein branches but no enhancement of the hepatic veins—is the most crucial. The time window between the arrival of contrast in the hepatic artery to filling of the hepatic veins is fairly narrow, and many hypervascular lesions are only visible during this time (Fig. 6). In most patients, effective arterial phase enhancement is achieved when the central lines of k-space are acquired about 10–15 seconds after the end of injection. However, transit times from the ante-cubital fossa to the hepatic artery have been shown to range from 8–32 seconds and an initial test dose of contrast with real time detection is recommended for optimal arterial phase imaging.

We use a 2 ml test bolus of Gd-DTPA followed by a minimum 20 ml saline flush injected at a rate of 4 ml/sec. A magnetization-prepared spoiled GRE T1w sequence (Turbo FLASH, TR 1000 msec TE 1.58 msec, inversion time 500 msec, FA 80°, BW 380 Hz/pixel, matrix 123×256, slice thickness 10 mm) is positioned over the abdominal aorta at the level of the diaphragm and a series of transverse images obtained at 1 second intervals. Using a user-defined region of interest positioned over the aorta, an enhancement curve is generated to determine peak enhancement. Based on an injection rate of 4 ml/sec the optimum delay between the start of injection and start of data acquisition is calculated as—the time to peak aortic enhancement *plus* the duration of Gd injection *minus* the interval between starting acquisition and acquisition of the central lines of "k" space.

Normal and Abnormal Enhancement

Lesions which have a predominantly arterial blood supply are best seen at the arterial phase after Gd because the normal liver shows relatively little enhancement in this phase (Fig. 6). Since most of the hepatic blood inflow (about 80%) arrives via the portal vein, parenchymal liver enhancement is maximum at the portal phase which occurs 20–30 seconds later. Hypovascular lesions are most conspicuous in the portal phase, but rim enhancement in the periphery of hypovascular tumors, which allows them to be distinguished from benign lesions, is seen best on arterial phase images, so both phases should be acquired in all patients (Fig. 7). The equilibrium phase occurs 2–3 minutes after injection. At this time contrast between normal, and abnormal tissues is poor and some lesions are no longer visible, but this phase is often helpful for characterization. When lesions with a large fibrous component such as cholangiocarcinomas or hemangiomas are suspected, further images should be obtained approximately 10 minutes after injection. At this stage such lesions are often more conspicuous due to gradual accumulation of Gd producing increasing enhancement (Fig. 8). For similar reasons, peritoneal tumor deposits and extra-hepatic inflammatory change are also best demonstrated on delayed FST1w images after Gd (Fig. 9).

TISSUE-SPECIFIC CONTRAST AGENTS

Two types of specific contrast media have been developed for liver MR—agents based on Gd or manganese chelates which shorten T1 relaxation time and target the hepatocytes, and superparamagnetic iron oxide (SPIO) particles which cause a marked shortening of T2* and are extracted by the reticulo-endothelial cells of the liver, spleen, and bone marrow. Non-hepatocellular tumors become more conspicuous after contrast enhancement because malignant lesions lack functioning Kupffer cells or hepatocytes, so their signal intensity is unchanged while the surrounding liver becomes either hyperintense (T1 agents) or hypointense (SPIO) (Fig. 10). Liver-specific contrast agents also help to distinguish between benign and malignant hepatocellular lesions because they are taken up by functioning hepatocytes and Kupffer cells in focal nodular hyperplasia (FNH), many liver cell adenomas, and in the regenerating nodules of cirrhosis (Fig. 11). Well-differentiated hepatocellular carcinoma (HCC) may also show contrast uptake but to a lesser extent.

HEPATOCYTE AGENTS

Three hepatocyte agents (gadobenate, gadoxetic acid, and mangafodipir) are currently available. All three agents are paramagnetic, producing T1 shortening and positive enhancement on T1-weighted images. They all have a greater relaxivity (the ability of a contrast agent to selectively increase the relaxation time of water protons in tissue) than the non-specific ECF agents. The relaxivity of contrast agents varies according to whether it is measured in saline, plasma, or in tissue. In the liver the estimated T1 relaxivities of ECF

Gd, gadobenate, gadoxetic acid, and mangafodipir are respectively 6.7, 30, 16.6, and 21.7 $mmol^{-1}$, sec^{-1}. T1w GRE imaging is recommended for all three agents. To improve the detection of sub-centimeter lesions the same T1w 3D VIBE sequence as is used with Gd-DTPA is recommended.

Gadobenate

Gadobenate (Gd-BOPTA, Multihance, Bracco) has a biphasic enhancement profile. In the first few minutes after injection the agent has an ECF distribution similar to the non-specific Gd chelates. Although gadobenate is mostly eliminated via renal excretion, approximately 3–5% is eliminated via the liver, resulting in increased contrast between normal liver (high signal) and tumor (low signal) on images obtained 40–120 minutes after injection (Fig. 12 and 13). Gadobenate in plasma has a T1 relaxivity almost twice that of the ECF Gd agents so effective dynamic imaging is achieved at a dose of 0.05 mmol/kg (half the usual dose for Gd-DTPA which is 0.1 mmol/kg).

Gadoxetic Acid

Gadoxetic acid (Gd-EOB-DTPA, Primovist, Schering) in plasma also has a higher T1 relaxivity than ECF Gd ($8.2 mmol^{-1}$, sec^{-1}, for gadoxetic acid compared with $5.9 mmol^{-1}$, sec^{-1} for Gd-DTPA). Like gadobenate it also has a biphasic enhancement profile, with an ECF distribution immediately after injection, but the proportion taken up into hepatocytes is much greater, about 50% of the injected dose (Fig. 14). Maximum contrast between normal and abnormal tissue occurs 10–40 minutes after injection (Fig. 15) and the recommended dose is 25 μmol/kg. The high rate of biliary excretion results in enhancement of the bile ducts in the late phase, so a cholangiogram can be obtained (Fig. 14).

Mangafodipir

Mangafodipir trisodium (Mn-DPDP, Teslascan, GE-Amersham) is more appropriately described as a metabolic contrast agent than a hepatocyte agent. Tissues with numerous mitochondria and active aerobic metabolism such as the liver, pancreas, kidneys, adrenal glands, gastrointestinal mucosa and myocardium all take up the agent. The manganese dissociates from its ligand and binds to intracellular macromolecules, after which it is eliminated by biliary and intestinal secretion in a similar way to dietary manganese. Mangafodipir in plasma has a similar T1 relaxivity to ECF Gd but it must be administered by slow injection (over 1–2 minutes), or infusion (2–3 ml per minute), to minimize adverse events which occur in approximately 7% of patients. The optimum window for lesion detection is between 15 minutes and 2 hours, but some metastases and HCC may be more conspicuous on 24 hour images due to abnormal retention of the contrast agent in HCC or delayed washout around the periphery of metastases (Fig. 16). Mangafodipir also shows positive enhancement of the biliary tree and produces cholangiographic images when combined with thin slice high-resolution T1w sequences (Fig. 17). This technique maybe used to confirm bile duct leakage following surgery when non-specific fluid collections are present on unenhanced images (Fig. 18).

RETICULO-ENDOTHELIAL SYSTEM (KUPFFER CELL) AGENTS

Two SPIO agents are available for liver MR, ferumoxides (AMI-25, Endorem, Guerbet) and ferucarbotran (SHU 555A, Resovist, Schering). The distribution of SPIO varies with particle size. In the size range of 30–200 nm approximately 80% of the injected dose is taken up by the normal liver. When SPIO particles are clustered within the macrophages, they induce local field inhomogeneities which lead to rapid spin dephasing and loss of signal in normal liver tissue on both T1w and T2w images. The effect is more pronounced on T2w images due to the high R2/R1 ratio of SPIO. Abnormal areas appear as areas of high signal intensity against a very low signal background liver, so tumor-to-liver contrast is considerably increased (Fig. 19).

Ferumoxides

Ferumoxides has a mean particle size of about 150 nm. There have been few efficacy-related dose-finding studies performed with ferumoxides, so the optimum dose is uncertain and doses of 10 and 15 µmol/kg are recommended in the U.S.A. and Europe respectively. Some recent studies showed a dose of 7.5 µmol/kg to be as effective as a 15 µmol/kg dose for detecting lesions in patients with and without diffuse liver disease at a field strength of 1.0T (Fig. 20). Whichever dose is used, ferumoxides is normally given as a dilute infusion over 30 minutes to minimize side effects, particularly back pain, although a recent multicenter study showed no increase in the incidence or severity of adverse events when undiluted ferumoxides was given by slow injection. Images are optimum 15–120 minutes from the end of injection.

Ferucarbotran

Ferucarbotran has a recommended dose of 7–10 µmol/kg and is given by bolus injection with very few and mild side effects. Although predominantly a T2* agent with a mean particle size of 60 nm, the preparation contains a proportion of very small particles (about 15 nm) which, in the first few minutes after injection when the particles are dispersed throughout the intravascular space, produce T1 enhancement. The blood half-life of ferucarbotran is about 3–4 minutes and as the particles are sequestered by the RE cells they become more clustered. This increases their susceptibility effects, and the loss of signal due to T2* shortening becomes the dominant contrast mechanism. At this time signal loss is apparent on T1w and T2w images. Ferucarbotran has a relaxivity 4–5 times higher than ECF Gd agents so T1w images obtained in the first 2–3 minutes after injection are similar to images obtained with Gd-DTPA (Fig. 21). However, the T1 effect is dose-dependent and since ferucarbotran has been marketed at only two pre-filled volumes the individual dose is variable. Patients weighing under 60 kg receive 0.9 ml whereas patients weighing 60 kg or more receive 1.4 ml—this equates to an individual patient dose in the range of 7–11 µmol/kg. T1 enhancement is similar to ECF Gd at the higher dose but liver and vessels have almost the same signal intensity at a lower dose. This produces a virtual "blank canvas" against which focal lesions are conspicuous and readily distinguished from adjacent vessels (Fig. 22). We regard T1w and T2w images after ferucarbotran as complementary and obtain T1w images about 15 and 45 seconds after contrast injection in all patients with suspected metastatic disease. T2w GRE images are acquired 10 minutes later when T2 enhancement is optimum.

Choice of Acquisition Sequence Parameters

T2w GRE sequences with optimized parameters are recommended for maximum lesion detection following SPIO. Signal loss is more pronounced on GRE than on spin echo sequences due to the greater sensitivity of GRE to susceptibility effects. Further, the contrast effect of SPIO is less on fast spin echo (FSE) images because multiple closely spaced refocusing pulses diminish the local field inhomogeneities induced by the SPIO particles. Magnetization transfer (MT) effects which reduce the SI of solid lesions are also a feature of FSE but not GRE sequences. As ETL increases, FSE becomes increasingly insensitive to SPIO, and MT effects become more pronounced so lesion-to-liver contrast may be particularly poor on long echo train breathhold FSE images following SPIO (Fig. 23). Breathhold sequences are desirable because respiratory artifacts are eliminated and scanning time is reduced. While GRE imaging meets this requirement and also maximizes the effect of SPIO, parameters must be optimized to minimize noise and maximize the signal from solid lesions. We compared the accuracy of four SPIO-enhanced breathhold sequences (three GRE sequences and one FSE sequence) using optimized parameters, for the detection of colorectal metastases. Enhanced FSE was no better than unenhanced images with accuracies of 82% and 81% respectively but the three GRE sequences achieved accuracies between 90%–93% and were significantly more sensitive than non-contrast images (Fig. 24). We further refined the best of the GRE sequences by reducing the slice thickness from 10 to 6 mm and applying fat suppression to improve the detection of sub-centimeter and surface lesions (Fig. 25). This sequence is also very valuable for depicting extra-hepatic and peritoneal tumor deposits which are well seen against the suppressed signal of fat and the reduced liver signal after SPIO (Fig. 26). The recommended sequence parameters are as follows: TR 148 msec, TE 14 msec, FA 30°, matrix 132×256, BW 65–80 Hz/pixel, 65% phase resolution combined with a 68–75% rectangular 280–400 mm FOV to achieve a 132×256 matrix and flow compensation. The low bandwidth is used to minimize noise and increase signal-to-noise ratio while flow compensation gradients minimize flow artifact. The maximum signal intensity of any tissue occurs at a specific FA known as the Ernst angle, so the FA for this sequence is derived from the average Ernst angle for hepatic metastases at a field strength of 1.5T and a T1 of 1,000 msec. At a FA of 30° metastases tend to have a higher signal than hemangiomas and cysts because their T1 values are different (approximately 1337 msec for hemangiomas and approximately 3143 msec for cysts). Although this feature may be helpful in distinguishing benign from malignant lesions, the signal intensity of non-solid benign lesions is more distinctive on unenhanced T2w images so these should be obtained in all patients (Fig. 27). Unenhanced heavily T2w images are invaluable for demonstrating the high water content of cysts and hemangiomas but hypervascular metastases or metastases following chemotherapy may also exhibit a very high signal on T2w images and be indistinguishable. When the location of an apparently benign lesion on unenhanced images is likely to influence patient management, Gd-enhanced imaging is required for reliable characterization (Fig. 28). For effective fat suppression we use a water excitation technique which selectively excites water protons using a binomial pulse sequence. With this approach 6–7 images are obtained during a breathhold period of 20 seconds.

DIAGNOSTIC VALUE OF CONTRAST AGENTS

Lesion Detection

Rapid sequential imaging after ECF Gd improves the detection of hypervascular lesions, particularly small HCCs. The added value of dynamic Gd-enhanced imaging for the detection of liver metastases is less well documented but with current techniques we see many metastases on Gd-enhanced VIBE images which are invisible on unenhanced T1w and T2w images (Fig. 29). We compared multi-slice helical CT at a slice thickness of 3.2 mm, 3D Gd-enhanced VIBE with an effective slice thickness of 2.5 mm, and SPIO-enhanced T2w GRE images at a slice thickness of 6 mm in 58 patients who underwent hepatic resection; both MR techniques were evaluated with unenhanced T1w and T2w sequences. The results of two independent observers were analyzed against the gold standard of surgery with intra-operative ultrasound and histopathology of the resected specimen sectioned at 3 mm intervals. For the detection of all lesions and for the sub-set of lesions 1 cm or smaller, SPIO was marginally more accurate and sensitive than Gd-enhanced MR and both MR techniques were significantly better than CT (Fig. 30). CT was also associated with the highest number of false positive calls and almost half of these were due to benign lesions being wrongly interpreted as metastases (Fig. 31).

There have been relatively few studies which have compared the different liver specific agents with each other or with helical CT, but all of these agents appear to improve lesion detection compared with unenhanced imaging. In the dynamic phase gadobenate and gadoxetic acid are equivalent to ECF Gd but more sensitive for the detection of small lesions when dynamic and delayed images are combined (Fig. 32). In phase 3 clinical trials, mangafodipir was shown to be more sensitive than CT but there is no evidence to suggest that it is better than ECF Gd for detecting liver metastases. In the first two hours after injection mangafodipir appears to have no advantage over unenhanced MR for HCC detection due to uptake in well-differentiated lesions, but imaging at 24 hours is probably more sensitive (Fig. 16).

SPIO-MR is currently regarded as one of the most accurate imaging methods for detecting small metastases. Sensitivity is similar to that of CTAP but accuracy is higher because CTAP produces more false positives. Several studies have shown SPIO-MR to be significantly more sensitive than non-contrast MR and helical CT and to improve on dynamic Gd-enhanced imaging for the detection of metastases. Studies comparing SPIO and Gd for the detection of HCC have produced conflicting results. In the authors' experience, diffuse infiltrating tumors are often best demonstrated with SPIO whereas small focal lesions are better seen on arterial phase Gd images (Fig. 33).

Lesion Characterization

Dynamic Gd-enhanced imaging is most valuable for characterizing liver pathology on the basis of its perfusion pattern, and should be regarded as the first choice technique for clinical MRI of the liver.

Regarding lesion characterization with gadobenate and gadoxetic acid, imaging at both the dynamic and delayed phases is recommended when a hepatocellular lesion is suspected, to demonstrate hepatocyte selectivity (Fig. 34). However, although hepatocellular lesions may show late hepatocyte-specific enhancement, this may be difficult to distinguish from non-specific delayed accumulation of contrast within the interstitial space of tumors which do not contain functioning hepatocytes (Fig. 35). Mangafodipir is limited in its ability to characterize lesions. Although its use reliably distinguishes between hepatocellular and most non-hepatocellular tumors, benign and malignant lesions may show similar enhancement patterns (Fig. 36). Uptake can be seen in all tumors of hepatocellular origin including HCC and has rarely been observed in neuroendocrine metastases.

Gadobenate may have a role in distinguishing FNH from adenoma. In a recent study of contrast media in histologically-confirmed hepatocellular lesions, adenomas showed little or no uptake of gadobenate on delayed images, while uptake and retention of mangafodipir and SPIO was consistently present. In FNH lesions, all three agents showed consistent uptake on delayed images.

SPIO enhancement is probably the most sensitive discriminator of benign and malignant hepatocellular lesions. Although hepatocellular tumors show varying degrees of SPIO uptake, a percentage signal intensity loss (PSIL) of greater than 40% on T2w post contrast images is almost always associated with benign disease (see Fig. 2, chap. 6). In order to measure PSIL, the same imaging sequence with identical parameters must be acquired before and after contrast. Unenhanced T2w images are necessary to distinguish benign non-hepatocellular lesions from metastases because cysts, hemangiomas, and metastases may all be highly hyperintense against the reduced signal intensity of background liver after SPIO. Most lesions can be correctly characterized by review of both pre- and post-contrast T2w images. A proportion of hemangiomas show a decrease in signal intensity after SPIO on T2w images (Fig. 37). This maybe explained by contrast in the vascular lakes that comprise hemangiomas, which is slow to clear due to sluggish flow. It has also been suggested that signal loss maybe due to uptake of SPIO particles in the macrophages or endothelial cells within hemangiomas.

DUAL CONTRAST MRI

Given the different contrast mechanisms of SPIO and ECF Gd and the different contributions of the two agents to the diagnosis of liver lesions, it would be expected that used in combination they could be even more effective. In a single examination the high sensitivity of SPIO for lesion detection can be combined with dynamic Gd-enhanced imaging which is able to characterize most lesions as benign or malignant. Further, the different magnetic properties of the two agents may lead to a synergistic increase in contrast between the reduced signal intensity of background liver after SPIO and the increased signal intensity of enhancing lesions after Gd (Fig. 38). The combined effects of SPIO and Gd may also improve the characterization of lesions, particularly nodules in cirrhosis which often show overlapping enhancement characteristics when either contrast agent is used alone. Well-differentiated HCC may show some uptake of SPIO, dysplastic nodules which are typically hypovascular are occasionally hypervascular and HCC which is typically hypervascular may be hypovascular. Much of this overlap is overcome when SPIO and Gd are used in combination (Fig. 39).

With the double contrast MRI technique the second agent can be injected immediately after acquisition of the images from the first agent. Gd injected before SPIO has no effect on subsequent SPIO-enhanced T2w images (Fig. 40). A "Gd-first" approach is useful to detect benign hepatocellular lesions which maybe isointense with adjacent liver on unenhanced and SPIO images. SPIO may then be administered for a specific diagnosis (see Fig. 4, chap. 6). SPIO produces a prolonged reduction in liver signal on both T1w and T2w images. Consequently, post-Gd lesion enhancement is more pronounced after prior injection of SPIO due to the reduced signal of background liver and hypervascular lesions are particularly conspicuous (Fig. 38). However, hypovascular lesions may be less conspicuous because Gd enhancement of liver parenchyma is less pronounced after SPIO. In studies using SPIO shortly followed by dynamic Gd-enhanced imaging in patients with late stage cirrhosis, significantly more HCCs (particularly lesions <1 cm) were detected with SPIO and Gd images combined compared with unenhanced or SPIO-enhanced images alone, although a few lesions were only visible with SPIO enhancement. The combined effects of SPIO and dynamic Gd-enhanced imaging also improved characterization of dysplastic nodules and HCC.

Although DCMR is probably the most sensitive approach for diagnosing liver tumors the additional costs and increased examination time requires the careful selection of only those patients whose clinical management maybe altered. We reserve the use of DCMR for three main applications: firstly, diagnostic problem cases when the results of MR with a single contrast agent are equivocal (Figs. 41 and 42), secondly as a "one-stop-shopping" approach in surgical patients who are candidates for hepatic resection or transplantation (see Fig. 18, chap. 5) particularly patients with co-existing benign and malignant lesions (Fig. 43) and to assess the resectability status of hilar cholangiocarcinoma in patients who are being considered for surgery (Fig. 44). Thirdly, DCMR is performed in patients with cirrhosis considered to be at high risk of developing HCC (see Fig. 36, chap. 9).

ILLUSTRATIVE FIGURES

Non-specific extra-cellular (ECF) gadolinium agents—Figures 1–9
Tissue-specific contrast agents—Figures 10, 11
Hepatocyte agents—Figures 12–18
Reticulo-endothelial system (Kupffer cell) agents—Figures 19–28
Diagnostic value of contrast agents—Figures 29–37
Dual contrast MRI—Figures 38–44.

REFERENCES

General Reviews

1. Reimer P, Scneider G, Schima W. Hepatobiliary contrast agents for contrast-enhanced MRI of the liver: properties, clinical development and applications. Eur Radiol 2004; 14:S59–S78.
2. Helmberger T, Semelka RC. New contrast agents for imaging the liver. Magn Reson Imaging Clin N Am 2001; 9:745–766.
3. Kim MJ, Kim JH, Lim JS, et al. Detection and characterization of focal hepatic lesions: mangafodipir vs. superparamagnetic iron oxide-enhanced magnetic resonance imaging. J Magn Reson Imaging 2004; 20:612–621.
4. Tang Y, Yamashita Y, Arakawa A, et al. Detection of hepatocellular carcinomas arising in cirrhotic livers: comparison of gadolinium-and ferumoxides-enhanced MR imaging. Am J Roentgenol 1999; 172:1547–1554.

ECF Gadolinium Chelates

5. Low RN. MR imaging of the liver using gadolinium chelates. Magn Reson Imaging Clin N Am 2001; 9:717–743.
6. Yamashita Y, Mitsuzaki K, Yi T, et al. Small hepatocellular carcinoma in patients with chronic liver damage: prospective comparison of detection with dynamic MR imaging and helical CT of the whole liver. Radiology 1996; 200:79–84.

Mangafodipir

7. Rummeny EJ, Torres CG, Kurdziel JC, et al. MnDPDP for MR imaging of the liver. Results of an independent image evaluation of the European phase 111 studies. Acta Radiol 1997; 38:638–642.
8. Kane P, Ayton V, Walters HL, et al. MnDPDP-enhanced MR imaging of the liver, correlation with surgical findings. Acta Radiol 1997; 38:650–654.
9. Bartolozzi C, Donati F, Cioni D, et al. Detection of colorectal liver metastases: a prospective multicenter trial comparing unenhanced MRI, MnDPDP-enhanced MRI, and spiral CT. Eur Radiol 2004; 14:14–20.
10. Scharitzer M, Schima W, Schober E, et al. Characterization of hepatocellular tumors: value of mangafodipir-enhanced magnetic resonance imaging. J Comput Assist Tomogr 2005; 29:181–190.
11. Lee VS, Rofsky NM, Morgan GR, et al. Volumetric mangafodipir-trisodium-enhanced cholangiography to define intrahepatic biliary anatomy. Am J Roentgenol 2001; 176:906–908.

Gadobenate

12. Petersein J, Spinazzi A, Giovagnoni A, et al. Focal liver lesion: evaluation of the efficacy of gadobenate dimeglumine in MR imaging of focal liver lesions: -a multicenter phase 3 clinical study. Radiology 2000; 215:727–736.
13. Kim YK, Lee JM, Kim CS. Gadobenate dimeglumine-enhanced liver MR imaging: value of dynamic and delayed imaging for the characterization and detection of focal liver lesions. Eur Radiol 2004; 14:5–13.
14. Grazioli L, Morana G, Krichin MA, Schneider G. Accurate differentiation of focal nodular hyperplasia from hepatic adenoma at gadobenate dimeglumine-enhanced MR imaging: prospective study. Radiology 2005; 236:166–177.

Gadoxetic Acid

15. Hamm B, Staks T, Muhler A, et al. Phase I clinical evaluation of Gd-EOB-DTPA as a hepatobiliary MR contrast agent: safety, pharmacokinetics, and MR imaging. Radiology 1995; 195:785–792.
16. Huppertz A, Balzer T, Blakeborough A, et al. Improved detection of focal liver lesions at MR imaging: multicenter comparison of gadoxetic acid-enhanced MR images with intraoperative findings. Radiology 2004; 230:468–478.
17. Huppertz A, Haraida S, Kraus A, et al. Enhancement of focal liver lesions at gadoxetic acid-enhanced MR imaging; correlation with histopathologic findings and spiral CT-initial observations. Radiology 2005; 234:4478–4678.

SPIO Agents

18. Scott J, Ward J, Guthrie JA, Wilson D, Robinson PJ. MRI of liver: comparison of CNR enhancement using high dose and low dose ferumoxide infusion in patients with colorectal liver metastases. Magn Reson Imaging 2000; 18:297–303.
19. Bluemke DA, Weber TM, Rubin D, et al. Hepatic MR imaging with ferumoxides: multicenter study of safety and effectiveness of direct injection protocol. Radiology 2003; 228:457–464.
20. Ward J, Guthrie JA, Wilson D, et al. Colorectal hepatic metastases, detection with SPIO-enhanced breathhold imaging: comparison of optimized sequences at 1.5T. Radiology 2003; 228:709–718.
21. Vogl T J, Schwarz W, Blume S, et al. Preoperative evaluation of malignant liver tumors: comparison of unenhanced and SPIO (Resovist)-enhanced MR imaging with biphasic CTAP and intraoperative U.S. Eur Radiol 2003; 13:262–272.
22. Helmberger T, Gregor M, Holzknecht N, et al. Comparison of dual phase helical CT with native and ferumoxide-enhanced magnetic resonance imaging in detection and characterization of focal liver lesions. Radiology 1999; 39:678–684.

Dual Contrast

23. Ward J, Robinson P. Combined use of MR contrast agents for evaluating liver disease. Magn Reson Imaging Clin N Am 2001; 9:767–783.
24. Bhartia B, Ward J, Guthrie JA, Robinson PJ. Hepatocellular carcinoma in cirrhotic livers: double-contrast thin-section MR imaging with pathologic correlation of explanted tissue. Am J Roentgenol 2003; 180:577–584.
25. Ward J, Guthrie JA, Scott DJ, et al. Hepatocellular carcinoma in the cirrhotic liver: double contrast MR imaging for diagnosis. Radiology 2000; 216:154–162.

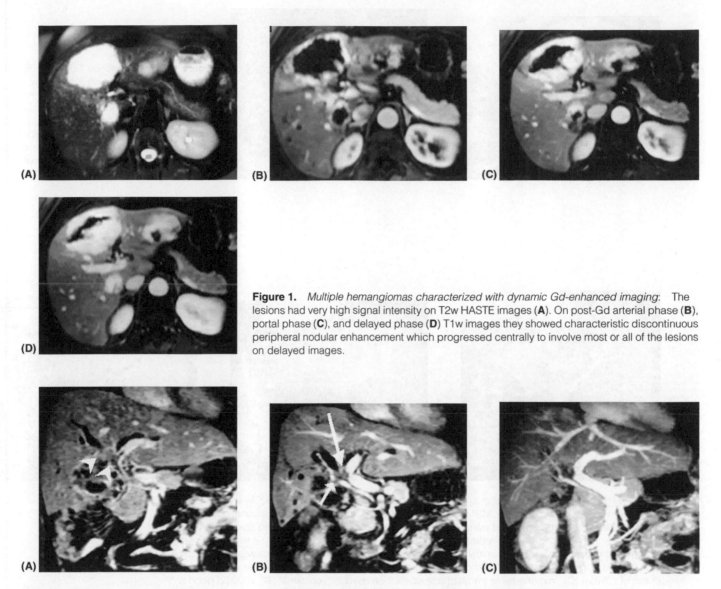

Figure 1. *Multiple hemangiomas characterized with dynamic Gd-enhanced imaging:* The lesions had very high signal intensity on T2w HASTE images (**A**). On post-Gd arterial phase (**B**), portal phase (**C**), and delayed phase (**D**) T1w images they showed characteristic discontinuous peripheral nodular enhancement which progressed centrally to involve most or all of the lesions on delayed images.

Figure 2. *Simultaneous soft tissue and vascular assessment in a patient with a surgically confirmed colorectal liver metastasis:* Coronal oblique post- Gd T1w images (**A** and **B**) showed tumor invading the common hepatic duct and right intrahepatic bile ducts (arrowheads), also involvement of the portal vein bifurcation (long arrow) and right hepatic artery (short arrow) which was replaced from the superior mesenteric artery. MIP image (**C**) derived from the same post-Gd sequence as (**A**) and (**B**) provided a comprehensive assessment of the vascular anatomy.

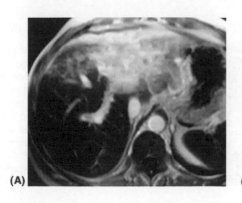

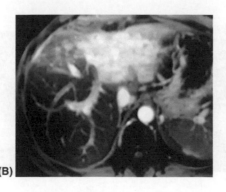

Figure 3. *Fat suppression accentuates gadolinium enhancement:* In a patient with an intrahepatic cholangiocarcinoma, identical Gd-enhanced in-phase T1w 2D GRE images were obtained without (**A**) and with (**B**) fat suppression. Measured lesion-to-liver contrast-to-noise ratios were 69 and 80 for images (**A**) and (**B**) respectively.

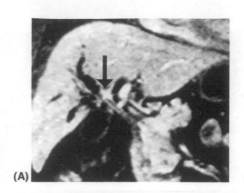

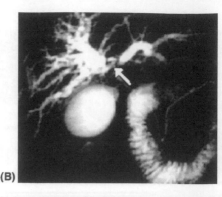

Figure 4. *High resolution 1.5 mm VIBE imaging*: In a patient with a surgically confirmed 1 cm hilar cholangiocarcinoma, delayed coronal oblique post-Gd T1w imaging (**A**) showed a 1 cm tumor (arrow) at the confluence of the right and left intrahepatic bile ducts. The lesion shown in (**A**) correlated with the point of obstruction (arrow) on the corresponding HASTE MRCP image (**B**).

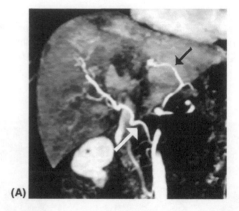

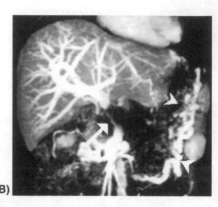

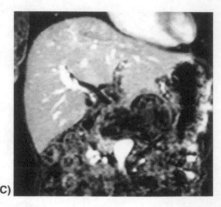

Figure 5. *High resolution VIBE imaging to evaluate the portal/mesenteric vasculature*: In a patient with a large pancreatic cystadenocarcinoma, MIP reconstruction derived from Gd-enhanced coronal oblique T1w images acquired at the arterial (**A**) and portal (**B**) phases of enhancement demonstrated aberrant arterial anatomy. The right hepatic artery was replaced from the SMA [white arrow in (**A**)] and the left hepatic artery arose from the left gastric artery [black arrow in (**A**)], the portal/mesenteric vein confluence was occluded [white arrow in (**B**)] and extensive varices were shown [arrowheads in (**B**)]. A single image with an effective slice thickness of 1.5 mm (**C**), from the same portal phase acquisition used to reconstruct (**B**), showed good soft tissue detail of the cystic tumor and adjacent parenchyma.

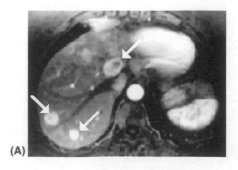

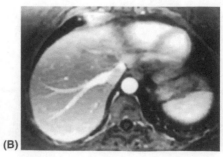

Figure 6. *Hypervascular neuroendocrine metastases*: Gd-enhanced T1w image obtained at the arterial phase of enhancement (**A**) showed three hyperintense metastases (arrows) which were no longer visible by the portal phase (**B**) when the background liver was maximally enhanced. Note optimal arterial phase enhancement on (**A**) as demonstrated by enhancement of the hepatic arteries and portal veins before the hepatic veins were opacified.

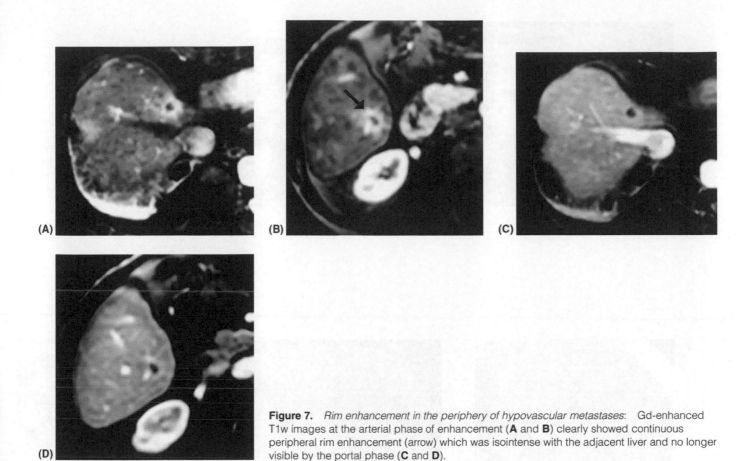

Figure 7. *Rim enhancement in the periphery of hypovascular metastases*: Gd-enhanced T1w images at the arterial phase of enhancement (**A** and **B**) clearly showed continuous peripheral rim enhancement (arrow) which was isointense with the adjacent liver and no longer visible by the portal phase (**C** and **D**).

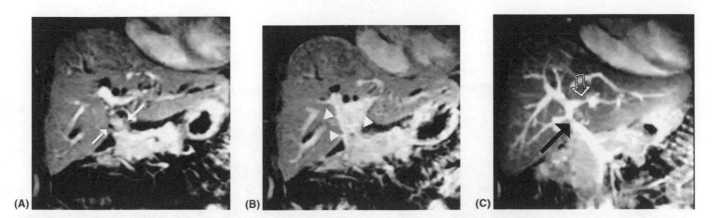

Figure 8. *Delayed enhancement in hilar cholangiocarcinoma*: Gd-enhanced portal phase coronal oblique T1w image (**A**) showed an ill-defined tumor at the liver hilum (arrows). On the corresponding image acquired 10 minutes later (**B**) more extensive tumor (arrowheads) was apparent due to intense delayed enhancement. MIP image (**C**) derived from the same acquisition as (**A**) showed narrowing of the distal main portal vein (black arrow) and left intrahepatic portal vein (open arrow) which corresponds with the tumor extent shown in (**B**).

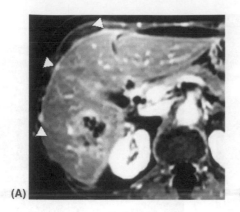

(A)

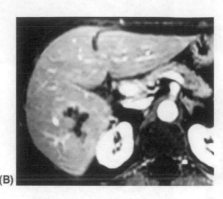

(B)

Figure 9. *Delayed enhancement in peritoneal tumor deposits from colon cancer.* T1w images obtained 10 minutes after Gd injection (**A**) clearly showed enhancing tumor deposits over the liver surface (arrowheads) which were not visible on the corresponding portal phase image (**B**).

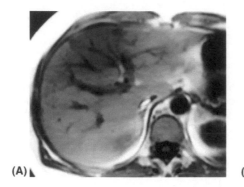

(A)

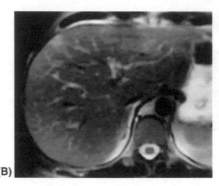

(B)

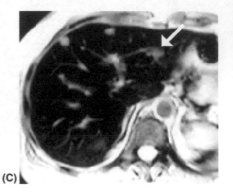

(C)

Figure 10. *Improved detection of metastatic colon cancer with SPIO:* Compared with unenhanced T1w (**A**) and HASTE (**B**) images, lesion-to-liver contrast was markedly improved on the post-SPIO fat-suppressed T2w GRE image (**C**). An additional 1 cm metastasis [arrow in (**C**)] was only visible after SPIO.

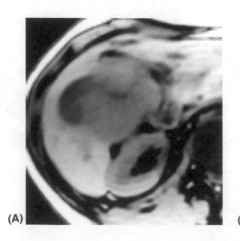

(A)

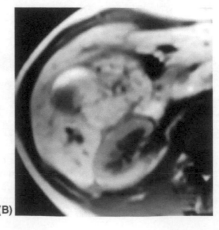

(B)

Figure 11. *Liver-specific contrast uptake in two patients with focal nodular hyperplasia (FNH):* An FNH lesion which was mildly hypointense to liver on unenhanced T1w imaging (**A**) showed uptake of contrast greater than that of normal liver on the corresponding image obtained after mangafodipir (**B**). Note contrast in the gallbladder on (**B**) due to biliary excretion. In a second patient, T2w images obtained before (**C**) and after SPIO (**D**), showed marked uptake of SPIO by the liver and the lesion. The characteristic central scar of FNH (arrow) was best depicted after SPIO. (*Continued*)

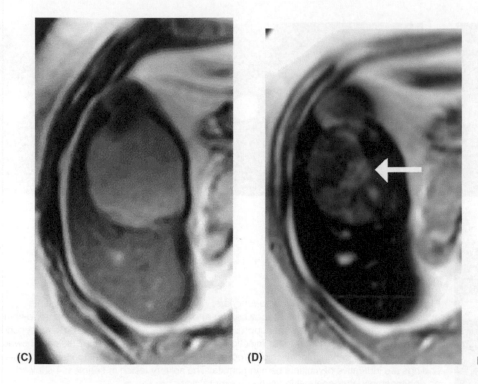

(C)

(D)

Figure 11. (*Continued*)

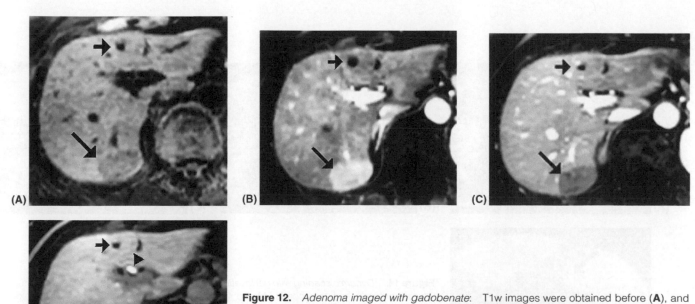

(A)

(B)

(C)

(D)

Figure 12. *Adenoma imaged with gadobenate*: T1w images were obtained before (**A**), and 15 seconds (**B**), 45 seconds (**C**), and 40 minutes (**D**) after bolus injection of gadobenate. The lesion (long arrow) showed marked enhancement at the arterial phase (**B**) which rapidly faded to hypointensity relative to the background liver by the portal phase (**C**). Compared with (**A**) there was marked enhancement of the normal liver parenchyma on delayed images (**D**) due to uptake by functioning hepatocytes, but little contrast uptake by the lesion. Note a simple cyst in segment four (short arrow) and enhancement of the CBD (arrowhead) due to biliary excretion.

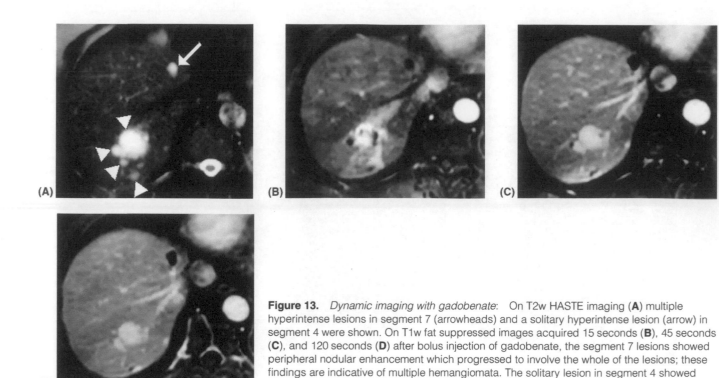

Figure 13.   *Dynamic imaging with gadobenate*:   On T2w HASTE imaging (**A**) multiple hyperintense lesions in segment 7 (arrowheads) and a solitary hyperintense lesion (arrow) in segment 4 were shown. On T1w fat suppressed images acquired 15 seconds (**B**), 45 seconds (**C**), and 120 seconds (**D**) after bolus injection of gadobenate, the segment 7 lesions showed peripheral nodular enhancement which progressed to involve the whole of the lesions; these findings are indicative of multiple hemangiomata. The solitary lesion in segment 4 showed no enhancement after contrast indicating a simple cyst.

Figure 14.   *Dynamic imaging with gadoxetic acid*:   Enhancement of the vascular structures on T1w images acquired 15 seconds (**A**) and 45 seconds (**B**) after bolus injection of gadoxetic acid was similar to that seen with extra-cellular Gd agents. On the corresponding image acquired 2 minutes after injection (**C**) most of the contrast had cleared from the intra-vascular space and enhancement of the normal liver parenchyma due to hepatocyte uptake was already apparent. Progressive enhancement of the normal liver was observed over time and tumor-liver contrast was optimum approximately 20 minutes after injection (**D**). Biliary enhancement was also seen at this time (arrow).

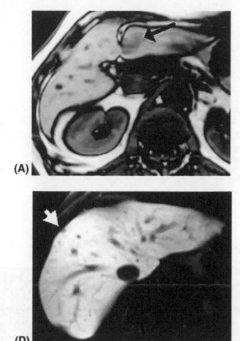

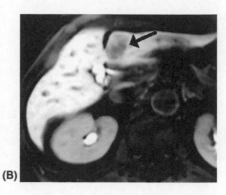

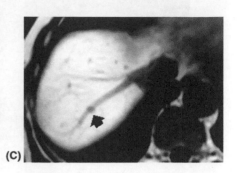

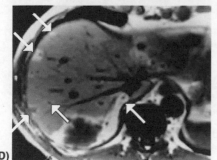

Figure 15. *Improved detection of metastatic colon cancer with gadoxetic acid:* Compared with the unenhanced T1w image (**A**), the contrast between the liver and tumor (long arrow) was dramatically increased on the corresponding image obtained 20 minutes after gadoxetic acid (**B**) when hepatocyte enhancement was maximum. Additional sub-cm lesions (short arrows) which were not visible on unenhanced sequences were shown on the 20 minute post-contrast T1w images (**C**, **D**) and confirmed by later enlargement on follow-up.

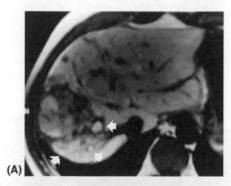

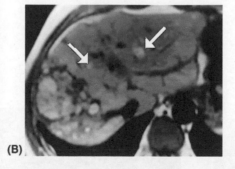

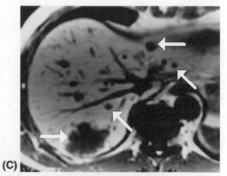

Figure 16. *Improved detection of tumor with 24-hour mangafodipir-enhanced imaging:* On T1w images obtained 20 minutes after mangafodipir (**A**), a large HCC with numerous peripheral nodules (short arrows) showed contrast uptake similar to that of background liver. On the corresponding image obtained 24 hours later (**B**), the liver parenchyma had returned to its base-line signal intensity; the previously detected lesions and several additional tumor nodules (long arrows) were then more conspicuous because of abnormal contrast retention by the HCC. In a different patient with colorectal cancer, multiple metastases (arrows) were seen with high lesion-to-liver contrast on 20 minute post-mangafodipir T1w images (**C**) when there was maximum enhancement of the background liver. However several additional small metastases (arrows) were well seen on T1w images obtained 24 hours later (**D**) because retained contrast medium in the compressed liver tissue at the periphery of the lesions is particularly conspicuous against the normal signal of the background liver. (Images courtesy of Dr. J. Healy).

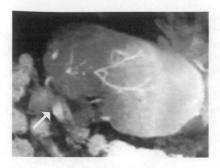

Figure 17. *Contrast cholangiogram*:   MIP image was derived from mangafodipir-enhanced T1w 3D GRE images at an effective slice thickness of 1.5 mm in a child with recurrent cholangitis following split liver transplantation. The mangafodipir-MR cholangiogram showed normal caliber of the intra-hepatic ducts and prompt flow across the bilio-enteric anastomosis (arrow).

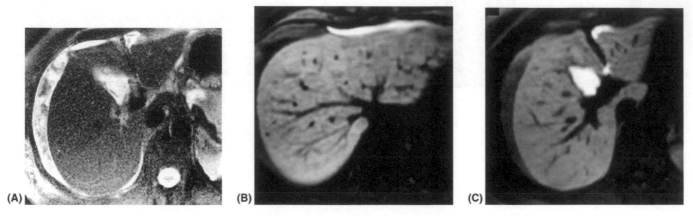

(A)   (B)   (C)

Figure 18. *Contrast cholangiography—bile duct leak following laparoscopic cholecystectomy*:   Unenhanced HASTE image (**A**) showed non-specific free fluid over the liver surface and in the gallbladder fossa. T1w images obtained 30 minutes after infusion of mangafodipir (**B**, **C**) demonstrated leakage of contrast into the gallbladder fossa and over the anterior surface of the left lobe, confirming a biliary leak.

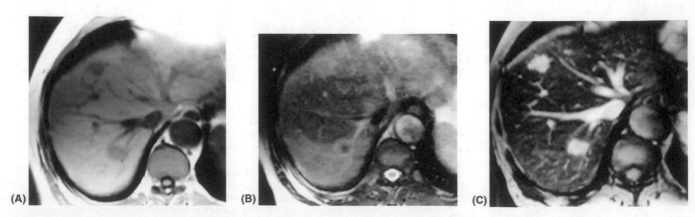

(A)   (B)   (C)

Figure 19. *Colonic metastases more conspicuous after SPIO*:   Compared with unenhanced T1w (**A**) and T2w (**B**) images, tumor-to-liver contrast was dramatically increased on T2w GRE images obtained after SPIO (**C**) due to a marked reduction in the signal intensity of the normal liver.

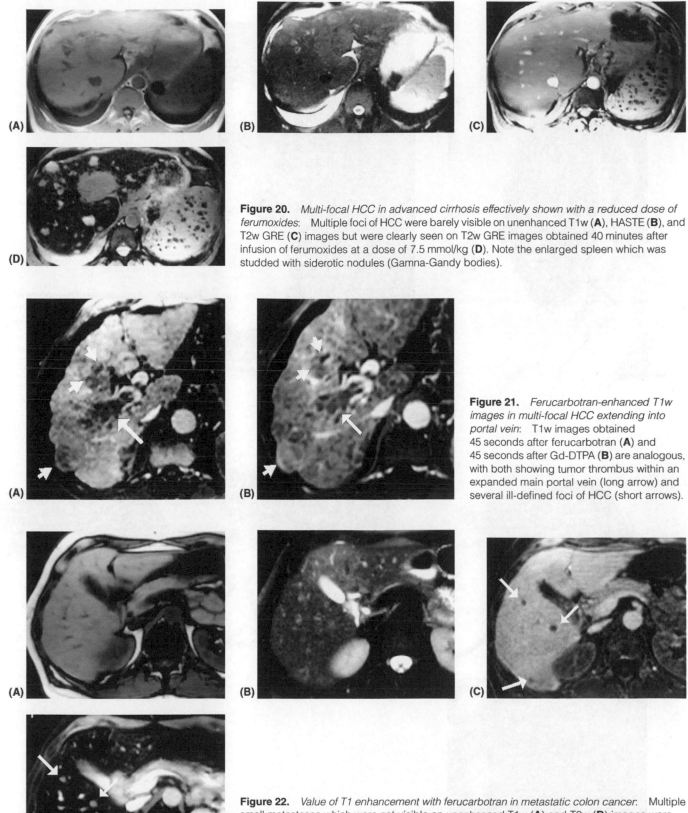

Figure 20. *Multi-focal HCC in advanced cirrhosis effectively shown with a reduced dose of ferumoxides:*   Multiple foci of HCC were barely visible on unenhanced T1w (**A**), HASTE (**B**), and T2w GRE (**C**) images but were clearly seen on T2w GRE images obtained 40 minutes after infusion of ferumoxides at a dose of 7.5 mmol/kg (**D**). Note the enlarged spleen which was studded with siderotic nodules (Gamna-Gandy bodies).

Figure 21. *Ferucarbotran-enhanced T1w images in multi-focal HCC extending into portal vein:*   T1w images obtained 45 seconds after ferucarbotran (**A**) and 45 seconds after Gd-DTPA (**B**) are analogous, with both showing tumor thrombus within an expanded main portal vein (long arrow) and several ill-defined foci of HCC (short arrows).

Figure 22. *Value of T1 enhancement with ferucarbotran in metastatic colon cancer:*   Multiple small metastases which were not visible on unenhanced T1w (**A**) and T2w (**B**) images were clearly seen (arrows) on T1w images (**C**) obtained 45 seconds after bolus injection of ferucarbotran. In (**C**) the lesions were hypointense relative to the background liver and vessels which were isointense due to the relatively weak T1 effect of the normal dose of iron oxide. The lesions were all well seen on T2w GRE images (**D**) obtained 10 minutes after (**C**).

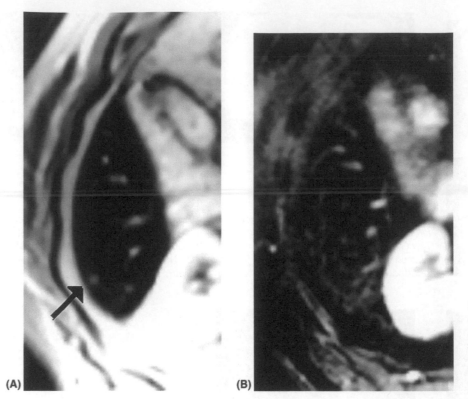

Figure 23. *Importance of the choice of pulse sequence for effective lesion detection after SPIO:* A 5 mm surgically confirmed metastasis (arrow) was well shown on SPIO-enhanced T2w GRE (**A**) but was not visible on the corresponding SPIO-enhanced FSE T2w image (**B**).

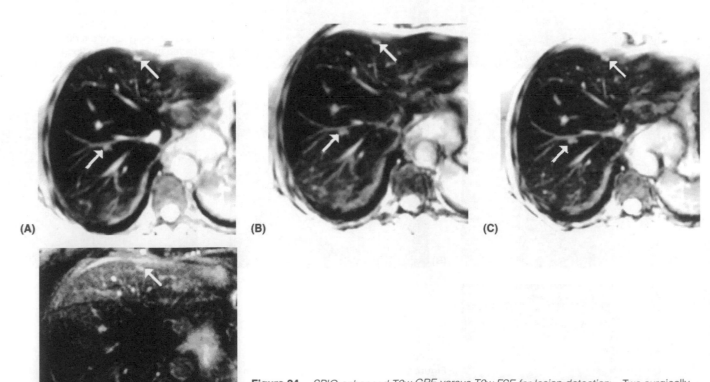

Figure 24. *SPIO enhanced T2w GRE versus T2w FSE for lesion detection:* Two surgically confirmed sub-cm metastases (arrows) were clearly seen on multi-echo data image combination (MEDIC) GRE sequence (**A**), T2w GRE with a TE of 11 msec (**B**), and T2w GRE with a TE of 15 msec (**C**) acquired after SPIO. Only one was visible on the corresponding SPIO-enhanced FSE T2w sequence (**D**).

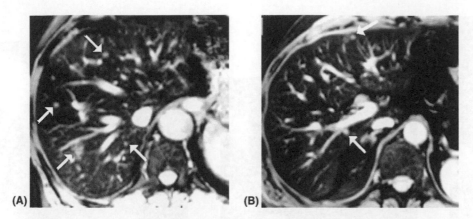

Figure 25. *Optimized T2w GRE sequence with fat suppression for improved visualization of small metastases:*   Multiple small colorectal metastases (arrows) were clearly shown on SPIO-enhanced T2w GRE images acquired with a 6 mm slice thickness and fat suppression (**A, B**).

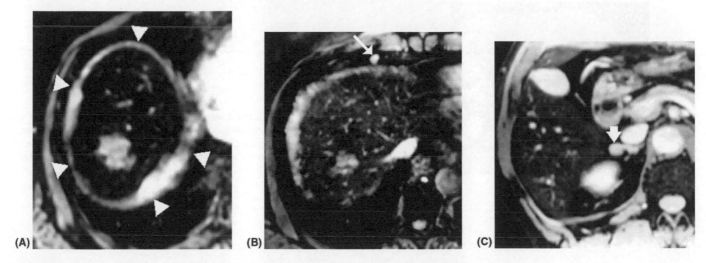

Figure 26. *Value of SPIO-enhanced T2w GRE images with fat suppression for detecting extra-hepatic disease:*   The high signal intensity of peritoneal disease (**A** and **B**) (arrowheads), lymphadenopathy (**B**) (long arrow), and adrenal metastasis (**C**) (short arrow) in three different patients was highly conspicuous on SPIO-enhanced T2w fat-suppressed GRE images against the reduced signal intensity of the liver and the suppressed signal of intra-abdominal fat.

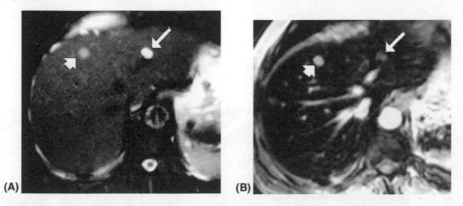

Figure 27. *Co-existent benign and malignant liver lesions after SPIO—importance of unenhanced heavily T2w images for lesion characterization:*   On unenhanced HASTE imaging (**A**) a simple cyst (long arrow) was well defined and strongly hyperintense while the metastasis (short arrow) was ill defined and only slightly hyperintense relative to the background liver. On SPIO-enhanced T2w GRE (**B**) the cyst had a relatively reduced signal intensity compared with (**A**) and was barely visible, while the metastasis was more conspicuous because of the 30⁰ flip angle chosen to maximize the signal from metastases. On post-Gd T1w images (not illustrated) the cyst showed no enhancement.

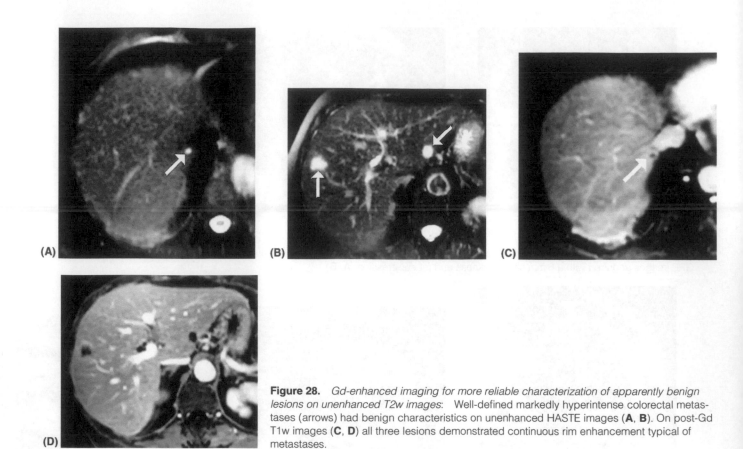

Figure 28. *Gd-enhanced imaging for more reliable characterization of apparently benign lesions on unenhanced T2w images:* Well-defined markedly hyperintense colorectal metastases (arrows) had benign characteristics on unenhanced HASTE images (**A**, **B**). On post-Gd T1w images (**C**, **D**) all three lesions demonstrated continuous rim enhancement typical of metastases.

Figure 29. *Metastatic pancreatic cancer:* Small sub-cm metastases which were not visible on unenhanced T1w (**A**) and T2w (**B**) images were well seen (arrows) on portal phase Gd-enhanced T1w images (**C**).

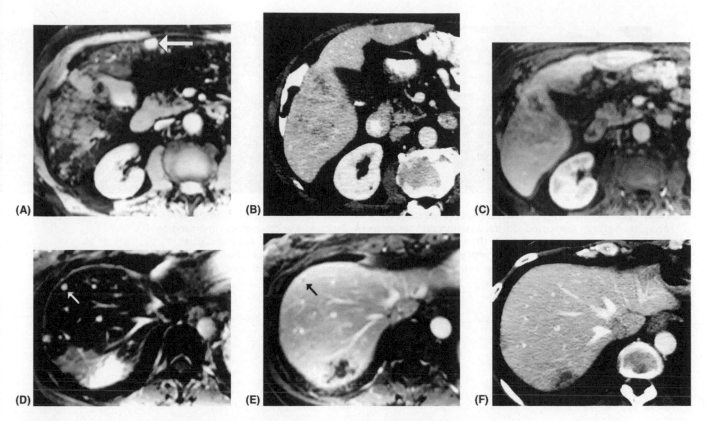

Figure 30. *Metastatic colon cancer—improved detection with SPIO:* A metastasis (long arrow) which was conspicuous on SPIO-enhanced T2w GRE image (**A**) was not detected by either of two observers on thin-slice helical CT (**B**) or Gd-enhanced T1w imaging (**C**). In a second patient a 1-cm lesion (short arrow) was well seen on SPIO-enhanced T2w GRE (**D**) and Gd-enhanced T1w imaging (**E**) but was not visible on thin-slice helical CT (**F**).

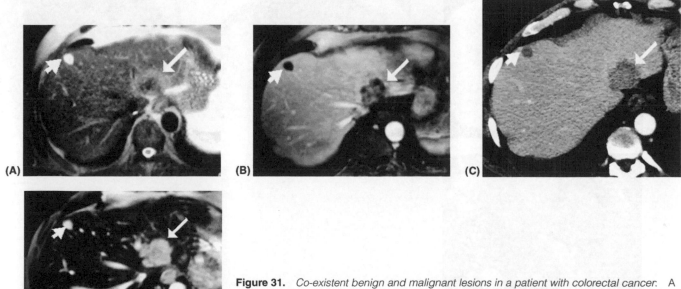

Figure 31. *Co-existent benign and malignant lesions in a patient with colorectal cancer:* A simple cyst (short arrow) and a metastasis (long arrow) had markedly different signal intensity characteristics on HASTE (**A**) and Gd-enhanced T1w (**B**) images, but the lesions had similar appearances on CT (**C**) and SPIO-enhanced T2w GRE imaging (**D**). The benign lesion was wrongly interpreted as a metastasis on CT but correctly characterized as benign on Gd- and SPIO-enhanced images viewed in combination with HASTE.

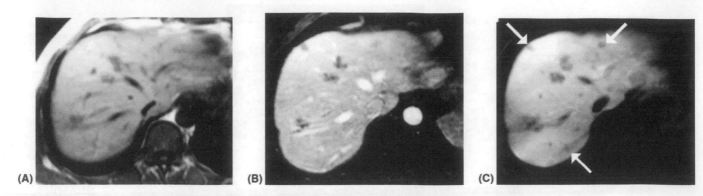

Figure 32. *Colorectal liver metastases—improved detection with gadobenate-enhanced dynamic and delayed imaging:* Compared with the unenhanced T1w image (**A**), lesion-to-liver contrast was improved on T1w images obtained at both the ECF (**B**) and hepatocyte (**C**) phases of enhancement. Additional small metastases (arrows) were only visible after contrast. Combined review of both phases of enhancement allows lesions which may be more clearly seen at the hepatocyte phase to be distinguished from vessels which show high signal at the early vascular phase.

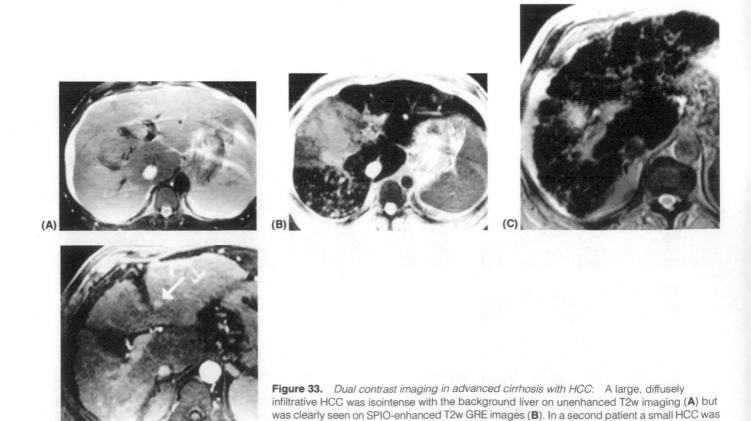

Figure 33. *Dual contrast imaging in advanced cirrhosis with HCC:* A large, diffusely infiltrative HCC was isointense with the background liver on unenhanced T2w imaging (**A**) but was clearly seen on SPIO-enhanced T2w GRE images (**B**). In a second patient a small HCC was difficult to distinguish from strands of fibrosis on SPIO-enhanced T2w GRE imaging (**C**) but was well visualized (arrow) on immediate post-Gd T1w images (**D**).

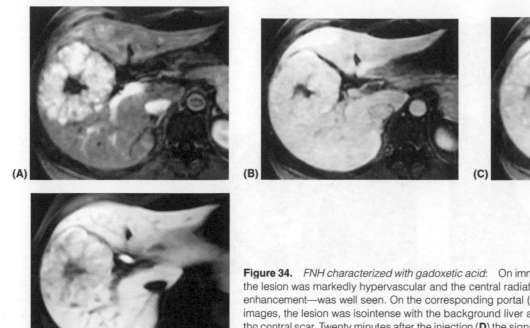

Figure 34. *FNH characterized with gadoxetic acid*: On immediate post-contrast T1w images the lesion was markedly hypervascular and the central radiating scar—which showed no enhancement—was well seen. On the corresponding portal (**B**) and equilibrium phase (**C**) images, the lesion was isointense with the background liver and there was no enhancement of the central scar. Twenty minutes after the injection (**D**) the signal intensity of the background liver was maximized, persistent isointense enhancement of the lesion was apparent and the non-enhancing scar and its radiations were particularly conspicuous.

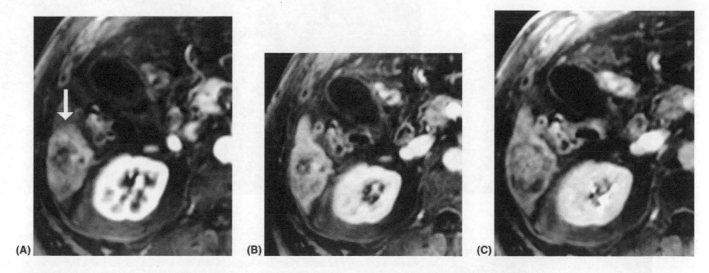

Figure 35. *Poorly differentiated HCC with delayed enhancement after gadobenate*: On arterial phase T1w images (**A**), the lesion (arrow) showed moderate inhomogeneous enhancement which faded to inhomogeneous isointensity by the portal phase (**B**). The equilibrium phase image (**C**) showed accumulation of contrast in the central part of the tumor and washout of contrast from the periphery (a feature which is characteristic of malignancy). This enhancement persisted at the later hepatocyte phase (**D**) due to non-specific accumulation of contrast within the interstitial space. Delayed enhancement of the interstitial space of metastases is frequently observed following injection of the non-specific ECF Gd chelates as demonstrated in a different patient with colorectal metastases (arrows) imaged 70 minutes after injection of Gd-DTPA (**E**). This example illustrates the importance of evaluating images at early and delayed phases of enhancement when a bi-phasic contrast agent is used. (*Continued*)

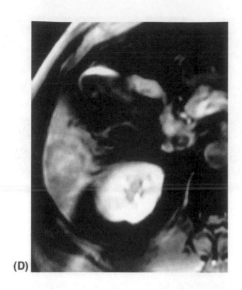

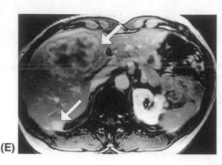

(D)

(E)

Figure 35. (*Continued*)

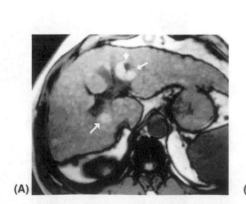

(A)

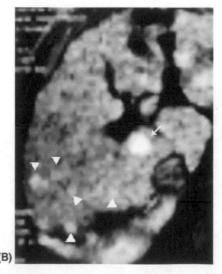

(B)

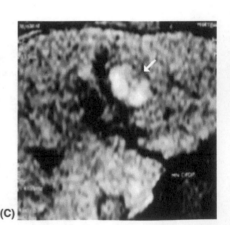

(C)

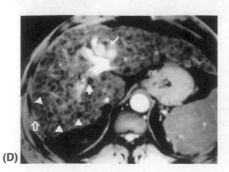

(D)

Figure 36. *Dysplastic nodules and HCC in advanced cirrhosis imaged with mangafodipir and SPIO:* Unenhanced opposed-phase T1w image (**A**) showed two hyperintense lesions (long arrows) in a diffusely nodular liver. The larger of the two lesions contained a hypointense fatty focus (short arrow) which was highly suggestive of HCC. The second lesion had MR signal characteristics that were consistent with either a dysplastic nodule or HCC. On mangafodipir-enhanced T1w images (**B**, **C**) both lesions (long arrows) exhibited uniform uptake of contrast with no distinguishing features. Multiple additional enhancing nodules were also seen (arrowheads). However on SPIO-enhanced T2w GRE images (**D**) the larger lesion showed no uptake of iron oxide confirming HCC (long arrow) while the second lesion showed considerable uptake consistent with a dysplastic nodule (short arrow). A third ill-defined lesion which also exhibited mangafodipir enhancement (open arrow) showed mixed uptake after SPIO and was likely to represent a focus of HCC developing in a dysplastic nodule. The other sub-cm nodules seen on (**C**) showed marked uptake of iron oxide indicating benign disease (arrowheads).

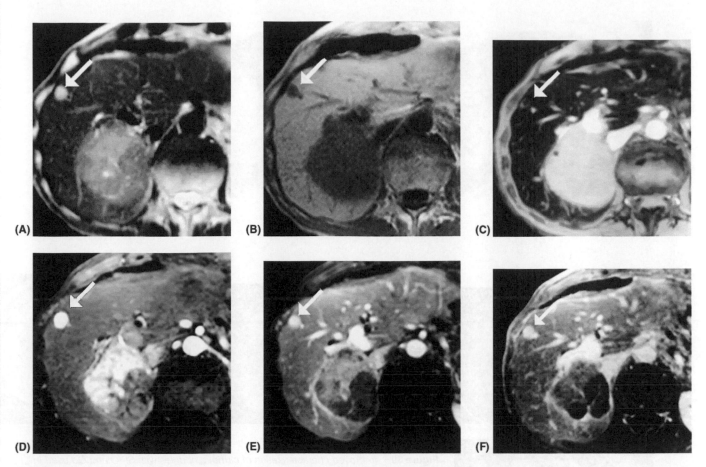

Figure 37. *Co-existent HCC and hemangioma: reduced signal intensity on T2w imaging after SPIO in a small hemangioma*:   The hemangioma (arrow) was well defined and hyperintense on unenhanced HASTE imaging (**A**) and hypointense on unenhanced in-phase T1w imaging (**B**). On SPIO-enhanced T2w GRE images (**C**) the hemangioma was barely visible due to uptake of SPIO particles. On Gd-enhanced arterial phase (**D**), portal phase (**E**) and delayed phase (**F**) T1w images the hemangioma demonstrated characteristic features with enhancement similar to that of the vessels at each phase of enhancement.

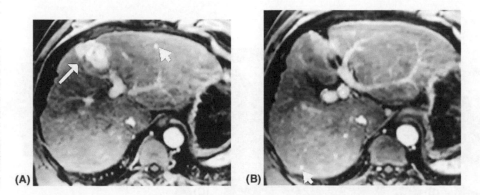

Figure 38. *Multiple HCCs in advanced cirrhosis*:   On T1w images obtained approximately 3 hours after SPIO infusion and 15 seconds from the end of Gd injection (**A**, **B**) a large HCC (long arrow) and two additional sub-cm lesions (short arrows) were highly conspicuous due to a synergistic increase in contrast between the early enhancing lesions after Gd and the reduced signal intensity of the background liver after SPIO. The lesions were visible on the previously acquired SPIO-enhanced T2w GRE images (**C**, **D**) but the smaller lesions were difficult to distinguish from adjacent vessels. (*Continued*)

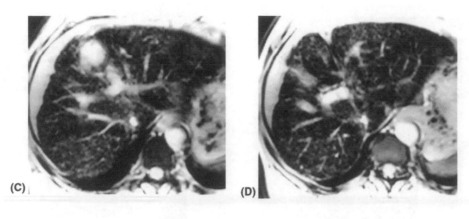

Figure 38.   (*Continued*)

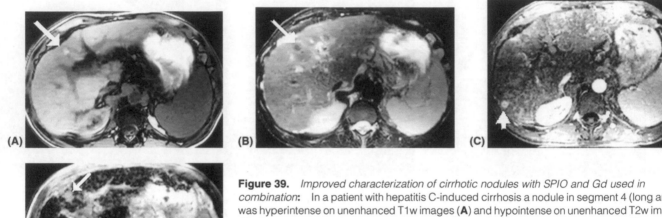

Figure 39.   *Improved characterization of cirrhotic nodules with SPIO and Gd used in combination:*   In a patient with hepatitis C-induced cirrhosis a nodule in segment 4 (long arrow) was hyperintense on unenhanced T1w images (**A**) and hypointense on unenhanced T2w images (**B**). The vascularity of the nodule shown on the post-Gd arterial phase T1w images (**C**) was little different from the adjacent liver, suggesting it was a dysplastic nodule. However, on SPIO-enhanced T2w GRE images (**D**) the nodule showed no uptake of SPIO, indicating its malignant nature. A second 10 mm HCC [short arrow in (**C**) and (**D**)] which showed characteristic enhancement with arterial phase hypervascularity (**C**) and no uptake of SPIO (**D**) was not visible on (**A**) or (**B**). Both lesions were histologically confirmed HCCs.

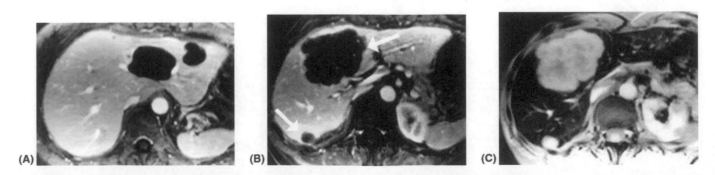

Figure 40.   *Effect of Gd injected prior to SPIO on subsequent SPIO enhancement:*   In a patient with co-existent benign and malignant lesions, portal phase Gd-enhanced T1w images showed two simple cysts on [non-enhancing in (**A**)] and two metastases with continuous rim enhancement [arrows in (**B**)]. The presence of Gd had no appreciable effect on the subsequent T2w GRE image (**C**) obtained approximately 100 minutes after Gd injection and 30 minutes after SPIO infusion.

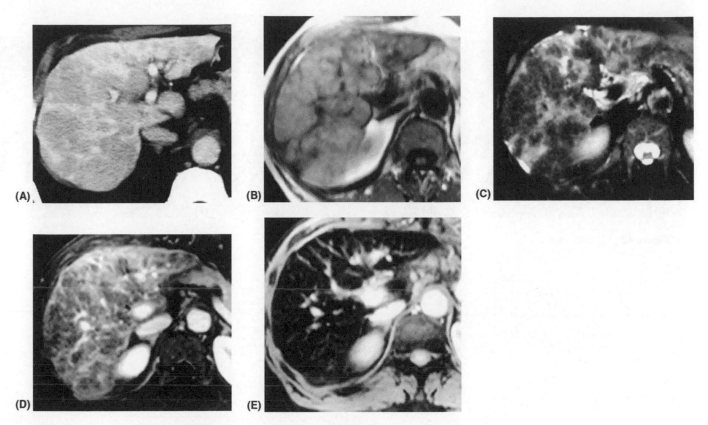

Figure 41. *Dual contrast imaging for lesion characterization after inconclusive Gd-enhanced imaging:* In a patient with extensive metastatic disease reported on CT and sonography, the CT (**A**), unenhanced T1w (**B**), unenhanced T2w (**C**), and portal phase post-Gd T1w (**D**) images all showed very abnormal liver architecture and inhomogeneous enhancement. On subsequent SPIO-enhanced T2w GRE imaging (**E**), a much more uniform appearance was shown indicating functioning liver tissue and benign disease in the areas of abnormal signal on unenhanced images. Biopsy confirmed hepatitis with patchy acute inflammatory change.

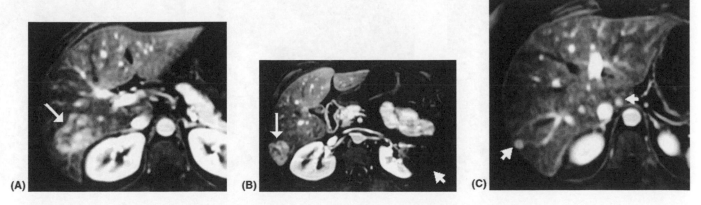

Figure 42. *Inconclusive lesion characterization following Gd—characterization improved with SPIO:* Probable liver metastases were reported on sonography and CT in a patient with malaise and a cystic tumor in the left kidney. Arterial phase Gd-enhanced T1w images (**A, B, C**) showed the two lesions found on sonography and CT (long arrows in **A** and **B**) and two previously undetected sub-cm lesions (short arrows in **C**) which were only visible on arterial-phase post-Gd images. All four liver lesions were hypervascular so a diagnosis of metastatic renal cell carcinoma was considered. However, since the renal mass [short arrow in (**B**)] had benign characteristics and synchronous liver metastases from renal carcinoma are rare, SPIO was given. On the SPIO-enhanced T2w GRE images (**D, E, F**) all of the liver lesions demonstrated a signal intensity loss greater than normal liver and were no longer visible indicating the presence of functioning Kupffer cells and allowing the diagnosis of benign hepatocellular lesions, histologically confirmed as FNH. (*Continued*)

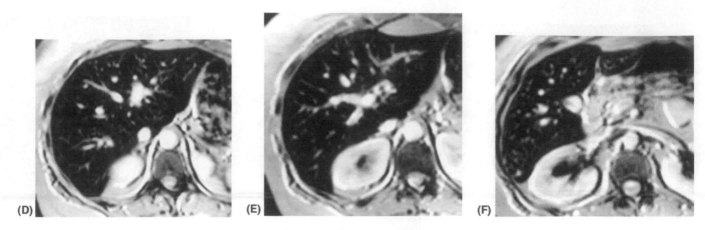

Figure 42.   (*Continued*)

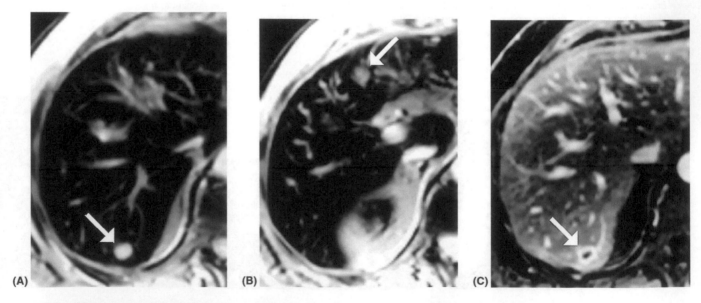

Figure 43.   *SPIO followed by Gd to detect and characterize co-existent benign and malignant lesions*:   In a surgical candidate, SPIO-enhanced T2w GRE images (**A**, **B**) showed two lesions (arrows) located in segments 4 and 7. On subsequent Gd-enhanced T1w images (**C**, **D**, **E**) the segment 7 lesion showed the characteristic continuous rim enhancement of a metastasis [arrow in (**C**)] while the lesion in segment 4 [arrow in (**D**) and (**E**)] demonstrated the typical discontinuous nodular and centripetal enhancement of a hemangioma. Lesion enhancement following Gd was particularly conspicuous due to the reduced signal of the background liver after SPIO. (*Continued*)

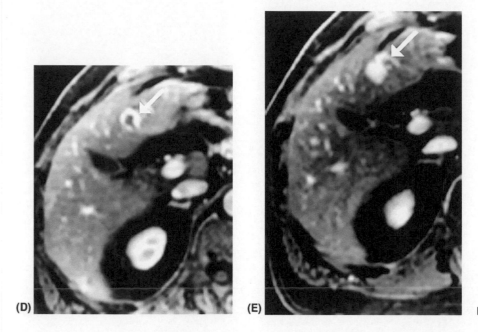

(D)   (E)   **Figure 43.**   (*Continued*)

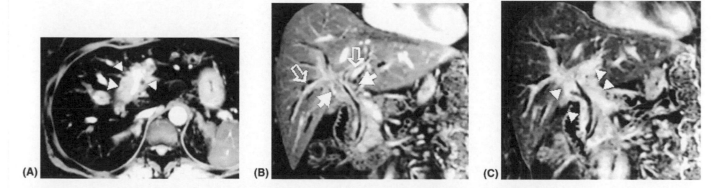

(A)   (B)   (C)

Figure 44.   *SPIO followed by Gd to assess operability of cholangiocarcinoma*:   SPIO-enhanced T2w GRE image (**A**) showed tumor encasing the origin of the left intrahepatic portal vein (arrowheads) but there was no evidence of intrahepatic metastases. Subsequent portal phase Gd-enhanced T1w image acquired at the portal phase of enhancement (**B**) and obtained along the length of the bile duct in the coronal oblique plane, showed the enhancing portal venous structures (open arrows) and an ill defined mass at the liver hilum (closed arrows). The corresponding T1w image acquired 10 minutes later (**C**) showed more extensive tumor along the entire length of the common bile duct and right and left hepatic ducts (arrowheads) due to a gradual accumulation of gadolinium within the lesion. Lesion enhancement was particularly conspicuous against the reduced signal intensity of the background liver following prior injection of SPIO.

CHAPTER 4

Normal and Variant Anatomy, and Imaging Artifacts

T his chapter covers the significant normal variations of vascular liver anatomy which the radiologist is likely to encounter, and gives an account of the common anomalies of perfusion and non-portal venous inflow effects, and also illustrates the likely location of lymph node deposits in patients with malignant liver tumors. Post-resection anatomy and image artifacts arising from therapeutic implants are also described.

HEPATIC ARTERIAL ANATOMY

About three quarters of patients show conventional arterial anatomy with the common hepatic artery (CHA) arising along with the splenic and left gastric arteries from the celiac axis. The CHA then divides to form the gastro-duodenal artery and the proper hepatic artery which itself divides to form the left and right hepatic arteries.

The most frequent variation is that in which the right hepatic artery (RHA) arises from the superior mesenteric artery (SMA). The variant RHA supplies part or the whole of the right lobe of the liver. An accessory or replaced RHA arising from the SMA can be recognized in axial sections because it lies posterior to the portal vein unlike the normally placed CHA which lies anterior to the vein.

Another fairly common anomaly is the origin of CHA from SMA. With this variation, the hepatic arteries may be anterior or posterior to the portal vein. Less common anomalies include the origin of the left hepatic artery (LHA) from the left gastric artery (LGA) or directly from the celiac axis. Combinations of these anomalies may also occur in the same patient.

Anomalous arterial anatomy is of no consequence in the healthy subject, but is critically important when trans-arterial chemotherapy or embolization of liver tumors is being considered. In the native liver, loss or reduction in arterial supply has little effect as long as the portal venous supply is maintained because of numerous collateral pathways by which arterial blood can reach the biliary tree. In the transplanted liver these collaterals do not exist, so a patent hepatic artery is essential to maintain the integrity of the biliary system. Unlike the rest of the liver parenchyma, the bile ducts receive their nutritive flow from the hepatic arterial route rather than from the portal venous system.

The arterial anastomosis used most frequently in liver transplantation is a direct end to end anastomosis of the donor CHA or celia\c artery directly onto the proper hepatic artery of the recipient. In cases where arterial anomalies or damage are present in either donor or recipient, a conduit or patch graft may be constructed.

VENOUS ANATOMY

The number, location, and orientation of the hepatic veins are a critical determinant of surgical anatomy of the liver (see below). The main hepatic veins are most readily identified in the axial plane, while the RAO coronal plane is optimum for demonstrating the main portal vein and its principal intrahepatic branches.

Anatomic anomalies of the portal veins are uncommon. The main portal branches to left and right lobes arise roughly perpendicular to the axis of the main portal vein at the hilum, with the left portal branch running in an antero-superior direction, the right portal vein in a postero-inferior direction, relative to the axial plane of the body.

The hepatic veins are less consistent in their anatomy. Although there are almost always three major venous trunks—right, middle, and left hepatic veins—any of them may branch within 1–2 cm of their entry into the inferior vena cava (IVC). If early branching causes difficulty in identification of hepatic veins in the axial plane, it is helpful to review axial sections at a more inferior level to identify the location of the gallbladder. At the superior aspect of the liver, the middle hepatic vein is the one which points in the same radial direction as the orientation of the gallbladder on more inferior slices.

The most common significant variation of hepatic venous anatomy is one or more accessory right hepatic veins (RHV) which may drain part or the whole of segments 5 and 6. In patients who are candidates for tumor resection, the existence of accessory hepatic veins may allow surgical procedures which would be otherwise impossible.

SEGMENTAL OR WEDGE-SHAPED SIGNAL INTENSITY CHANGES

Variations in parenchymal signal intensity with a regional or segmental distribution arise from several different causes, probably all mediated by the final common factor of local alterations in portal venous inflow. Regional edema or inflammation is manifested as an area of hypointensity on T1w and hyperintensity on T2w images (see chapter eight). Areas of liver parenchyma affected by patchy fatty change show signal differences between in-phase and opposed-phase T1w images (see chapter seven). Segmental or regional hyperintensity on T1w images may also be associated with cholestasis. This appearance is most often seen in patients with biliary obstruction, and in such cases the area which appears hyperintense on unenhanced T1w images also shows more marked dilatation of the bile ducts than the remaining liver. No signal difference is apparent on T2w imaging in these patients, but the T1 hyperintensity persists on post-Gd sequences.

PERFUSION

The development of dual phase, and more recently multiple phase post-contrast CT and MRI techniques has enabled the recognition of focal and regional anomalies of perfusion in the liver. These anomalies arise from disturbances in the balance of arterial and portal venous inflow to areas of the liver. Because the liver sinusoids receive blood from both arterial and portal venous branches, occlusion of one inflow source is normally compensated by increased inflow from the remaining source. Most commonly, branch portal vein obstruction or occlusion results in locally increased arterial inflow which is manifested as locally increased enhancement of the parenchyma during the arterial-dominant phase of post-contrast acquisition on CT and MRI. These anomalies have been described as transient hepatic attenuation differences (THADs) on CT and transient hepatic intensity differences (THIDs) on MRI and may be interpreted as arterio-portal shunts. Perfusion anomalies of this type are found in 10–15% of multiphase CT or MR examinations. The main causes are as follows:

Hilar or Intrahepatic Tumor Causing Obstruction of Portal Vein Branches

Lobar portal vein obstruction is most often associated with primary malignancy, either cholangiocarcinoma (which tends to constrict the portal vein branches) or hepatocellular carcinoma (which characteristically invades the lumen of the veins). Obstruction of portal branches at segmental and subsegmental level is commonly seen with metastatic disease. Whenever a THID is seen in a patient who is at risk of metastatic disease, a meticulous search should be made for a small tumor associated with the perfusion anomaly.

Localized Portal Hypoperfusion Not Associated with Tumor

In some cases thrombosed portal vein branches can be visualized on venous phase imaging, but most commonly the cause of the portal hypoperfusion is not detectable. However, the mechanism of arterio-portal shunting has been confirmed on angiographic studies, and in some cases, follow up imaging shows resolution of the THID or progression to segmental or subsegmental atrophy of the parenchyma. The incidence of small peripheral THIDs is considerably higher in cirrhotic patients than in those with normal liver parenchyma, so in the context of a search for hepatocellular carcinoma, the perfusion pattern of the liver must be carefully reviewed.

Traumatic Arterio-Portal Shunts

Although intrahepatic vascular thrombosis, fistula formation, and arterio-portal shunting can be a consequence of either blunt or penetrating liver trauma, by far the commonest perfusion artifact from this group of causes results from percutaneous needle biopsy. Few systematic post-biopsy studies have been performed, but evidence from pre and post-biopsy CT imaging suggests that a substantial proportion of patients (38% in one series) develop focal areas of abnormal perfusion and arterio-portal shunting, which can be confirmed on arteriography, at the typical sites of percutaneous biopsy in the right lobe. On dynamic post-Gd MRI, these biopsy artifacts typically show a small central area of hemorrhage or thrombosis, surrounded by an area of arterial hyper-perfusion. In some cases there is sufficient local edema or inflammatory reaction to produce focal hypointensity on unenhanced T1w and hyperintensity on T2w images.

Non-Portal Venous Inflow to the Liver

Perfusion anomalies often arise in those areas of the liver parenchyma which receive venous inflow from non-portal sources, discussed in more detail below.

Increased Arterial Perfusion in the Presence of Normal Portal Inflow

This pattern is typically associated with hyperaemic reaction in the liver parenchyma associated with adjacent inflammatory disease, for example acute cholecystitis or sub-hepatic abscess.

MRI Appearances

THIDs which are caused by local portal vein obstruction or arterio-portal shunting from other causes generally appear as wedge-shaped areas of increased enhancement during the arterial-dominant phase after contrast, with the apex of the wedge pointing towards the liver hilum and the base lying on the liver surface. This is the common type of THID described above. Post-biopsy THIDs have a more specific appearance. The THIDs associated with inflammatory disease tend to be ill-defined and show a non-segmental distribution.

NON-PORTAL VENOUS INFLOW TO THE LIVER

In most subjects, the whole of the liver parenchyma receives portal venous inflow, and post-contrast enhancement is uniform in the portal phase. However, in a significant minority of patients, portal venous inflow into small areas of parenchyma adjacent to the liver surface is replaced by venous drainage from other sources. These variants are manifest in two ways—they are common sites of focal fatty sparing or of focal fatty change which appear as areas of relative hypointensity on opposed-phase T1w imaging (see chapter seven), and they may also appear on post-Gd T1w imaging as areas of early enhancement. This perfusion pattern differs from the THIDs described above since there is no increase in the arterial supply to the affected area—the enhancement appears early because the pathway of venous filling is shorter than with the main portal circulation, so these areas enhance several seconds ahead of the main portal inflow. The main sites of non-portal venous inflow are as follows:

Para-Umbilical Veins—The Veins of Burow and the Inferior Vein of Sappey

These veins run roughly parallel with the umbilical vein remnant in the ligamentum teres and in the falciform ligament, draining venous blood from the anterior abdominal wall. Whereas the umbilical vein itself, when it reopens in some patients with portal hypertension, traverses the parenchyma of the left lobe from the fissure for the falciform ligament to enter the left main branch of the portal vein, the small para-umbilical veins empty directly into the liver parenchyma adjacent to the falciform ligagment.

The Superior Veins of Sappey

These veins drain part of the right hemi-diaphragm in the region of the median arcuate ligament of the liver and typically enter the liver parenchyma adjacent to the falciform ligament. They may communicate with the internal thoracic and superior epigastric veins.

Cholecystic Veins

These veins comprise the normal venous drainage of the gallbladder, and empty into the adjacent liver parenchyma.

Parabiliary Veins

These small veins form a plexus around the bile duct and are responsible for the appearance of cavernous transformation in some patients with occlusion of the main portal vein. The parabiliary veins drain into the liver parenchyma adjacent to the porta hepatis.

Capsular Veins

These small veins draining the liver capsule, particularly over the diaphragmatic surface, normally empty into the inferior phrenic vein, but in patients with obstruction or occlusion of the superior vena cava, these veins can form collaterals draining systemic blood into the liver, usually the superior aspect of segment 4. Dilated capsular veins are also seen in some patients with chronic Budd-Chiari syndrome, but in these cases the widespread subcapsular abnormality of perfusion forms just one aspect of a global disturbance in liver blood flow.

Post-Operative Venous Anomalies

Following surgery to the stomach or duodenum, some patients develop anomalous venous inflow to the liver from the right gastric or pancreatico-duodenal veins. Angiographic studies have confirmed the abnormal venous anatomy, which may be manifest as THIDs in contrast-enhanced MRI.

MRI Appearances

Probably the most common of these THIDs arises from the drainage of para-umbilical veins at the anterior surface of segment 4 immediately adjacent to the falciform ligament. Less commonly, para-umbilical venous inflow causes a THID to the left side of the falciform ligament on the anterior surface of segment 3. Inflow from the superior vein of Sappey typically creates a THID on either left or right side of the falciform ligament, a little way in toward the porta hepatis. Drainage from the cholecystic veins goes into segments 4 or 5 on either side of the gallbladder fossa and THIDs from the parabiliary plexus are shown on the posterior surface of segments 2 and 4, or on the anterior surface of segment 1 at the porta hepatis. Collateral inflow from capsular veins typically occurs over the bare area of the liver or in the superior aspect of segment 4.

As well as contributing to unusual perfusion patterns and THIDs, any of these veins may become enlarged to form porto-systemic collaterals with reversed flow in patients with portal hypertension.

LYMPHATIC DRAINAGE FROM THE LIVER

Most of the deep and superficial parenchymal liver lymphatics drain to the porta hepatis and into the nodes ranged along the vessels and ducts in the lesser omentum. From there, the main drainage is into the celiac nodes. The liver parenchyma adjacent to the bare area, which typically includes parts of segments 8 and 4, but sometimes includes parts of segments 7 or 2, drains via diaphragmatic lymphatics into the phrenic nodes which lie just superior to the diaphragm and adjacent to the right cardiophrenic angle. MR examinations which cover the whole of the liver will also include the typical lymph node metastasis sites at the porta hepatis, celiac, and phrenic nodal groups.

POST-RESECTION ANATOMY

The exceptional facility of the liver parenchyma to regenerate after injury allows very extensive resection with little loss of long-term functional capacity. A useful guide is that after resection of 80% of the liver parenchyma, the residual fragment will hypertrophy to about 80% of the original size of the whole organ. The regenerative capacity of the residual fragments, however, does depend on the absence of underlying diffuse liver disease, the integrity of the vascular supply, and on effective biliary drainage of the liver residue. The range of current surgical procedures is wide, and new approaches continue to be developed, so it is impossible to describe all the variations of post-operative anatomy. Mainstream procedures include left and right hemi-hepatectomy in which removal of left and right lobe respectively is accompanied by preservation of the main portal vein and usually also the common hepatic and common bile ducts. Tumors which extend across the hepatic hilum may require extended left or extended right hepatectomies (trisectionectomies). With these procedures the residual liver may consist only of segments 6 and 7 (left trisectionectomy) or segments 2 and 3 (right trisectionectomy) with segment 1 either remaining or separately resected. These more extensive procedures usually require biliary reconstruction with drainage into a Roux loop.

Following resection, liver anatomy may be more difficult to interpret, but the key features are the same as in the native liver—the position of the portal vein, IVC, and hepatic veins, and the falciform ligament and the gallbladder fossa. Particularly when the residual hepatic veins show early branching, the segmental anatomy of the hypertrophied liver remnant may be difficult to recognize, so it is especially helpful to know from the surgical team whether the middle hepatic vein has been excised. Metallic clips used over the cut surface of the liver and in the region of the vessels of the hilum may cause minor difficulty with image artifacts and small areas of hematoma or fibrotic residues may persist, particularly at sites of wedge resection near the liver surface. Low signal on T2w imaging and lack of enhancement on post-Gd T1w imaging help to discriminate benign surgical residues from possible recurrent tumor.

ARTIFACTS FROM CLIPS, STENTS, COILS, ETC.

A discussion of the safety aspects of MR in relation to metallic implants is outside the scope of this book. Readers are reminded that every MR department must undertake safety procedures, including screening all patients for metallic implants. A recent review and reference source is given by Shellock and Crues (2004).

The technology of stents and other therapeutic implants continues to evolve rapidly, so it is impossible (and unsafe) to predict the effect of new devices on the diagnostic quality of MR images on the upper abdomen. The following comments and illustrations provide only a general guide to the types and severity of artifacts associated with metallic implants.

Plastic stents are magnetically inert, and are visualized on MR only as a result of their effect on adjacent vessel walls or by fluid in the lumen (see examples in chapter 13). While the metallic alloys used in the manufacture of surgical clips, stents, coils, and other implants are now often chosen to minimize ferromagnetic properties, the effect of these objects on MR imaging is not always predictable, and occasionally the artifacts produced can be so severe as to seriously disrupt the diagnostic value of the images. As usual with liver MR, the choice of sequence is most important; the image artifact produced by metallic objects is significantly less when using sequences which are insensitive to susceptibility effects.

Surgical clips are not usually problematic. Occasionally, clips clustered around a site of hepatic resection may hamper the recognition of recurrent tumor near the resection margin, but with an appropriate combination of sequences and contrast agents, this can usually be overcome (see also chapter 12). Similarly, the alloys used for TIPS usually show sufficient ferromagnetic activity to create a signal void around the prosthesis, but not enough to disrupt visualization of the adjacent vessels. Metallic biliary tract stents are less predictable, with some devices producing quite extensive artifacts. Similar artifacts can arise from caval filters. Much more severe artifacts may arise from metallic embolization coils used to treat aneurysms or arteriovenous malformations or fistulae arising in the branches of the visceral circulation in the upper abdomen. Chemotherapy ports may be placed in the subcutaneous tissues of the abdominal wall and these often contain a sufficient mass of metal to produce a major artifact on MRI even when the ferromagnetic properties of the alloys used are very weak.

ILLUSTRATIVE FIGURES

Hepatic arterial anatomy— Figures 1–6
Venous anatomy— Figures 7–14
Segmental and perfusion anomalies— Figures 15–19
Biopsy-related perfusion anomalies— Figures 20–23
Lymph node abnormalities— Figures 24–32
Post-resection anatomy— Figures 33–34
Artifacts from clips, stents, coils, etc.— Figures 35–46

REFERENCES

1. Michels NA. Blood supply and anatomy of the upper abdominal organs. Philadelphia: J B Lippincott, 1955.
2. Gabata T, Matsui O, Kadoya M, et al. Segmental hyperintensity on T1-weighted MRI of the liver: indication of segmental cholestasis. J Magn Reson Imaging 1997; 7:855–857.
3. Lee SJ, Lim JH, Lee WJ, et al. Transient subsegmental hepatic parenchymal enhancement on dynamic CT: a sign of postbiopsy arterioportal shunt. J Comput Assist Tomogr 1997; 21:355–360.
4. Ueda K, Matsui O, Kadoya M, et al. Pseudolesion in segment IV of the liver on MRI: prevalence and morphology in 250 cirrhotic livers compared with 250 normal livers. J Comput Assist Tomogr 1999; 23:63–68.
5. Hashimoto M, Heianna J, Tate E, et al. Small veins entering the liver. Eur Radiol 2002; 12:2000–2005.
6. Breen DJ, Rutherford EE, Lee-Elliott C, et al. Intrahepatic arterioportal shunting and anomalous venous drainage: understanding the CT features in the liver. Eur Radiol 2004; 14:2249–2260.
7. Shellock FG, Crues JV. MR procedures: biological effects, safety, and patient care. Radiology 2004; 232:635–652.

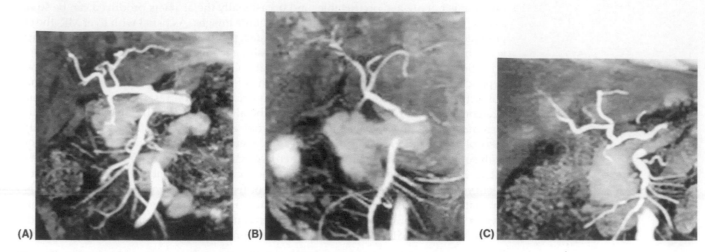

Figure 1. *Conventional arterial anatomy:*   Post-Gd T1w MIP images in three different patients (**A**, **B**, **C**) showing CHA arising from the celiac axis and giving rise to left and right hepatic arteries, and no visible supply to the liver from the SMA.

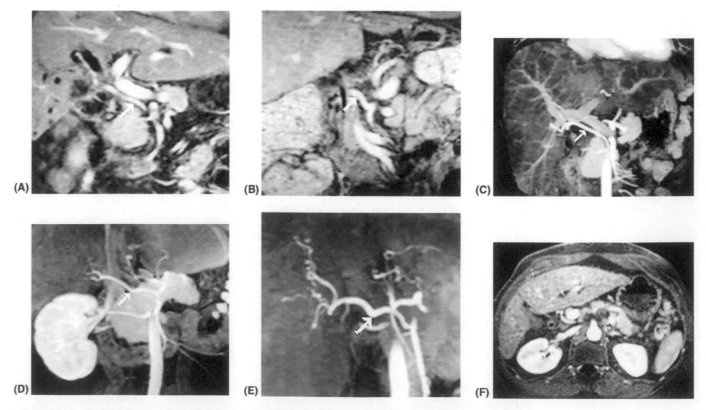

Figure 2. *Common variant arterial anatomy—RHA from SMA:*   Post-Gd T1w coronal slices (**A**, **B**) or MIP images (**C**, **D**, **E**) from five different patients, each showing an accessory or replaced RHA (arrows) arising from the SMA. Post-Gd axial image from a different patient (**F**) showed the typical position of the replaced RHA posterior to the portal vein—hepatic arteries from the celiac axis pass anterior to the portal vein.

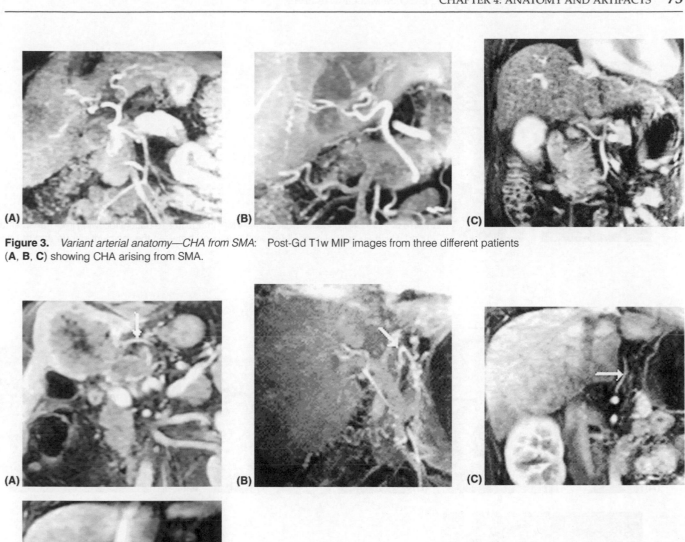

Figure 3. *Variant arterial anatomy—CHA from SMA*:   Post-Gd T1w MIP images from three different patients (**A**, **B**, **C**) showing CHA arising from SMA.

Figure 4. *Variant arterial anatomy—LHA from LGA*:   Post-Gd T1w coronal slice (**A**) and MIP images (**B**) in two different patients, showing the LHA (arrows) arising from the LGA. In a different patient the LGA [arrow in (**C**)] gives origin to the LHA [arrow in (**D**)].

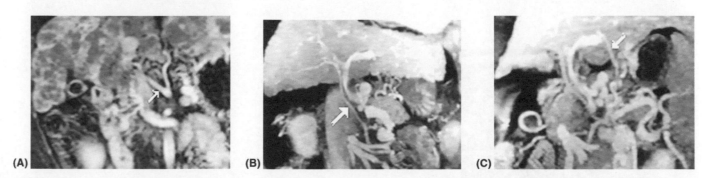

Figure 5. *Other arterial anomalies*:   Post-Gd T1w MIP images showing anomalous origin of the CHA (arrow) directly from the celiac axis (**A**). In a different patient the RHA (arrow) arose from the SMA (**B**) while the LHA (arrow) arose from the celiac axis (**C**).

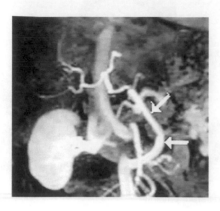

Figure 6. *Arterial conduit:* Post-Gd T1w MIP image from a patient following liver transplantation during which an arterial conduit (arrows) was used between the recipient's aorta and the donor.

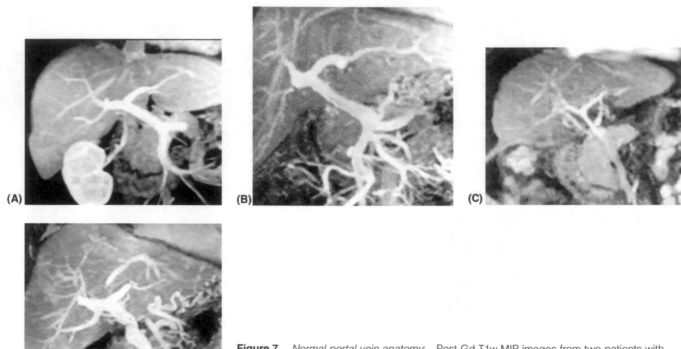

(A) **(B)** **(C)**

(D)

Figure 7. *Normal portal vein anatomy:* Post-Gd T1w MIP images from two patients with normal portal vein orientation and branching (**A**, **B**) and a third patient with chronic liver disease and with normal branching anatomy, but a very small portal vein (**C**). In a fourth patient following successful liver transplantation, post-Gd T1w coronal MIP image showed a minor (normal) degree of irregularity in the caliber of the vein following end-to-end anastomosis between donor and recipient portal veins.

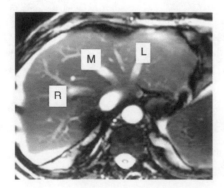

Figure 8. *Normal hepatic veins:* Axial true FISP image showing the normal orientation of the left (L), middle (M) and right (R) hepatic veins.

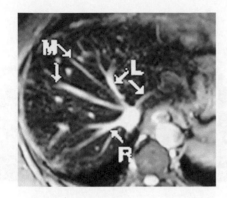

Figure 9. *Early branching of hepatic veins:* Axial HASTE image showing branching of the right hepatic vein (R) close to its termination in the IVC, also two middle (M) and two left (L) hepatic veins.

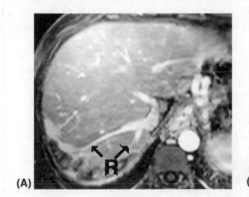

(A)

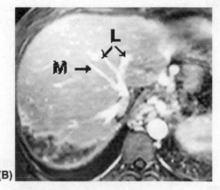

(B)

Figure 10. *Early branching of hepatic veins:* Post-Gd T1w axial images (**A**, **B**) showing branching of both left (L) and right (R) hepatic veins close to their termination in IVC, and a single middle hepatic vein (M); also note large varices around the gastroesophageal junction.

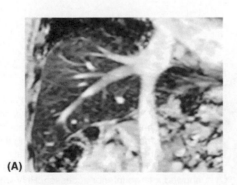

(A)

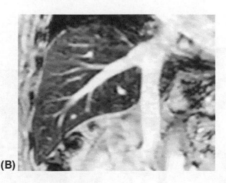

(B)

Figure 11. *Normal branching of right hepatic vein:* Post-SPIO T2w coronal images (**A**, **B**) showing the typical distribution of the RHV.

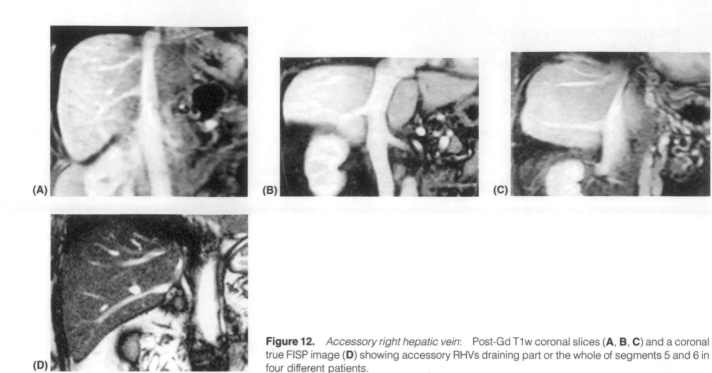

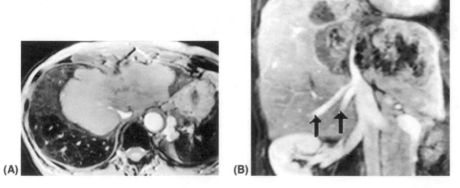

Figure 12. *Accessory right hepatic vein:* Post-Gd T1w coronal slices (**A**, **B**, **C**) and a coronal true FISP image (**D**) showing accessory RHVs draining part or the whole of segments 5 and 6 in four different patients.

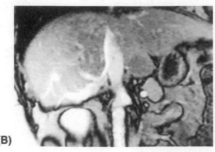

Figure 13. *Surgical advantage with accessory right hepatic vein:* In a patient with extensive hepatic metastases, post-SPIO T2w axial imaging (**A**) showed extensive involvement of left and right lobes with tumor surrounding the IVC superiorly. However, post-Gd T1w coronal imaging (**B**) showed the presence of two inferior accessory RHVs (arrows) which allowed surgical resection of the tumor with the preservation of segments 5 and 6.

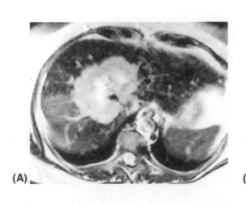

Figure 14. *Surgical advantage with accessory right hepatic vein:* In another patient extensive metastatic tumor surrounding the IVC was shown on post-SPIO T1w axial imaging (**A**). Post-Gd T1w coronal imaging (**B**) showed a large inferior accessory RHV which allowed surgical resection of the tumor with preservation of segments 5 and 6.

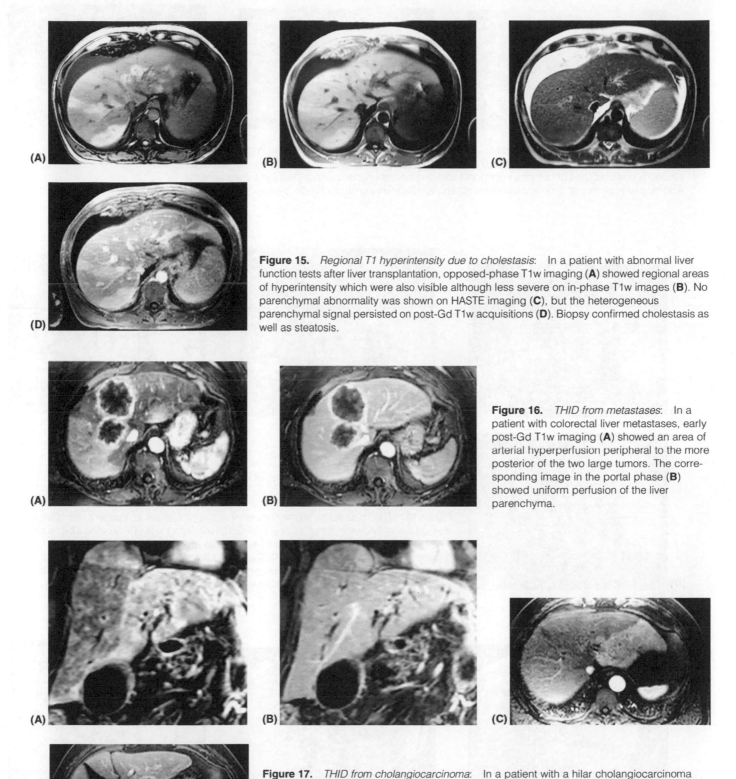

Figure 15. *Regional T1 hyperintensity due to cholestasis*: In a patient with abnormal liver function tests after liver transplantation, opposed-phase T1w imaging (**A**) showed regional areas of hyperintensity which were also visible although less severe on in-phase T1w images (**B**). No parenchymal abnormality was shown on HASTE imaging (**C**), but the heterogeneous parenchymal signal persisted on post-Gd T1w acquisitions (**D**). Biopsy confirmed cholestasis as well as steatosis.

Figure 16. *THID from metastases*: In a patient with colorectal liver metastases, early post-Gd T1w imaging (**A**) showed an area of arterial hyperperfusion peripheral to the more posterior of the two large tumors. The corresponding image in the portal phase (**B**) showed uniform perfusion of the liver parenchyma.

Figure 17. *THID from cholangiocarcinoma*: In a patient with a hilar cholangiocarcinoma mainly affecting the left lobe, post-Gd T1w imaging in the RAO coronal plane showed increased arterial perfusion to the left lobe (**A**). The corresponding portal phase image (**B**) showed uniform perfusion of all the liver parenchyma. In a different patient with HCC, the early post-Gd T1w image (**C**) showed increased arterial perfusion to segment 2. Note the absence of contrast from the hepatic veins although some contrast has refluxed into the IVC. At a more inferior level, portal phase imaging (**D**) showed a well-encapsulated HCC involving the posterior aspect of segments 2 and 3.

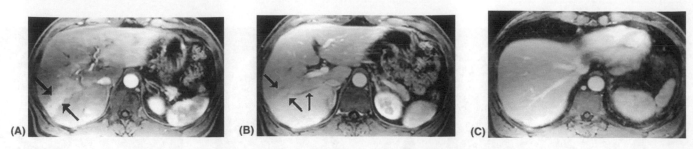

Figure 18. *THID from venous occlusion:*   An early post-Gd T1w image (**A**) showed an irregular area of arterial hyperperfusion crossing segment 7 (arrows). The corresponding portal phase image (**B**) showed subsegmental branches of both the right portal vein and the right hepatic vein to be thrombosed (arrows). A portal phase section at a more cranial level (**C**) showed the main right hepatic vein to be enhancing normally.

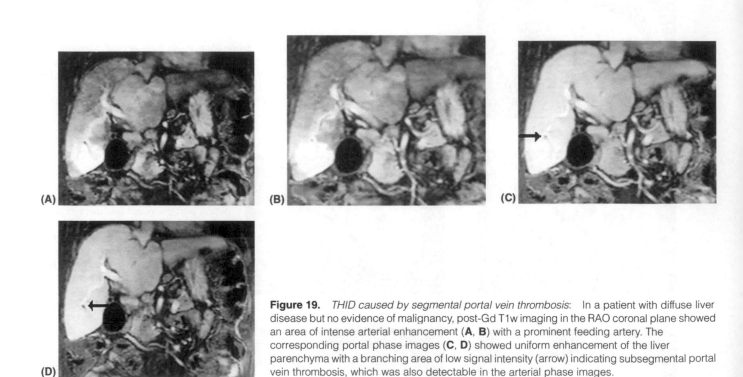

Figure 19. *THID caused by segmental portal vein thrombosis:*   In a patient with diffuse liver disease but no evidence of malignancy, post-Gd T1w imaging in the RAO coronal plane showed an area of intense arterial enhancement (**A**, **B**) with a prominent feeding artery. The corresponding portal phase images (**C**, **D**) showed uniform enhancement of the liver parenchyma with a branching area of low signal intensity (arrow) indicating subsegmental portal vein thrombosis, which was also detectable in the arterial phase images.

Figure 20. *Artifact from needle biopsy:*   In a patient with advanced cirrhosis and portal hypertension, the site of a liver biopsy performed 6 days previously produced a linear area of low signal on unenhanced T1w imaging (**A**) which was hyperintense on T2w imaging (**B**). On post-Gd T1w imaging (**C**), the area of hemorrhage at the biopsy site showed persistently low signal, but an area of increased enhancement was highlighted around it.

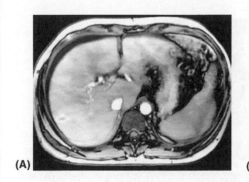

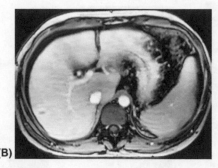

Figure 21. *Artifact from needle biopsy:* In a patient who had undergone biopsy of the right lobe, post-Gd T1w imaging in arterial (**A**) and portal (**B**) phases showed the low signal intensity of the central hemorrhage surrounded by a hypervascular rim due to arterio-portal shunting.

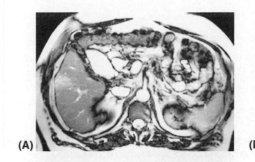

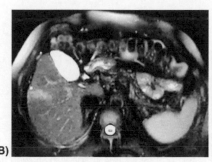

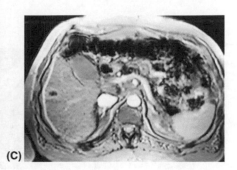

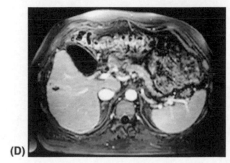

Figure 22. *Artifact from needle biopsy:* Another patient with chronic liver disease underwent needle biopsy of the right lobe. Subsequent MR showed an ill-defined area of hyperintensity on both true FISP (**A**) and HASTE (**B**) imaging. Unenhanced GRE T2w images (**C**) resolved the lesion to a central area of low signal surrounded by a rim of hyperintensity. Post-Gd T1w imaging in the portal phase (**D**) showed similar central low signal surrounded by a reactive hypervascularity.

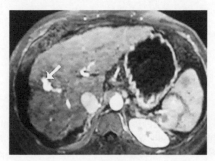

Figure 23. *Post-biopsy AV fistula:* Following needle biopsy of the right lobe in a patient with advanced cirrhosis, post-Gd T1w imaging in the arterial dominant phase showed an irregular vascular malformation approximating with the site of previous biopsy (arrow).

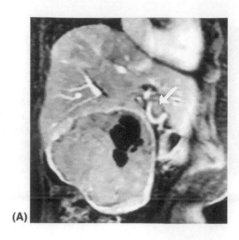
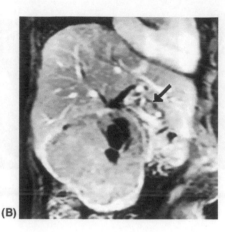

Figure 24. *Porta hepatis lymph node metastases*: In a patient with a large colorectal metastasis to the right lobe, post-Gd T1W imaging in arterial (**A**) and portal (**B**) phases in RAO coronal projection showed enlarged lymph nodes adjacent to the hepatic artery and portal vein (arrows).

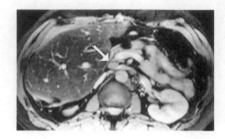

Figure 25. *Porta hepatis lymph node metastasis*: In a patient with colorectal liver metastases, this post-SPIO T2w image also showed an enlarged porto-caval lymph node (arrow).

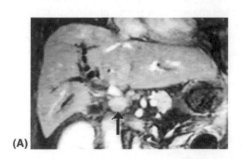
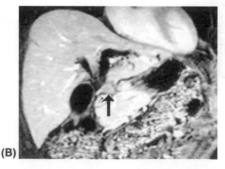

Figure 26. *Porta hepatis lymph node metastases*: In two patients with malignant tumors causing biliary obstruction, post-Gd T1w imaging in the RAO coronal plane also showed enlarged lymph nodes at the porta hepatis (arrows).

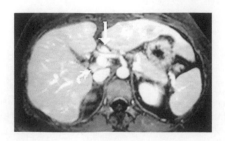

Figure 27. *Hypervascular nodal metastases*: Portal phase post-Gd T1w image in a patient with melanoma metastatic to the liver also showed hypervascular lymph nodes anterior to the hepatic artery (straight arrow) and in the porto-caval space (curved arrow).

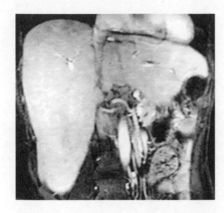

Figure 28. *Non-malignant enlargement of porta hepatis nodes:* In a patient with primary biliary cirrhosis but no malignancy, post-Gd T1w imaging in RAO coronal plane showed multiple enlarged nodes in the porta hepatis, a fairly common accompaniment of PBC.

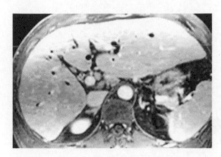

Figure 29. *Non-malignant enlargement of porta hepatis nodes:* In another patient with no evidence of malignancy but this time with primary sclerosing cholangitis (PSC), axial post-Gd T1w imaging showed multiple enlarged nodes in the porta hepatis, a well-recognized feature of PSC in the absence of malignant change.

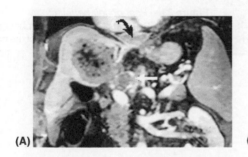
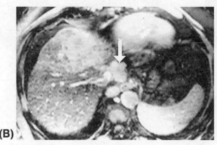
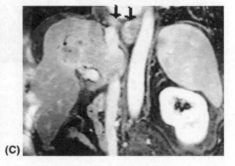

(A) (B) (C)

Figure 30. *Porta hepatis and phrenic lymph node metastases:* In a patient with colorectal liver metastases, post-Gd T1w imaging (**A**) showed enlarged nodes at the porta hepatis (straight arrow), and also enlarged nodes in the phrenic group just superior to the diaphragm (curved arrow). Axial T2w image in the same patient (**B**) showed the position of the enlarged nodes (arrow) in the axial plane. In another patient with metastatic liver disease, post-Gd T1w imaging in RAO coronal plane (**C**) showed phrenic lymph node metastases (arrows).

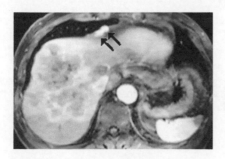

Figure 31. *Hypervascular phrenic lymph node metastases:* In a patient with colorectal liver metastases, axial post-Gd T1w imaging showed hypervascular lymph node metastases in the phrenic group (arrows).

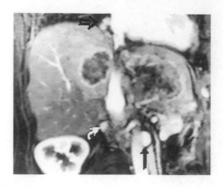

Figure 32. *Hypervascular lymph node metastases*: In another patient with colorectal liver metastases, post-Gd T1w imaging in RAO coronal plane showed hypervascular lymph node deposits in para-aortic (straight arrow), para-caval (curved arrow), and phrenic (open arrow) nodal groups.

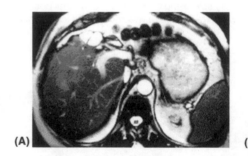 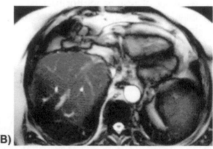

(A) (B)

Figure 33. *Post-op left hepatectomy* FISP images (**A**, **B**) showed the typical morphology of the liver remnant following removal of the left lobe.

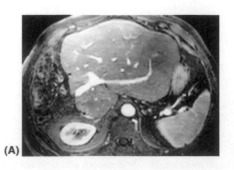 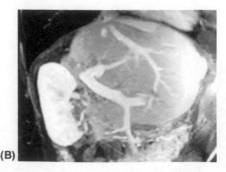

(A) (B)

Figure 34. *Post-op extended right hepatectomy*: Post-Gd T1w axial (**A**) and coronal MIP (**B**) images in two different patients following extended right hepatectomy showed the typical configuration of the residual segments 1, 2, and 3.

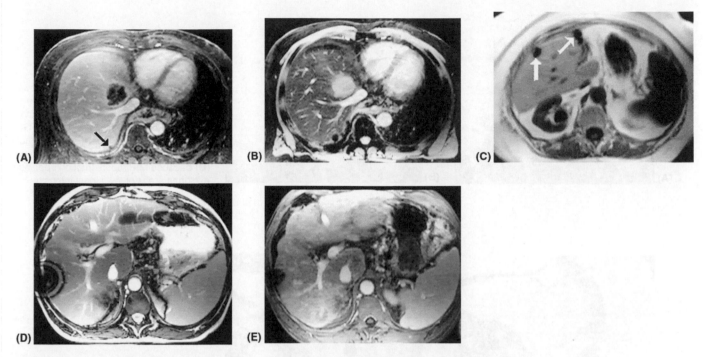

Figure 35. *Surgical clip artifacts:*   In a patient with recurrent colorectal metasasis just anterior to the right hepatic vein, post-Gd T1w VIBE image (**A**) showed a small area of signal loss on the posterior liver surface (arrow) caused by a surgical clip. The size of the artifact was much greater on the post-SPIO T2w image obtained at the same level (**B**). In another post-resection patient, unenhanced SE T1w imaging (**C**) showed areas of signal drop-out caused by surgical clips on the liver surface (arrows). In third patient with a large metallic clip placed on the lateral aspect of the right lobe of the liver, true FISP imaging (**D**) showed a substantial artifact, but on post-Gd T1w VIBE imaging (**E**) the artifact was much smaller.

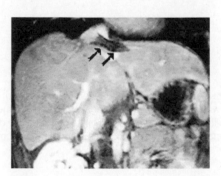

Figure 36. *Artifact from TIPS:*   In a patient with Budd-Chiari syndrome caused by a web adjacent to the IVC, a metal stent was inserted through the web and across the insertion of the left hepatic vein into the IVC. Post-Gd T1w image in RAO coronal plane showed the full length of the stent as a well-defined area of signal loss (arrows).

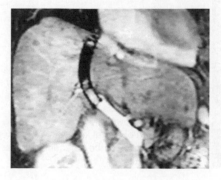

Figure 37. *Artifact from TIPS:*   Following insertion of a TIPS between the right main branch of the portal vein and the middle hepatic vein in a patient with resistant ascites, post-Gd T1w imaging in the RAO coronal plane showed the full length of the stent as a well-defined area of signal drop-out. The artifact created by the stent was sufficient to obliterate almost completely the signal from blood within it, but a little Gd enhancement within the lumen was visible near the lower end of the TIPS.

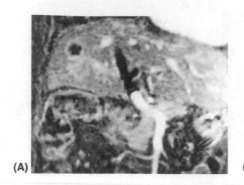 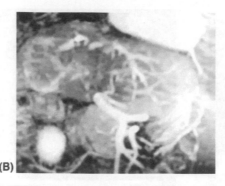

(A) (B)

Figure 38. *Artifact from TIPS:* Following placement of a TIPS between the main portal vein and the right hepatic vein, the typical area of signal drop-out was visible on post-Gd T1w coronal imaging (**A**). Note that the artifact was not visible on the corresponding MIP image (**B**) because MIP reconstruction specifically excludes areas of low signal intensity.

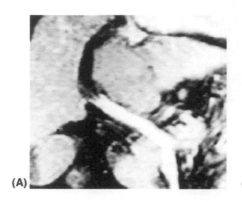 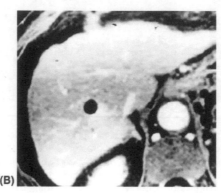

(A) (B)

Figure 39. *Artifact from TIPS:* Post-Gd T1w imaging in coronal (**A**) and axial (**B**) planes showed the typical well-defined signal drop-out caused by a TIPS between the portal vein and right hepatic vein.

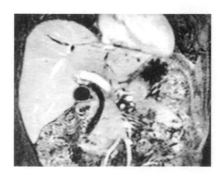

Figure 40. *Artifact from metallic biliary stent:* A metallic stent was placed in the bile duct of a patient with malignant obstruction. Post-Gd T1w imaging in the RAO coronal plane showed the full length of the stent. Note that the artifact was sufficient to obscure the wall of the common bile duct, but did not interfere with visualization of the portal vein, nor did it obscure the adjacent anatomy in the liver, pancreas, and duodenum.

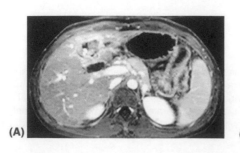 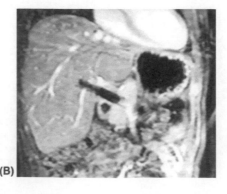

(A) (B)

Figure 41. *Artifact from metallic biliary stent:* Post-Gd T1w images in axial (**A**) and coronal (**B**) planes in a patient with a metallic stent placed across a malignant biliary obstruction showed the stent as a clearly defined area of signal loss without interfering with visualization of the adjacent vascular and hepatic anatomy.

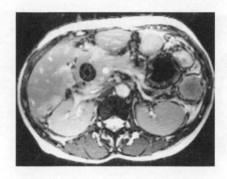

Figure 42. *Artifact from metallic biliary stent:* In another patient with malignant biliary obstruction, a similar metallic stent produced an artifact on true FISP imaging which was approximately double the size of the artifact created by the same stent on post-Gd T1w images.

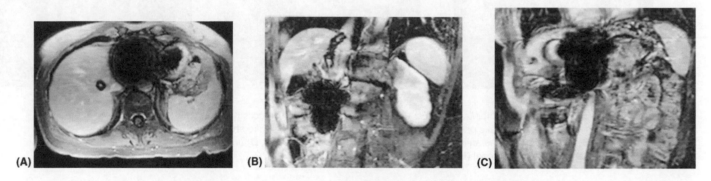

(A) (B) (C)

Figure 43. *Different artifacts from TIPS and metallic biliary stents:* In a patient with both a TIPS and a metallic biliary stent, post-Gd T1w imaging in axial (**A**) and coronal (**B, C**) planes showed the typical TIPS artifact as a well-defined area of signal loss along the shunt between the IVC and right portal branch. A much larger and less well-defined artifact arose from the biliary tract stent, sufficient to obliterate local anatomic landmarks.

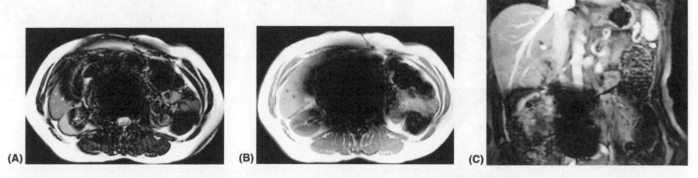

(A) (B) (C)

Figure 44. *Artifact from IVC filter:* In a patient with a metallic caval filter placed following multiple pulmonary emboli, the artifact created by the filter produced a very disruptive effect on both true FISP (**A**) and on unenhanced T1w (**B**) imaging in the axial plane. On post-Gd T1w imaging obtained in the RAO coronal plane (**C**), the artifact was much less obtrusive.

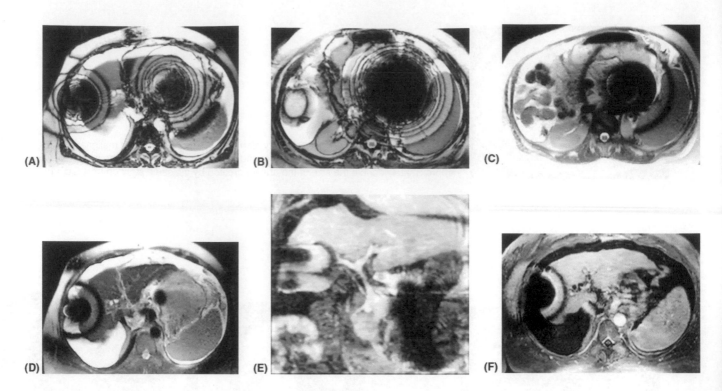

Figure 45. *Artifacts from metallic embolization coils*:   In a patient with embolization coils placed in the right lobe of the liver and in a pancreatic pseudo-aneurysm, large disruptive artifacts were shown in axial true FISP images (**A**, **B**). The severity of the artifact was less marked on HASTE images (**C**, **D**) and post-Gd T1w imaging (TE1.8msec) obtained in coronal (**E**) and axial (**F**) planes.

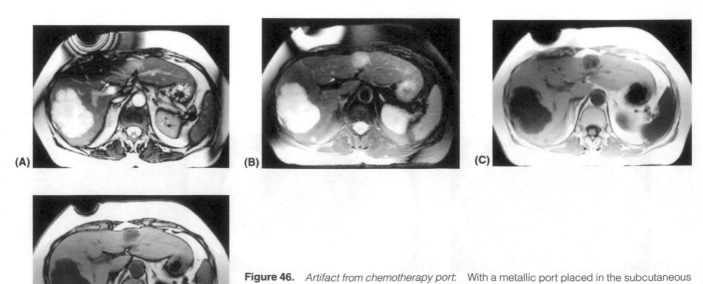

Figure 46. *Artifact from chemotherapy port*:   With a metallic port placed in the subcutaneous tissues of the right costal margin, a substantial artifact was shown on true FISP imaging (**A**) with a little less artifact on the HASTE image at the same level (**B**). On unenhanced T1w images, the artifact appears slightly larger on the in-phase image (**C**) than on the opposed-phase image (**D**) because of the longer TE used for the in-phase acquisition.

CHAPTER 5

Cysts and Cyst-Like Lesions of the Liver

T his chapter discusses the MR imaging and related clinical aspects of those liver lesions which appear mainly or entirely cystic on sonography and CT. The differential diagnosis of cysts and metastases is covered here, but see also chapter 11.

SIMPLE LIVER CYSTS

Simple liver cysts are probably developmental anomalies. They contain serous fluid and are bounded by a thin fibrous wall lined by epithelium of biliary type, but they do not communicate with the biliary tree. Cysts may be of any size but are asymptomatic unless they are large enough to compress adjacent vessels or bile ducts, or when they are complicated by infection or hemorrhage. Cysts can be solitary, but the incidental discovery of several cysts of sub-centimeter size is quite common. Multiple larger cysts are less frequent, but still not rare, and occasional patients have numerous cysts of small size scattered through the liver.

On MRI, the typical liver cyst is round or ovoid, with a well-defined edge and watery contents producing homogeneous very high signal on T2w and very low signal on T1w images. No enhancement is seen with gadolinium. Internal septation is an atypical and infrequent feature. Larger cysts are prone to internal hemorrhage, resulting in the contents showing increased signal on T1w imaging, and irregular solid components may appear. Similar signal changes can be produced by infection within a cyst. Occasionally a fluid-fluid level may develop after hemorrhage.

POLYCYSTIC DISEASE

The liver is affected in about 40% of patients with adult polycystic renal disease, and in a few cases only the liver is affected. The pancreas is also involved in a small minority of cases. Presentation usually results from the effects of gross liver enlargement causing increasing abdominal girth, pain from stretching of the liver capsule, compression effects on the inferior vena cava or hepatic veins, sometimes leading to Budd-Chiari syndrome, or pain from hemorrhage into cysts. Most patients have normal liver function, but a minority are associated with hepatic fibrosis leading eventually to liver failure.

MRI shows considerable liver enlargement with replacement of much of the normal parenchyma by multiple cysts, showing similar characteristics to those of simple cysts described above. Variations in signal intensity between the cysts may indicate recent or previous episodes of hemorrhage.

OTHER DEVELOPMENTAL CYSTS

The spectrum of fibrocystic disease of the liver and biliary tract includes congenital hepatic fibrosis, adult polycystic liver disease, Caroli's disease and choledochal cysts. In some cases, these disorders co-exist with varying degrees of expression. Choledochal cysts are usually extrinsic to the liver and so distinct from intrahepatic cystic lesions, while even the localized intrahepatic forms of Caroli's disease usually show a readily recognizable appearance of saccular dilatation of bile ducts which may be segmental, lobar or may affect the whole of the liver. The typical MR appearance is that of dilated ducts showing irregular caliber, sometimes with an enhancing central dot which represents a portal vein branch surrounded by the dilated ducts.

Ciliated foregut cyst is a rare entity, recently described, which is manifest as a solitary, unilocular liver cyst, lined by primitive epithelium similar to that of bronchogenic cysts. The lesions reported have been in a sub-capsular location and 2–3 cm in size. The fluid content is mucinous, sometimes with internal hemorrhage as well, so typically shows mild hyperintensity on T1w and marked hyperintensity on T2w images.

HYDATID CYSTS

Infestation with the parasite Echinococcus granulosus occurs when ingested ova pass through the intestinal wall and enter the portal circulation to reach the liver. Uncomplicated liver hydatids may be asymptomatic, or present with right upper quadrant pain or liver enlargement. More dramatic presentations are associated with intraperitoneal rupture of a liver hydatid, or with dissemination of disease via the biliary tree or portal venous system.

MRI features of an uncomplicated liver hydatid include a multi-layered wall which typically shows low signal on both T1w and T2w images, resulting from a combination of fibrous capsule with varying degrees of calcification. The fluid content shows high signal on T2w imaging but may be either hypo- or hyperintense on T1w images. Rim enhancement is typically seen with gadolinium. The presence of daughter cysts around the periphery of the lesion is an inconstant but characteristic finding, and detachment of the membrane resulting in the "water lily" appearance is also highly characteristic.

CYSTADENOMA AND CYSTADENOCARCINOMA

Cystadenoma is a rare neoplasm usually presenting in middle-aged women which is slowly growing and thought to be pre-malignant. Presentation is usually by pressure effects, particularly pain and local intrahepatic bile duct obstruction. The lesions are solitary but may be loculated. The cysts are lined by a cuboidal or mucin-secreting epithelium and their fluid content is proteinaceous, haemorrhagic, and often mucinous or gelatinous. The presence of mesenchymal stroma around the cyst lining is a pre-malignant feature, which is sometimes only detectable at histology. Increased wall thickness and more extensive solid components are also associated with malignant change, but the features overlap so surgical excision is the preferred treatment.

MRI shows a cystic, often multi-locular but solitary lesion. The wall is often thicker than that of a simple cyst and usually shows nodular components which enhance after gadolinium. Internal septation is common and the septa may also enhance. The fluid contents show high signal on T2w and variable signal on T1w images, depending on mucin content and hemorrhage.

HAMARTOMA AND BILIARY ADENOMA

Biliary hamartomas or micro-hamartomas, also known as von Meyenburg complexes, are developmental anomalies arising in embryonic bile ducts, and are a common incidental finding in liver imaging. The lesions may be round or ovoid, but are often angular in shape and usually of sub-cm size (rarely larger than 1.5 cm). These lesions may be solitary but are not uncommonly multiple, and occasionally miliary. They are often located on or near the liver surface. Histology shows a lining of biliary epithelium and watery fluid contents with a varying degree of fibrous stroma. Like simple cysts, they remain stable on follow up examination.

Typical MRI appearances are of a small angular lesion with high signal on T2w and low signal on T1w images. Most of these lesions show no enhancement after gadolinium, but others show a thin rim of persisting enhancement which correlates histologically with a layer of compressed liver tissue around the lesion. Biliary adenoma is a somewhat similar lesion with a predominantly solid matrix which may show signal characteristics close to that of normal liver and in some cases a homogeneous blush appears on post-gadolinium images, an appearance difficult to distinguish from metastatic disease in some cases (see chapter 11).

Mesenchymal hamartoma is an uncommon developmental neoplasm seen in infancy. The lesions are composed of varying proportions of cystic and solid stromal elements, but usually present as a single multiloculated cystic mass. The fluid content shows watery signal on unenhanced images, while the nodular walls and septa enhance after gadolinium.

DIFFERENTIAL DIAGNOSIS OF CYSTS AND CYST-LIKE LESIONS

Differential diagnosis of cysts and related lesions arises in two distinct clinical scenarios—firstly, the distinction of benign lesions from small metastases in patients with known or suspected malignancy; and secondly the choice between surgical and conservative management of large cystic lesions.

Cysts etc. vs. Metastases

Benign simple cysts commonly co-exist with metastases, and are usually readily distinguishable. The most distinctive features of simple cysts are their clear-cut margin, their very low signal on T1w images, their lack of enhancement on post-Gd T1w images, and their uniformly bright signal on T2w images, so the most useful sequences for making this distinction are T2 sequences with a long echo train and long TE, and post-Gd T1w images. The great majority of metastases show less marked hyperintensity on T2w images, particularly FSE and HASTE sequences in which magnetization transfer effects further magnify the signal difference between cysts and tumors. Tiny cysts are particularly conspicuous on HASTE imaging, owing to the lack of motion artifact and the superior spatial resolution compared with FSE sequences (see Chapter 2).

Although most metastases are solid when untreated, larger lesions often develop central necrosis. Particularly after chemotherapy, this effect may be so marked as to produce a cyst-like appearance, while metastases from neuroendocrine primaries are frequently necrotic at the initial presentation. Untreated metastases, even when central necrosis produces watery signal from the contents, will almost always have an enhancing rim on post-Gd images, but occasionally after chemotherapy small metastases may appear completely cystic yet still show viable tumor on histologic examination after resection.

There is undoubted overlap between the signal characteristics of small simple cysts and biliary hamartomas. The latter may be distinguished by their angular shape, but either lesion may also be round or ovoid. Since neither lesion has clinical import, the distinction is of only academic interest. Those hamartomas which show rim enhancement are more problematic, but again the angular shape and intense high signal of the contents, in relation to the small size of the lesions, is helpful. Further, the peripheral enhancement—unlike that seen with hemangiomas—persists as a rim on delayed images. However, biliary adenomas of sub-cm size may show very similar signal intensity and enhancement characteristics to those of small metastases, and are only recognisable at histology.

Differential Diagnosis of Larger Cystic Lesions

Larger lesions which show the imaging characteristics of simple cysts may be treated conservatively, with pressure symptoms being treated by aspiration or laparoscopic fenestration. Lesions with a wall of discernible thickness which enhances, particularly if there are nodular components, should be regarded as potentially malignant; the distinction between cystadenoma and cystadenocarcinoma cannot be reliably made by imaging.

If the cyst contents are iso- or hyperintense on T1w images, indicating the presence of blood or mucin, the possibility of malignancy again has to be raised, even though some of these lesions will turn out after excision to be haemorrhagic simple cysts, benign cystadenomas, or ciliated foregut cysts.

With an appropriate clinical background, hydatid disease needs to be considered if a solitary cystic lesion shows an enhancing rim. The low signal capsule may be a pointer, and the presence of daughter cysts or the water lily sign is virtually pathognomonic. Uncomplicated hydatids may be less distinctive on imaging, and complement fixation tests for hydatid antigens are then vital.

ILLUSTRATIVE FIGURES

Simple cysts—Figures 1–4
Liver cysts with hemorrhage or infection—Figures 5–8
Polycystic disease—Figures 9,10
Choledochal cysts—Figures 11,12
Ciliated foregut cyst—Figure 13
Hydatid cysts—Figure 14
Cystadenoma/cystadenocarcinoma—Figures 15–17
Biliary adenoma/hamartoma/von Meyenberg complex—Figures 18–19
Mesenchymal hamartoma—Figures 20,21
Cysts in chronic liver disease—Figures 22,23
Differential diagnosis-cyst versus metastasis—Figures 24,25
Coexisting cysts and metastases—Figures 26,28
Cystic/necrotic metastases—Figures 27, 29–33
Cystic residues from RFA—Figure 34
Differential diagnosis of large atypical cysts—Figures 35–37

REFERENCES

1. Mortele KJ, Ros PR. Cystic focal liver lesions in the adult: differential CT and MR imaging features. Radiographics 2001; Jul-Aug; 21(4):895–910.
2. Vuillemin-Bodaghi V, Zins M, Vullierme MP, et al. Imaging of atypical cysts of the liver. Study of 26 surgically treated cases. Gastroenterol Clin Biol 1997; 21:394–399.
3. Vilgrain V, Silbermann O, Benhamou JP, et al. MR imaging in intracystic hemorrhage of simple hepatic cysts. Abdom Imaging 1993; 18:164–167.
4. Dranssart M, Cognet F, Mousson C, et al. MR cholangiography in the evaluation of hepatic and biliary abnormalities in autosomal dominant polycystic kidney disease: study of 93 patients. J Comput Assist Tomogr 2002; 26:541–552.
5. Murakami T, Imai A, Nakamura H, et al. Ciliated foregut cyst: radiologic features. Radiology 1990; 175:475–477.
6. Algidere AM, Aytekin C, Coskun M, et al. MRI of hydatid disease of the liver: a variety of sequences. J Comput Assist Tomogr 1998; 22:718–724.
7. Taorel P, Marty-Ane B, Charasset S, et al. Hydatid cyst of the liver: comparison of CT and MRI. J Comput Assist Tomogr 1993; 17:80–85.
8. Luo TY, Itai Y, Eguchi N, et al. Von Meyenburg complexes of the liver: imaging findings. J Comput Assist Tomogr 1998; 22:372–378.
9. Semelka RC, Hussain SM, Marcos HB, et al. Biliary hamartomas: solitary and multiple lesions shown on current MR techniques including gadolinium enhancement. J Magn Reson Imaging 1999; 10:196–201.

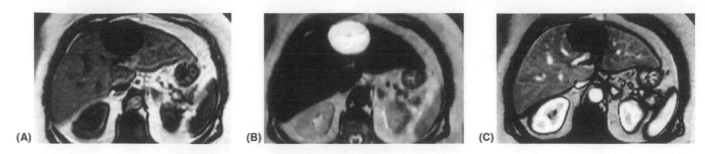

Figure 1. *Solitary liver cyst*: The lesion is round, the wall showed no appreciable thickness, the contents showed uniformly low signal on T1w images (**A**), uniformly high signal on T2w imaging (**B**) and the post-Gd T1w image (**C**) showed no enhancement in the wall or around the lesion.

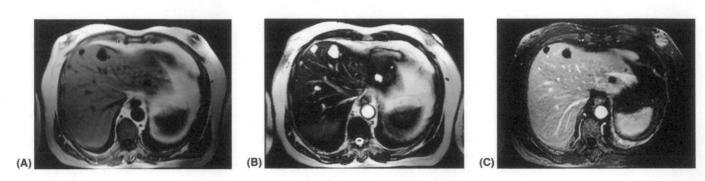

Figure 2. *Multiple simple cysts*: Several lesions in the same section showed similar characteristics of low signal on unenhanced T1w imaging (**A**), high signal on the true FISP image (**B**), and no enhancement on the post-Gd T1w image (**C**).

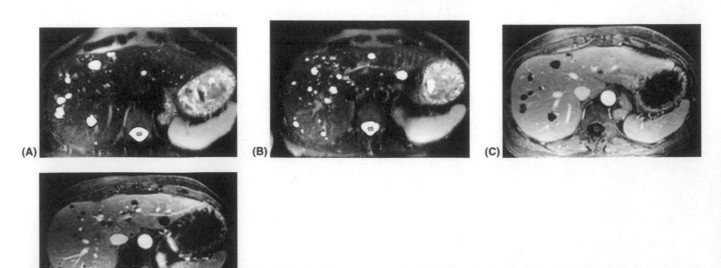

Figure 3. *Multiple simple cysts*: Sections at two levels through the liver showed several small lesions with uniformly high signal on the HASTE images (**A**, **B**) and uniformly low signal on the post-Gd T1w images with no enhancement of the wall of the cysts (**C**, **D**).

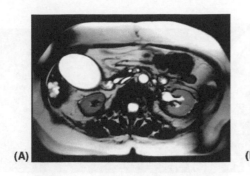

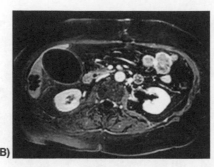

(A)

(B)

Figure 4. *Multiloculated cyst:* True FISP (**A**) and post-Gd T1w (**B**) images showed a well-defined loculated lesion in segment 5 with a thin, non-enhancing wall and contents of uniform watery signal (the larger cyst-like structure is the gallbladder).

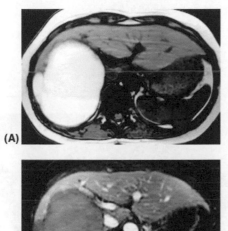

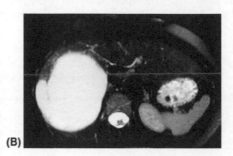

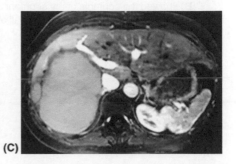

(A)

(B)

(C)

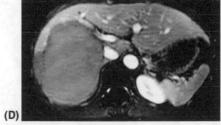

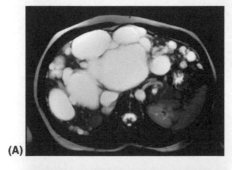

(D)

Figure 5. *Multi-loculated simple cyst with hemorrhage:* Unenhanced images showed a large cyst with a few septa and small peripheral nodular components adjacent to the cyst wall. The fluid within the cyst showed high signal on both T1w (**A**) and HASTE images (**B**). Early and delayed post-Gd T1w images (**C**, **D**) showed no enhancement in the cyst wall or contents.

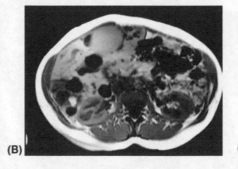

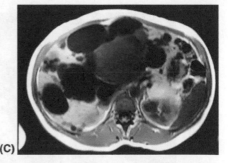

(A)

(B)

(C)

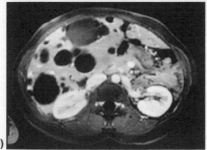

(D)

Figure 6. *Multiple simple cysts with hemorrhage:* HASTE image (**A**) showed multiple cysts all with uniformly high signal fluid content. Unenhanced T1w images at two levels (**B**, **C**) showed two of the cysts had increased signal intensity compared with the remaining cysts, indicating recent hemorrhage or infection. Post-Gd T1w image (**D**) showed no tumoral enhancement in the cyst walls.

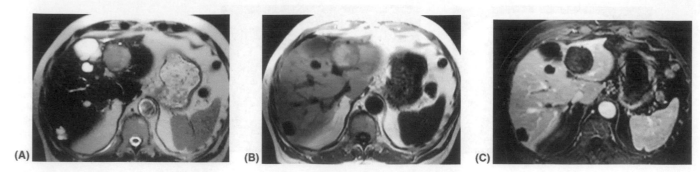

Figure 7. *Multiple cysts with hemorrhage*:   The true FISP image (**A**) showed several cysts with hyperintense contents typical of watery fluid, but also a cyst in segment 3 with much lower signal. Unenhanced T1w image (**B**) showed the contents of the segment 3 cyst to be slightly hyperintense and heterogeneous. Post-Gd T1w image (**C**) showed no enhancement in the wall of any of the cysts. The appearance was unchanged from an examination 5 years before.

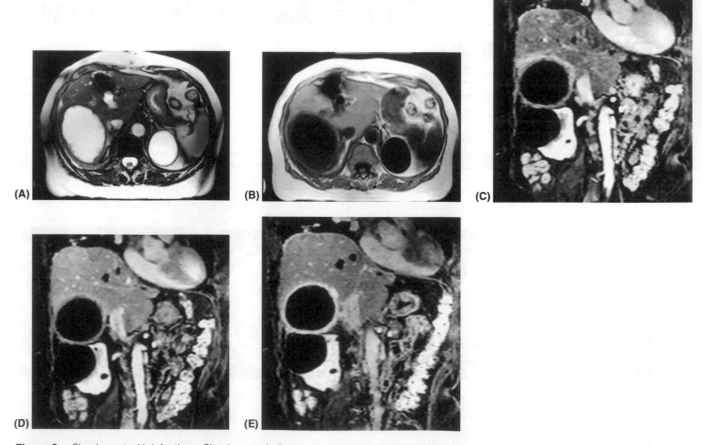

Figure 8. *Simple cyst with infection*:   Simple cysts in liver and kidneys had previously been noted in this elderly patient who re-presented with septic symptoms. True FISP image (**A**) showed a large cyst arising in the right lobe of the liver with a nodular wall and contents which although hyperintense were less bright then those of the simple renal cyst shown on the left. Unenhanced T1w imaging (**B**) again showed a markedly hypointense left renal cyst while the contents of the large liver cyst were less hypointense. Post-Gd T1w coronal images in arterial, venous and delayed phases (**C, D, E**) showed no enhancement in the cyst contents but an intensely enhancing capsule best seen on the delayed images. Note the difference in character between the wall of the infected hepatic cyst and the uninfected cysts elsewhere in the liver and in the right kidney in (**C, D, E**).

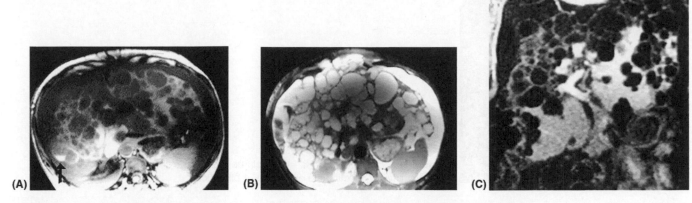

Figure 9. *Polycystic disease:* Unenhanced images showed the liver was largely replaced by cysts showing hypointensity on T1w and hyperintensity on T2w images (**A**, **B**). The patient also had ascites and one of the cysts near the posterior aspect of the right lobe [arrow in (**A**)] contained a little hemorrhage. Post-Gd T1w coronal image (**C**) showed normal enhancement of the residual liver parenchyma between the cysts, and a patent portal vein.

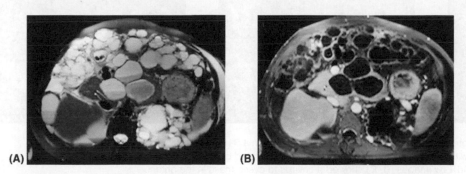

Figure 10. *Polycystic disease with hemorrhage:* T2w image (**A**) showed replacement of much of the liver tissue with cysts of varying sizes. Three of the centrally placed cysts showed fluid-fluid levels indicating hemorrhage with a hematocrit effect. Post-Gd T1w image (**B**) showed normal enhancement of the residual liver tissue. Note cystic replacement of the left kidney.

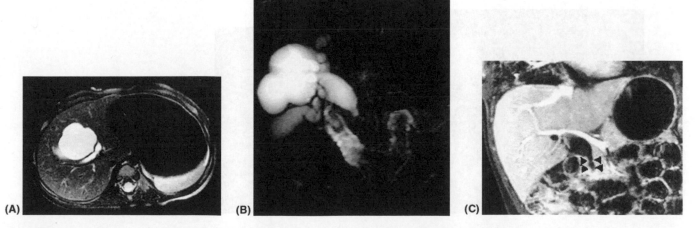

Figure 11. *Choledochal cyst:* HASTE image showed a lobulated cystic structure close to the liver hilum (**A**). HASTE MRCP in RAO projection (**B**) showed a lobulated dilatation of the main ducts with tapering of the common bile duct at the level of the pancreas. Post-Gd RAO coronal T1w image (**C**) showed the cylindrical dilatation of the common bile duct with tapering at pancreatic level (arrowheads).

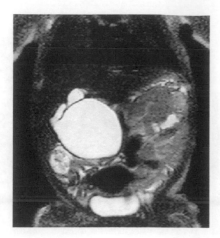

Figure 12. *Choledochal cyst:* Coronal true FISP image showed cystic dilatation mainly affecting the extra-hepatic bile duct.

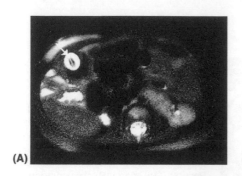 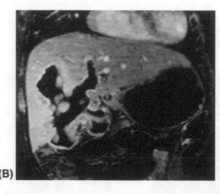 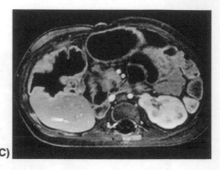

(A) (B) (C)

Figure 13. *Ciliated foregut cyst:* After previous surgical drainage of a cystic mass in a 9-month-old infant, the HASTE image (**A**) showed a cystic cavity with irregular nodular walls adjacent to the inflated balloon of a drainage catheter (arrow). Coronal and axial post-Gd T1w images (**B**, **C**) showed a collapsed cystic mass in the anterior segments of the right lobe with a degree of enhancement in the nodular wall of the cyst. Histology of the subsequent resection specimen showed a ciliated foregut cyst.

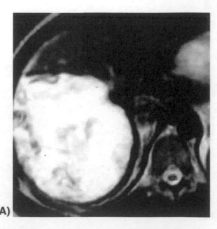 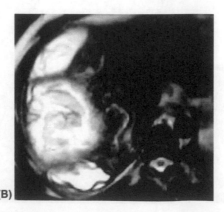

(A) (B)

Figure 14. *Hydatid cyst:* Axial T2w images at two levels (**A**, **B**) showed a multi-loculated cyst with hyperintense contents and the characteristic infolded membrane ("water-lily sign"). Post-Gd portal phase axial and coronal T1w images (**C**, **D**) showed the margin of the cyst to be iso- or hypointense to adjacent liver, indicating an inactive fibrotic cyst wall. (*Continued*)

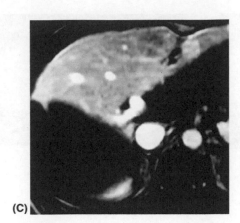

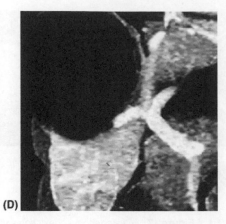

(C)

(D)

Figure 14. (*Continued*)

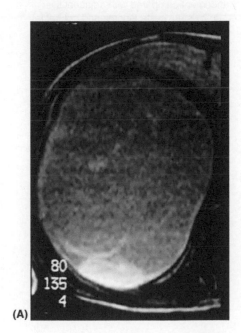

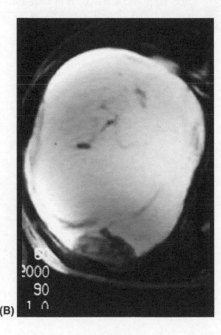

(A)

(B)

Figure 15. *Cystadenoma*: Unenhanced T1w and T2w images (**A**, **B**) showed a unilocular cystic mass with watery fluid contents, a little septation and a tumor nodule on the posterior wall.

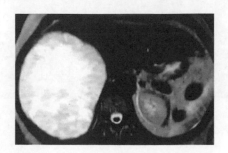

Figure 16. *Cystadenocarcinoma*: The internal papillary structure of the solid elements of this tumor was best seen on the T2w image. The mass appeared uniformly hypointense on unenhanced T1w images.

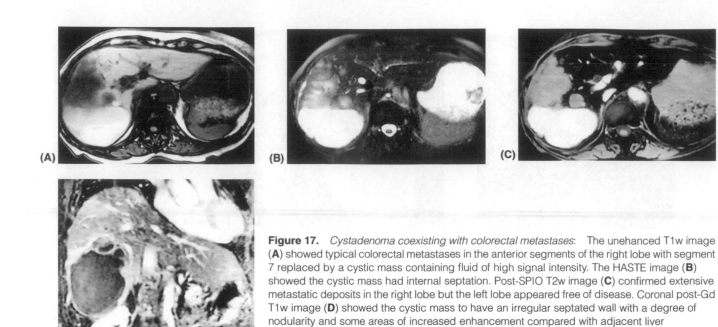

Figure 17. *Cystadenoma coexisting with colorectal metastases*: The unehanced T1w image (**A**) showed typical colorectal metastases in the anterior segments of the right lobe with segment 7 replaced by a cystic mass containing fluid of high signal intensity. The HASTE image (**B**) showed the cystic mass had internal septation. Post-SPIO T2w image (**C**) confirmed extensive metastatic deposits in the right lobe but the left lobe appeared free of disease. Coronal post-Gd T1w image (**D**) showed the cystic mass to have an irregular septated wall with a degree of nodularity and some areas of increased enhancement compared with adjacent liver parenchyma. Resection pathology confirmed co-existent cystadenoma and colorectal metastases.

Figure 18. *Von Meyenberg complex*: HASTE imaging (**A**) showed a sub-cm lesion close to the lateral surface of the right lobe. The lesion showed faint rim enhancement on post-Gd T1w portal phase imaging (**B**) and no in-filling on delayed imaging (**C**).

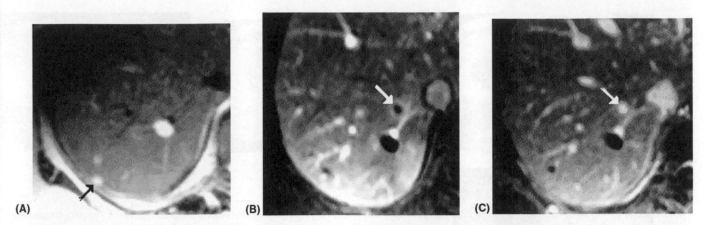

Figure 19. *Biliary adenoma*: T2w image (**A**) showed three hyperintense lesions including one on the surface (arrow). Post-Gd T1w images in arterial and delayed phases (**B**, **C**) showed the two deeper lesions to have no enhancement, typical of small cysts, while the surface lesion had enhanced in parallel with the adjacent liver. Note also a small metastasis [arrows in (**B**) and (**C**)] which was not visible on the unenhanced images. Surgery confirmed benign cysts, a 7 mm metastasis, and a 4 mm sub-capsular biliary adenoma.

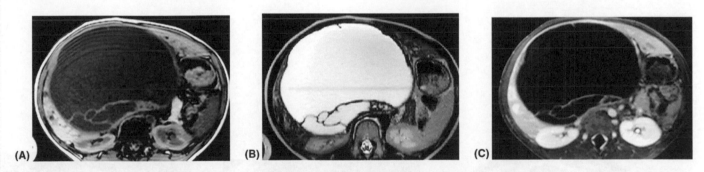

Figure 20. *Mesenchymal hamartoma*: Unehanced T1w and T2w images (**A**, **B**) in an 8-year-old child showed a unilocular but septated cystic mass with the cyst contents giving the signal intensity of watery fluid. The cyst wall was irregular in thickness and showed areas of hypointensity on both T1w and T2w images indicating local fibrosis. Post-Gd T1w image (**C**) showed minimal enhancement of the cyst wall.

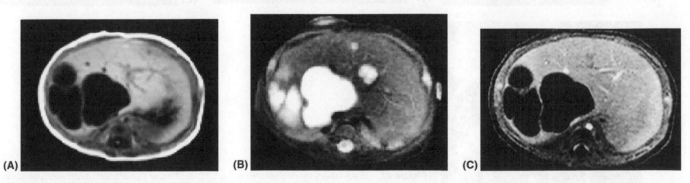

Figure 21. *Mesenchymal hamartoma*: A 6-week-old infant presented with a multilocular cystic mass with the contents showing the signal intensity of watery fluid on both T1w and T2w images (**A**, **B**). Post-Gd T1w imaging showed no appreciable tumor enhancement (**C**).

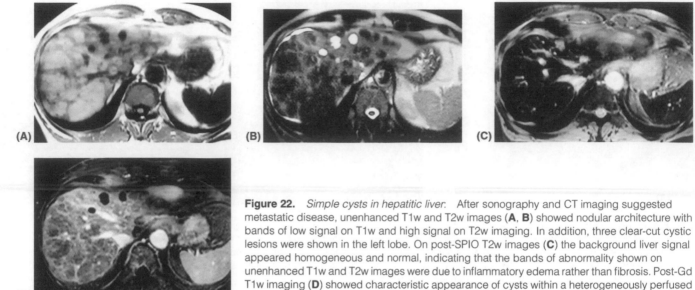

Figure 22. *Simple cysts in hepatitic liver.* After sonography and CT imaging suggested metastatic disease, unenhanced T1w and T2w images (**A**, **B**) showed nodular architecture with bands of low signal on T1w and high signal on T2w imaging. In addition, three clear-cut cystic lesions were shown in the left lobe. On post-SPIO T2w images (**C**) the background liver signal appeared homogeneous and normal, indicating that the bands of abnormality shown on unenhanced T1w and T2w images were due to inflammatory edema rather than fibrosis. Post-Gd T1w imaging (**D**) showed characteristic appearance of cysts within a heterogeneously perfused liver. Biopsy confirmed acute-on-chronic hepatitis.

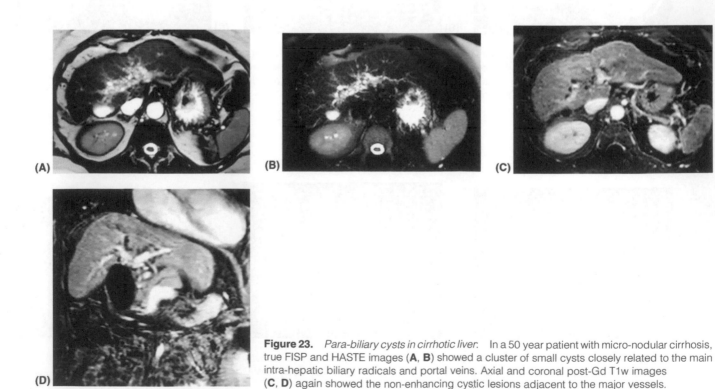

Figure 23. *Para-biliary cysts in cirrhotic liver.* In a 50 year patient with micro-nodular cirrhosis, true FISP and HASTE images (**A**, **B**) showed a cluster of small cysts closely related to the main intra-hepatic biliary radicals and portal veins. Axial and coronal post-Gd T1w images (**C**, **D**) again showed the non-enhancing cystic lesions adjacent to the major vessels.

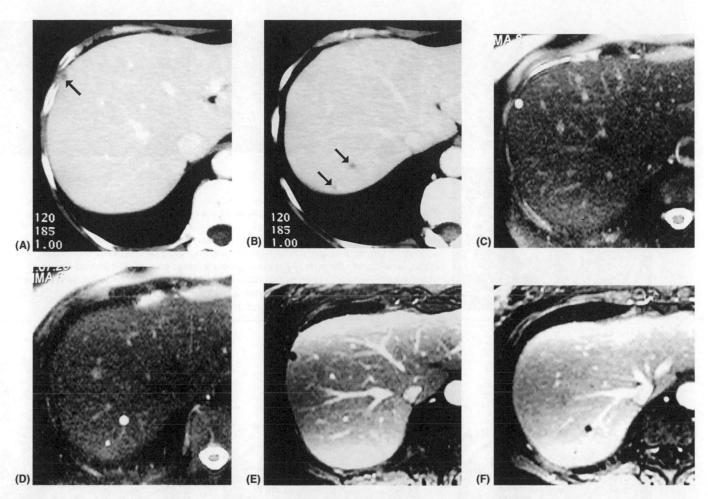

Figure 24. *Cysts or metastases?*: CT (**A**, **B**) in a patient with a primary colorectal carcinoma showed three small indeterminate liver lesions (arrows). The lesions were markedly hyperintense on T2w imaging (**C**, **D**) and showed no enhancement of the rim or contents on post-Gd T1w images (**E**, **F**). Diagnosis—simple cysts, confirmed on surveillance.

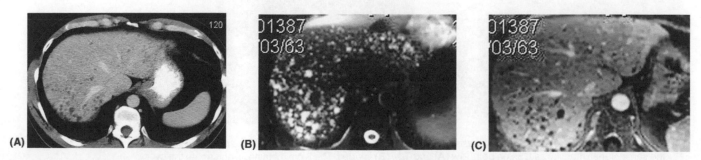

Figure 25. *Cysts or metastases?*: CT (**A**) showed numerous small lesions in a patient with established melanoma, initially diagnosed as metastases. The lesions all showed intensely bright signal on T2w images (**B**) and no enhancement on post-Gd T1w images (**C**). Diagnosis—multiple cysts, confirmed on surveillance.

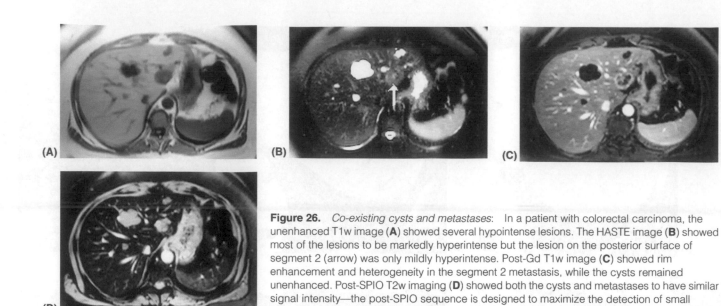

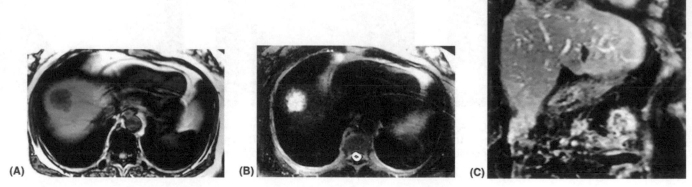

Figure 26. *Co-existing cysts and metastases*: In a patient with colorectal carcinoma, the unenhanced T1w image (**A**) showed several hypointense lesions. The HASTE image (**B**) showed most of the lesions to be markedly hyperintense but the lesion on the posterior surface of segment 2 (arrow) was only mildly hyperintense. Post-Gd T1w image (**C**) showed rim enhancement and heterogeneity in the segment 2 metastasis, while the cysts remained unenhanced. Post-SPIO T2w imaging (**D**) showed both the cysts and metastases to have similar signal intensity—the post-SPIO sequence is designed to maximize the detection of small metastases, and is ineffective in distinguishing between cysts and tumors.

Figure 27. *Necrotic colorectal metastasis*: A 4 cm mass close to the surface of the right lobe was moderately hypointense on T1w images (**A**) with a fairly well-defined margin. The T2w image (**B**) showed an irregular edge but the contents were largely of fluid density. Coronal post-Gd T1w image (**C**) showed the typical heterogeneous enhancement of colorectal metastasis.

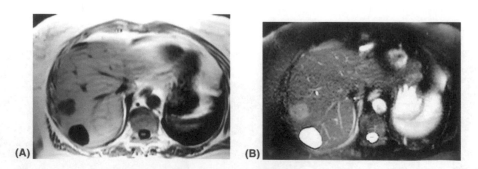

Figure 28. *Co-existing cyst and metastasis*: The clear-cut 4-cm cyst lying posteriorly in the right lobe showed the same signal intensity as CSF on both T1w (**A**) and T2w (**B**) images. The 3 cm metastasis anterior to the cyst was mildly hypointense on T1w and hyperintense on T2w images. Post-Gd T1w imaging showed no enhancement in the cyst, while the metastasis showed heterogeneous central enhancement in the early phase (**C**) with more marked rim enhancement on the venous phase image (**D**). (*Continued*)

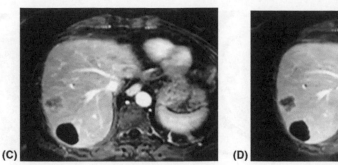

(C)   (D)   **Figure 28.** (*Continued*)

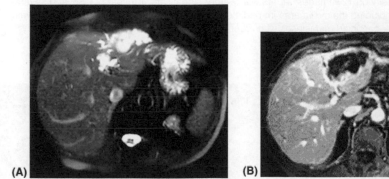

(A)   (B)   (C)

Figure 29. *Metastasis from mucin-secreting carcinoma*:   T2w imaging (**A**) showed a multi-loculated cystic mass lying anteriorly in the left lobe. Post-Gd T1w image (**B**) showed just a little patchy enhancement within the lesion and a more vascular tumor rim. Post-SPIO T2w image (**C**) showed the full extent of the tumor.

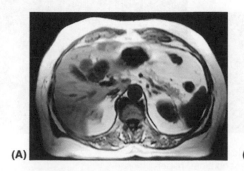
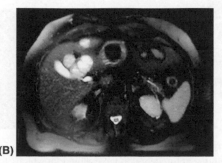
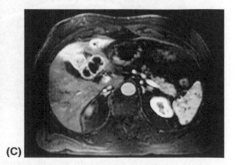

(A)   (B)   (C)

Figure 30. *Cystic metastases*:   The T1w image (**A**) showed multi-loculated cystic lesions occupying part of the left lobe with varying degrees of hypointensity. The HASTE image (**B**) showed the largely fluid but heterogeneous contents of the lesions. Post-Gd T1w image showed intense enhancement of the periphery of the lesions with a little central enhancement in the more solid components, and also a peripheral THID at the anterior aspect of segment 4. Histology confirmed metastases of neuro-endocrine origin.

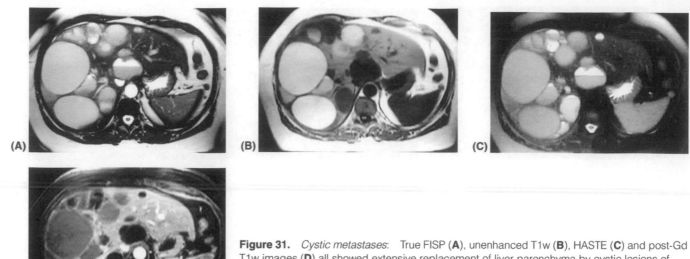

Figure 31.   *Cystic metastases*:   True FISP (**A**), unenhanced T1w (**B**), HASTE (**C**) and post-Gd T1w images (**D**) all showed extensive replacement of liver parenchyma by cystic lesions of varying sizes. The signal intensity of the cysts varied, some with high signal on T1w and less hyperintensity on T2w images, others with watery signal similar to that of CSF, and several lesions—including the cystic area immediately anterior to the aorta—exhibiting fluid levels. Diagnosis—carcinoid metastases with recent and old hemorrhage in some of the lesions.

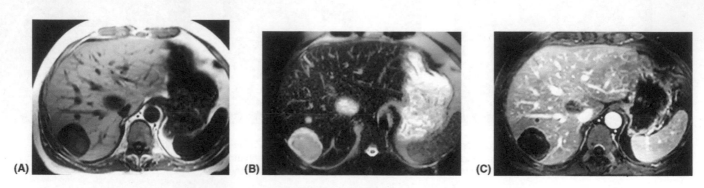

Figure 32.   *Necrotic metastases*:   T1w and HASTE images (**A**, **B**) showed two lesions in segment 7 and one adjacent to the inferior vena cava. All three lesions were markedly hyperintense on T2w and hypointense on T1w imaging, with heterogeneity of the wall of the segment 1 lesion and a filling defect or cast of necrotic material in the larger segment 7 lesion. Post-Gd T1w images (**C**) showed typical ring enhancement in both segment 7 lesions and patchy enhancement within the segment 1 lesion. Histology—metastases from a gastrointestinal stromal tumor (GIST).

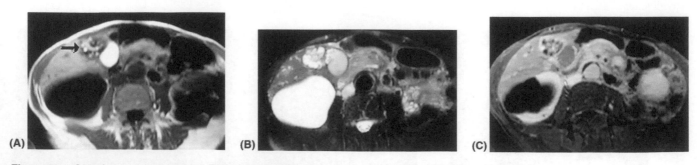

Figure 33.   *Complex cystic metastasis*:   The T1w image (**A**) showed a multiloculated cystic mass with mostly hyperintense contents (arrow) lying immediately anterolateral to the gallbladder which also contained hyper-intense bile. The large cyst lying posteriorly arose from the upper pole of the right kidney. T2w image (**B**) showed the multi-loculated and heterogeneous consistency of the multi-cystic liver lesion. Post-Gd T1w imaging (**C**) showed marked enhancement around the periphery and within the septa of the multi-cystic mass, and also showed enhancement of the thickened gallbladder wall. Diagnosis—carcinoma of the pancreas with necrotic liver metastasis.

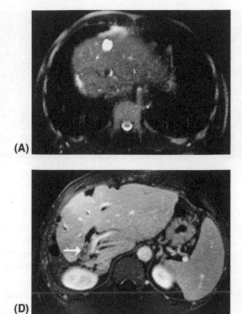
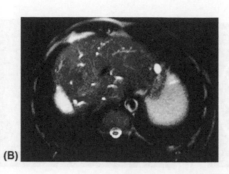
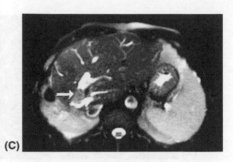
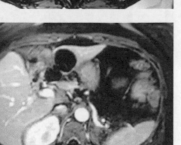

Figure 34. *Cystic residues after RF ablation:*   Following right hemi-hepatectomy and ablation of superficial lesions in the residual left lobe, HASTE images at two levels showed clear-cut peripheral lesions with contents having the same signal intensity as CSF (**A**, **B**). HASTE image at hilar level (**C**) showed duct dilatation caused by an endo-luminal recurrence of colorectal metastases (arrow). Post-Gd T1w image at the same level (**D**) showed the heterogeneous enhancement of the endo-luminal tumor (arrow). Note the lack of enhancement around the peripheral ablation sites, indicating successful sterilization of these tumors.

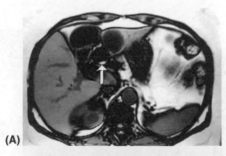
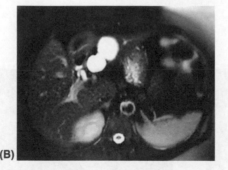
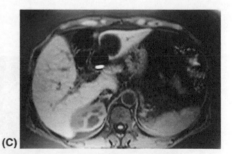

Figure 35. *Differential diagnosis of atypical cyst:*   Opposed-phase T1w image without fat suppression (**A**) showed a bi-locular cyst in segment 3. The posterior element contained a small amount of high signal material (arrow). The HASTE image (**B**) showed both loculi to have a smooth wall and no internal structure. Unenhanced VIBE image with fat suppression (**C**) again showed a small area of high signal content within the more posterior element of the cystic mass, suggesting recent bleeding. Post-Gd T1w image (**D**) showed no enhancement or nodularity of the cyst walls. Differential diagnosis—hemorrhage within a simple biliary cyst, or cystadenoma? Repeat examination after 6 months showed some further enlargement of the lesions so resection was carried out. Histology revealed cystadenoma with mesenchymal stroma (Edmondson's tumor).

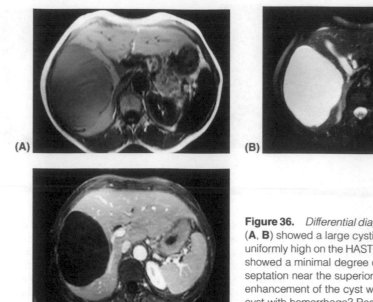

(A)

(B)

(C)

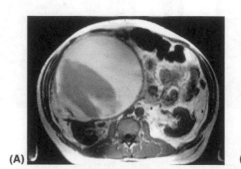

(D)

Figure 36. *Differential diagnosis of atypical large cyst:* Unenhanced T1w and HASTE images (**A, B**) showed a large cystic lesion replacing much of the right lobe. Note the fluid content was uniformly high on the HASTE image but only mildly hypointense on the T1w image. The cyst wall showed a minimal degree of nodularity. A HASTE image at a more cranial level (**C**) showed septation near the superior margin of the cyst. Post-Gd T1w imaging (**D**) showed no enhancement of the cyst wall or septa. Differential diagnosis—cystadenoma or simple biliary cyst with hemorrhage? Resection histology showed a simple biliary cyst containing old hematoma.

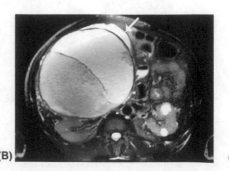

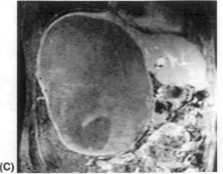

(A)

(B)

(C)

Figure 37. *Differential diagnosis of atypical large cyst:* T1w and HASTE images (**A, B**) showed a large cystic mass containing fluid which was hyperintense on both T1w and T2w images, but also included a large solid component. Note the relatively thick wall of the cyst with areas of nodularity best seen on the HASTE image. The gallbladder (arrow) was stretched over the anterior surface of the cyst. Post-Gd T1w imaging showed a minor degree of enhancement in the cyst wall but no enhancement of the contents. Differential diagnosis—cystadenoma or simple cyst with hemorrhage? Resection histology showed considerable hemorrhage within a solitary bile duct cyst with an unusually thick fibrotic wall.

CHAPTER 6

Solid Masses in the Non-Cirrhotic Liver

T his chapter reviews the clinical and MR imaging aspects of those focal benign and malignant lesions in the non-cirrhotic liver which appear largely or entirely solid on sonography and CT, excluding metastatic disease which is covered in chapters 10–12. Some aspects of their differentiation from metastatic disease are discussed here, but see also chapter 11.

FOCAL NODULAR HYPERPLASIA

Incidence

After hemangioma, focal nodular hyperplasia (FNH) is the second most commonly found benign malformation of the liver. It occurs most frequently in women of child-bearing age, is rare in children, and although it is not uncommon in older women, the lesions are then usually smaller and fewer in number. In about 20% of cases, multiple lesions are found. FNH occurs also in men, but with a much lower frequency—about one tenth of that in women. One substantial series of male patients showed the lesions to be smaller on average than those in women, to occur at an older average age, to be always solitary, and to show more atypical appearances on imaging. In female patients, it is not rare for FNH to co-exist with other benign malformations, particularly cysts, and hemangiomas, and an increased incidence in association with fatty change is also recognized.

Cause

The cause of FNH remains speculative. The typical vascular supply is by a dominant central artery, and this supports the view that FNH may be a hyperplastic response to a local vascular malformation. Because of the incidence in women of reproductive age, an association with female sex hormones has been proposed. Although occasional cases have enlarged during pregnancy, a systematic study has shown no consistent change in the size of lesions before and after pregnancy, and no association with oral contraception has been shown for FNH as a whole. However, the recently described variety of telangiectatic FNH, which has been found only in females, has almost always been associated with oral contraception.

Pathology

Pathology of the typical FNH lesion shows it to be composed of hepatocytes and Kupffer cells with rudimentary bile ductules which do not communicate with the biliary tree in the rest of the liver. The majority of lesions over about 3 cm size, and some of the smaller ones, contain a central "scar" containing blood vessels, fibrosis, and myxoid tissue. The blood supply is predominantly arterial and a central feeding artery may be seen within the scar. A minor degree of fat deposition is not uncommon, and rare instances of intra-lesional hemorrhage and calcification have been described. Malignant change does not occur.

The recently described telangiectatic variety of FNH probably accounts for less than 10% of lesions. The pathology is different from the typical FNH in that the lesions contain thin plates of hepatocytes with dilated sinusoids which are fed directly by smaller arteries. Blood-filled spaces may occur centrally, and areas of focal hemorrhage or necrosis are seen much more often than in the typical solid FNH. These lesions often show an inflammatory component, are commonly multiple, and may be associated with similar telangiectatic malformations in other organs. A recent analysis of the structure of cellular proteins in these lesions suggested that they should be classified as atypical adenomas rather than as FNH.

MRI Appearances

The lesions are usually round or ovoid when small, but larger lesions may be lobulated. The lesions are typically well-defined with clear-cut margins, although no capsule is present. FNH is usually isointense or slightly hypointense on T1w, and isointense or slightly hyperintense on T2w images, although a minority of lesions show more marked hyperintensity on T2w images. Most lesions are homogeneous apart from the "scar" which often takes the form of a central stellate area but may be quite extensive with septa extending well out into the periphery of the lesion, or smaller, appearing as a rounded central nodule. The signal intensity in the scar is lower on T1w and higher on T2w images than the rest of the lesion.

After gadolinium, small lesions show homogeneous enhancement in the arterial phase which is usually quite intense. This washes out fairly quickly, so that the lesion becomes only mildly hyperintense or sometimes isointense with surrounding liver during the venous phase. With larger lesions the arterial blush may be heterogeneous, particularly if a large central scar is present. On delayed images, the lesions may either retain contrast to a greater extent than surrounding liver, or may wash out further, returning to their pre-contrast T1w appearance.

Because the biliary radicles within FNH do not communicate with the rest of the biliary tree, hepatocyte specific contrast agents are retained in the parenchyma of these lesions for longer than in the adjacent liver. Delayed images after mangafodipir, gadobenate, or gadoxetic acid typically show persistent hyperintensity (less commonly, iso-intensity) compared with adjacent liver.

The central scar, which contains no hepatocytes, shows little or no enhancement in the arterial phase, but may enhance as early as the venous phase, although more typically the scar enhancement appears on images delayed by a few minutes. At this stage the scar often shows a higher signal than the rest of the lesion.

Uptake of super-paramagnetic iron oxide (SPIO) contrast is a characteristic feature of FNH. However, the degree of uptake may be less than in the surrounding liver, so the lesions become more easily visible on T2*w images after SPIO than on pre-contrast images. Visual assessment may be misleading and in order to confirm uptake of SPIO by the lesion, it is important to measure the change in signal intensity before and after SPIO, using the same T2*w sequence. The percentage signal intensity loss in normal liver parenchyma is usually 70–90%, while that in FNH is usually in the 40–70% range. Loss of signal from the parenchyma of the lesion accentuates the visibility of the central scar, which may become apparent for the first time only after SPIO contrast. The degree of uptake of SPIO is variable, with some FNHs—particularly small lesions—taking up more contrast than the surrounding liver, and so becoming hypointense. The uptake in some large lesions is heterogeneous, probably resulting from their greater proportion of fibrous tissue or central "scar".

The telangiectatic variant of FNH often shows atypical features. Over half of these lesions show areas of increased signal on unenhanced T1w images, possibly related to sinusoidal dilatation or foci of fat deposition. Signal intensity on T2w images is greater than with the typical solid FNH, and may approach the degree of hyperintensity usually associated with hemangiomas. Telangiectatic FNH is more commonly lobulated in shape and heterogeneous in structure than the typical FNH, and the central scar is rarely present. Although these lesions mostly show an intense arterial blush following gadolinium, the hyperintensity is heterogeneous, and more persistent than with the typical solid FNH.

Atypical Features of FNH

1. Many small lesions, and occasional large ones, do not show a central scar
2. Fat content is occasionally sufficient to recognize on chemical shift imaging
3. Occasional lesions show hyperintensity on T1w and hypointensity on T2w images
4. The composition of the central scar varies; when the scar is densely fibrotic with little myxoid and vascular tissue, it may appear hypointense on T2w images, and show little or no late enhancement after gadolinium

5. Rare cases have been described in which the lesions did not show arterial hyperintensity on post-Gd T1w images
6. Rare cases of a "pseudocapsule" around FNH lesions have been described.

Differential Diagnosis of FNH

FNH rarely produces clinical symptoms or signs, and even with large lesions, liver function tests are usually normal. FNH is most often discovered incidentally during the imaging investigation of patients with unrelated disorders. Once detected, the lesions must be differentiated from other solid liver tumors, particularly malignancies, in order to allow appropriate management. If a confident diagnosis of FNH can be made by imaging, no treatment is required apart from surveillance. Solid lesions which are discovered in the livers of patients who are otherwise well and who have no history of prior malignancy, are virtually always benign, and FNH is by far the most common pathology. In such cases, if the morphology, signal characteristics, and enhancement with gadolinium follow the typical pattern described above, the diagnosis is virtually certain, and a substantial (40% or more) drop in signal intensity of the lesion following SPIO contrast is sufficient to confirm its benign hepatocellular nature.

With atypical imaging features, or when FNH is suspected in patients with a history of malignancy, the behavior of the lesions with tissue specific contrast agents becomes critically important, and the diagnosis is unsafe without their use. Although some liver metastases appear similar to FNH on unenhanced images, and show hypervascularity in the arterial phase of post-Gd enhancement, the rate of washout from these lesions is usually faster than is seen with FNH. Hypervascular metastases are more likely than FNH to be hypointense on unenhanced T1w and markedly hyperintense on T2w images. However, the key feature is that metastases do not extract tissue-specific contrast agents—they become strikingly hyperintense to liver following SPIO contrast, and they do not show prolonged retention of T1 agents as is seen with FNH.

The imaging features of FNH do overlap with those of hepatocellular carcinoma (HCC) but this is rarely problematic since the clinical setting is usually indicative. Well-differentiated varieties of HCC may show some uptake of tissue specific contrast agents, and are also commonly hypervascular in the arterial phase after gadolinium. However, in the presence of advanced cirrhosis FNH-like nodules are rarely found—a large hypervascular nodule in a cirrhotic liver is virtually always HCC, while in the absence of cirrhosis, HCCs are usually several centimeters in size by the time of presentation. HCCs are often heterogeneous and a well-defined capsule is present which shows low signal on unenhanced images and delayed enhancement after gadolinium. The arterial blush is usually heterogeneous and fades fairly rapidly. It is unusual for these lesions to show significant accumulation of tissue specific contrast agents, and more often they take up none at all. Patients are often male, usually of fairly advanced years and almost always present with relevant symptoms, particularly abdominal pain, jaundice, weight loss or anemia.

Differential diagnosis of the telangiectatic variant of FNH is more problematic since the imaging features are more variable and the incidence and behavior of this lesion is as yet not well understood. The spectrum of imaging appearances overlaps with that of benign hemangioma, and it may also mimic malignancy. The behavior of these lesions with tissue specific contrast agents is not well-established, so excision or needle biopsy may be required in these rare cases.

ADENOMA

Liver cell adenoma is an uncommon benign neoplasm of hepatocyte origin. Most adenomas occur in female patients during the reproductive years, and there is a strong association with oral contraceptive use. Cases of liver adenoma in men may be linked with the use of anabolic steroids. In most cases adenomas are solitary, but a minority of patients have multiple lesions and when more than 10 lesions are present, the condition is described as "adenomatosis"—often, but not always, associated with glycogen storage disease.

Like FNH, uncomplicated adenomas rarely present clinically. When adenomas are discovered incidentally, their imaging appearances may overlap with those of FNH to a degree which makes diagnosis difficult, but most cases show specific features which allow a distinction to be made. The majority of adenoma patients present clinically with symptoms arising from hemorrhage or pressure effects. The possibility of malignant transformation has been raised by a single case report, but the risk of hemorrhage justifies active treatment of larger lesions once the diagnosis is made.

Histologically, the lesions are made up of hepatocytes which quite commonly contain fat deposits and sometimes show increased glycogen content. Unlike FNH, portal tracts are absent and there are no biliary radicles. Perhaps because the blood supply is less well-established than in FNH, hemorrhage, and necrosis are relatively common, particularly in larger lesions. Kupffer cells are present to a varying degree. In contrast with FNH, a central scar is not a recognized feature, but adenomas often have a pseudocapsule of compressed liver tissue surrounding the lesion.

MRI Appearances

The lesions are rounded or lobulated and often show a heterogeneous structure. The majority are mildly hyperintense on T2w imaging, the remainder isointense. Lesions may be isointense or hypointense on T1w images, but hyperintensity on in-phase T1 is quite common owing to the presence of fat or glycogen. The fat content is usually sufficient to show a distinct change in signal between in-phase and opposed-phase T1w images. The capsule, when present, is usually hypointense on both T1w and T2w images. Instances have also been described of increased iron deposition, producing hypointensity on both T1w and T2w imaging.

The presence of hemorrhage or post-haemorrhagic necrosis within the lesion produces the usual signal changes of hyperintensity on both T1w and T2w images from recent bleeding, and more marked hypointensity on T1w and hyperintensity on T2w images with later liquefaction of the hematoma. On post-Gd T1w imaging most lesions show a homogeneous arterial blush fading to become isointense except for late capsular enhancement, but a minority of lesions show relatively poor vascularity. Uptake of tissue specific contrast agents is also less consistent than with FNH; although most adenomas will show uptake of SPIO and mangafodipir, uptake of gadobenate is absent or much less marked.

Differential Diagnosis

When the diagnosis of adenoma is made, surgical treatment should be considered even for uncomplicated lesions because of the significant risk of later hemorrhage, and the smaller risk of malignant change. Although the imaging appearances may overlap with those of FNH, adenomas are more likely to show increased signal on unenhanced T1w images, heterogeneity on T2w images, a peripheral pseudocapsule but no central scar, and sufficient fat content to show a signal change on chemical shift imaging. A history of exposure to oral contraceptives or anabolic steroids is more likely with adenoma and multiple lesions are most often associated with glycogen storage disorders. Liver cell adenoma is not recognized in the context of cirrhosis, and the differentiation from metastases follows the approach described above for FNH.

Adenomas presenting with hemorrhage need to be distinguished from other liver lesions which present with acute hemorrhage. Bleeding from HCCs is usually associated with advanced tumor in older patients with established cirrhosis, while patients with bleeding adenomas are usually young women with normal or near normal liver function. This distinction is important, since patients with bleeding adenoma may require surgical resection, while the results of surgery for haemorrhagic HCC are uniformly poor. Large hemangiomas which may rarely bleed will usually be distinguished from adenoma by their typical imaging features, but will typically also come to surgery. Hemorrhage into liver metastases is uncommon and usually associated with widespread disease. Hemorrhage into liver cysts is most common with polycystic disease, but even with bleeding into a single cyst the underlying nature of the lesion should be apparent.

HEMANGIOMA

Incidence

Hemangioma is the most frequently encountered benign neoplasm of the liver. It is about three times more common in women than in men, and usually solitary although multiple lesions are not uncommon. Only in exceptional cases is a liver hemangioma responsible for symptoms, so these lesions are almost always found incidentally. In these circumstances we need to distinguish them from other, more significant, pathologies—particularly malignant liver tumors. Although hemangiomas are composed partly of blood vessels, percutaneous biopsy carries no particular hazard and may be performed. However, biopsy is rarely needed since the imaging findings are definitive in the majority of cases, and even with atypical presentations imaging is usually indicative of the diagnosis.

Pathology

Histology shows a variable mixture of abnormal blood vessels and vascular spaces with a stroma of fibrous tissue, and sometimes other mesenchymal elements are present. The relative proportion of vascular spaces, interstitium, and dense fibrosis is variable between lesions, even when they are small, and this variability may account for the atypical imaging characteristics seen in a minority of cases. Larger lesions may contain phleboliths or other dense calcifications, areas of fibrosis may coalesce to produce cartilage-like elements, and sometimes central areas of liquefaction are present. The lesions are usually very sharply defined, though not encapsulated. Small lesions are often round or oval, but larger lesions are usually irregular or geographic in shape. Their size is very variable, lesions of a few millimeters being quite common, while occasionally large lesions may replace a substantial proportion of the liver parenchyma.

Presentation

Imaging surveillance of patients already diagnosed shows that in the adult population hemangiomas remain stable in the vast majority of cases, so they appear to pose no threat to health. Adverse clinical events associated with these lesions are all rare. They include right upper quadrant pain associated with capsular involvement, spontaneous rupture with intraperitoneal bleeding, intra-lesional hemorrhage, local compression of bile ducts, compression of the inferior vena cava, and one possible case of malignant change has been reported. A few cases have also been described in which abdominal symptoms arose from pedunculated lesions developing on the liver surface, and rare instances of rapid enlargement during pregnancy have been recorded.

MRI Appearances

Typical imaging appearances include uniform hyper-echogenicity on sonography, hypo-attenuation on unenhanced CT, and a characteristic discontinuous, nodular, and usually peripheral early enhancement after contrast, with gradual infilling of the center of the lesion best seen on images delayed by 5–15 minutes. On unenhanced MRI, the typical lesion is sharply defined with a geographic or rounded shape, hypointense on T1w and strongly hyperintense on T2w images. Small lesions usually appear homogeneous, larger lesions are often heterogeneous, usually with central irregular areas of even greater hyperintensity on T2w and hypointensity on T1w images. On T2w imaging the lesions may be as bright as CSF, but are more often a little less intense. However, their marked hyperintensity is maintained to a greater degree than most metastases with increasing T2 weighting.

Typical T1 enhancement with gadolinium follows the same pattern as already described for CT. Early phase images show peripheral enhancement which is typically nodular and discontinuous. After the first pass phase, the nodular enhancement fades slowly to converge with the signal intensity of venous blood, then maintains this level of signal. Meanwhile the remainder of the lesion shows gradual increase in signal intensity over the next few minutes to produce a uniform blush of the same intensity as in the hepatic veins and IVC. The rate of enhancement is variable—in some patients the peripheral nodular component appears with the arterial dominant phase, while in other cases nodular enhancement begins in the portal phase. Infilling of the central part of the lesion is sometimes seen in the first 30 seconds after injection, whereas in other cases complete infilling may take 5–15 minutes. Particularly with larger lesions, there is often a central, relatively avascular area which enhances much less than the rest of the lesion or in some cases not at all; this component typically shows more marked hypo- and hyperintensity on T1w and T2w images respectively than the rest of the lesion.

The behavior of hemangiomas with SPIO contrast is complex. The lesions contain few—if any—functioning Kupffer cells, so there should be no intracellular accumulation of SPIO. However, the intravascular spaces within these lesions often accumulate enough SPIO contrast at an appropriate degree of dilution to create a significant T1-enhancing effect, which persists longer in the lesion than in the surrounding liver parenchyma, so as with gadolinium, the lesions show persisting increase in signal on delayed T1w images. The SPIO content may also cause reduced signal on delayed T2w images (see chap. 3).

Atypical Hemangiomas

Although the majority of hemangiomas show the characteristics described above, several atypical variants are recognized.

1. Enhancement may be very slow, heterogeneous, and incomplete even on delayed images. This is usually seen with large lesions, but even lesions of 1–3 cm may show this feature. It is postulated that the rate of enhancement varies with the size of the vascular spaces in the lesion—those with large vascular lakes enhance slowly, while with smaller vascular spaces the enhancement is more rapid
2. The degree of hyperintensity on T2w imaging is variable and in some cases with diffuse sclerosing histology the lesions may be much less intense than CSF. Diagnosis then relies on contrast enhancement, which may be slower than usual, but still eventually reaches isointensity with blood vessels
3. Rapid uniform enhancement is common, particularly with lesions smaller than 2 cm. Unlike hypervascular metastases, the enhancement in small hemangiomas fades slowly, in parallel with the vascular compartment. The presence of central or peripheral bright dots in the early phase of enhancement is another helpful feature in differentiating from malignancy
4. In rare cases, the pattern of enhancement may be heterogeneous or centripetal rather than centrifugal, but the early enhancement remains nodular and discontinuous
5. Occasionally, local arterioportal shunting is associated with a hemangioma so that a THID develops around the lesion.

Co-Morbidities

The simultaneous existence of hemangioma and FNH in the liver appears to occur more often than would be expected by chance, suggesting a common thread in the development of these lesions. Rarely, a large number of hemangiomas may co-exist, producing a peliosis-like appearance.

Although hemangiomas are occasionally found in the livers of patients with late stage cirrhosis, their frequency in this population is less than would be expected. It is postulated that the fibrotic reaction to liver damage tends to obliterate benign malformations such as hemangiomas which are soft and pliable.

The presence of diffuse fatty change in the liver increases the difficulty of diagnosing hemangioma because it produces increased echogenicity on sonography and reduced attenuation on unenhanced CT, so hemangiomas may be undetectable, although contrast enhancement should distinguish them from the surrounding tissue. Fatty change does not influence the T2 characteristics of the lesions on unenhanced MRI, but they may be invisible on opposed-phase T1w images, while remaining clearly defined on in-phase T1w images. The enhancement pattern with gadolinium remains unchanged. In some cases a rim of focal fatty sparing remains around the periphery of the lesion so that a hemangioma which is otherwise invisible on unenhanced CT or opposed-phase T1w images is shown by the halo of normal liver surrounding the lesion (see chap. 7).

Hemangiomas typically remain stable over sequential observations, but distinct enlargement has been shown to occur only in a tiny minority, including one case during pregnancy.

Differential Diagnosis

Occasionally small metastases, particularly those which are hypervascular, produce clear-cut lesions with bright signal on T2w imaging. Some metastases show a uniform early enhancement with gadolinium, and others show gradual centripetal enhancement over several minutes. All these features overlap with those seen in hemangiomas, but the differentiation can almost always be made with careful review of the behavior of the lesions at different T2 weightings, and close attention to the enhancement pattern. With larger lesions, the morphology is also helpful.

Although most malignant tumors show hyperintensity, they remain distinctly less intense than hemangiomas. Both liver parenchyma and solid tumors are susceptible to magnetization transfer effects, so the difference between benign malformations and tumor is greater on T2w sequences using a long echo-train (FSE or HASTE) and when TE is increased to add greater T2 weighting, this difference is magnified. However, a small minority of hemangiomas show a relatively weak T2 hyperintensity, and some metastases have a high fluid content producing exceptionally high signal on T2w images. In these cases the enhancement pattern with gadolinium is usually decisive. The key feature of hemangiomas is the discontinuous nodular form of the early enhancement, while metastases—even those with delayed infilling due to central necrosis—show a continuous rim of enhancement at the periphery of the lesion. Small hemangiomas which show a uniform early blush may be distinguished from metastases by the maintenance of their enhancement in parallel with the vascular compartment, while metastases typically show rapid washout of contrast following the early enhancement.

Very large hemangiomas, particularly those with heterogeneous internal structure, and patchy enhancement, need to be distinguished from HCC, fibrolamellar hepatoma, and intrahepatic cholangiocarcinoma. There may be considerable overlap between the characteristics of these lesions on unenhanced T1w and T2w images, but there are several useful clues. Firstly, hemangiomas even when large have a very clearly defined outline. The geographic shape is a pointer—malignancies are usually round, oval or diffuse. A further useful morphological pointer is that with benign malformations, the intrahepatic vessels appear undisplaced while large malignancies produce a distinct mass effect on the surrounding structures. Even when large, the marked T2 hyperintensity of hemangiomas is striking, and the enhancement, although it may be incomplete and heterogeneous, still typically shows the nodular, discontinuous, and peripheral pattern. Intrahepatic cholangio-carcinoma and FLH may both show central "scars" with delayed or absent enhancement, but the early peripheral enhancement of these tumors is continuous and more uniform than is seen with hemangioma.

ANGIOMYOLIPOMA

Mixed mesenchymal tumors containing a variable proportion of smooth muscle, blood vessels, fat, and fibrous tissue occur as a rare incidental finding in patients, usually female, whose livers are usually otherwise normal. The signal characteristics on MRI are variable owing to the inconstant histologic make-up of the lesions. With a predominant fat content, the lesions may mimic a lipoma, showing substantial signal loss in fat suppression sequences, while in other cases a lesser fat content may be demonstrated by signal variation between in-phase and opposed-phase T1w images. As with angiomyolipomas elsewhere in the body, the vascularity is variable with some lesions showing marked arterial phase enhancement with gadolinium, while others are hypovascular.

PERIPHERAL CHOLANGIOCARCINOMA

The more common hilar and extra-hepatic cholangiocarcinomas present with biliary obstruction as a primary feature, and these lesions are discussed in chapter 13. A small proportion of cholangiocarcinomas present as an intra-parenchymal mass, often with no associated duct obstruction. Satellite lesions are present in a substantial minority of cases, but the appearance on unenhanced imaging is often similar to that of metastatic disease. The discovery of a solitary mass in a patient with no known primary site should raise the suspicion of intrahepatic cholangiocarcinoma.

MRI Appearances

Imaging appearances vary according to the composition of the tumors. Unlike the more common hilar and extrahepatic tumors, peripheral cholangiocarcinomas usually contain a substantial proportion of acinar tissue, as well as a fibrous matrix. Characteristically, in the post-Gd arterial and portal venous phases the lesions show a strongly enhancing rim of glandular tissue with a hypovascular center. Peripheral washout with delayed and prolonged enhancement of the central fibrotic area is seen on later images. In-drawing of the liver capsule adjacent to the tumor is a well-recognized and useful distinguishing feature, since it hardly ever occurs in patients with untreated metastatic disease. Unlike HCC, cholangiocarcinoma does not show an enhancing capsule, and the margins of the mass may be ill-defined.

Differential Diagnosis

Metastasis from colorectal cancer may show similar morphology to intrahepatic cholangiocarcinoma. Large solitary metastases are uncommon and very unlikely in the absence of a known primary site. Fibrolamellar HCC may show similar appearances to peripheral cholangiocarcinoma. Helpful distinguishing features of FLH are its arterial hypervascularity and the typical presence of a stellate central scar of fibrous tissue showing little or no enhancement on delayed images. Conventional HCC may be distinguished by its arterial hypervascularity and the presence of a fibrous capsule.

HEPATOCELLULAR CARCINOMA IN THE NON-CIRRHOTIC LIVER

Although HCC most commonly develops against a background of cirrhosis (see chap. 9) a minority of HCCs occur in non-cirrhotic livers. In the Western world, most of these cases may be regarded as truly sporadic—i.e., they occur in livers which are otherwise histologically normal—but others will show evidence of chronic hepatitis B or hepatitis C infection, not amounting to cirrhosis. The fibrolamellar variant of HCC has distinctive features and is described further below.

Sporadic HCC occurs most often in patients over 50 years old and more often in males than females. The lesion usually presents with right upper quadrant pain, sometimes with jaundice, or with systemic symptoms of malignancy. Serum alpha-fetoprotein measurements are elevated in a little over half of the cases. The tumors are usually large at the time of presentation and most often solitary, sometimes with satellite lesions. The histology is typically well or moderately well differentiated, and these lesions tend to take a more indolent course than HCC in cirrhosis. The preferred treatment is by surgical resection when technically feasible, and survival, whether treated or untreated, is better than with HCC in cirrhosis.

MRI Appearances

Imaging typically shows a large solitary mass, satellite lesions are not uncommon, but multifocal presentation is unusual. Tumors are almost invariably heterogeneous and commonly show areas of hemorrhage and necrosis. Calcification and focal fatty areas are well recognized features. Because the tumors are often large at presentation, imaging may show local pressure effects, in particular the dilatation of lobar or segmental intrahepatic ducts, and altered perfusion caused by occlusion or compression of portal vein branches. Lymph node metastases are found at presentation more frequently than with HCC in cirrhosis.

MRI typically shows a large heterogeneous tumor which is mostly hypointense on T1w images, but areas of hyperintensity may indicate intra-tumoral hemorrhage. Opposed-phase and in-phase imaging may show areas of focal fat within the lesion. T2w images show a heterogeneously or occasionally diffusely hyperintense mass. Recent hemorrhage may produce ill-defined areas of hyperintensity on T1w images, while haemosiderin deposits from previous hemorrhage can be identified as foci of hypointensity on both T1w and T2w images. Post-gadolinium images typically show heterogeneous enhancement which is most marked in the arterial phase, with rapid washout resulting in the lesion returning to hypointensity on portal phase and delayed images. An enhancing capsule is often present. Direct invasion of the portal and hepatic vein branches is rarely a feature at presentation and seems to occur much later, relative to the size of the tumor, than with HCC in the cirrhotic liver.

FIBROLAMELLAR HCC

Fibrolamellar hepatocellular carcinoma (FLH) is sufficiently different in its demographics, histology, imaging appearances, and prognosis to make it worthwhile identifying this tumor separately. FLH is a disorder of young people, occurring most commonly in the 2nd and 3rd decades. Males and females are equally often affected. There is no association with underlying cirrhosis or hepatitis.

The histology shows cords or plates of malignant eosinophilic hepatocytes separated by parallel strands or sheets of fibrous tissue. Microvascular invasion is uncommon. Serum AFP is typically normal, and the abnormal hepatocytes within the lesion do not contain the AFP inclusions which are typical of HCC in cirrhosis. The lesions tend to be slow growing and have usually reached a substantial size (typically over 10 cm) at the time of presentation. Lymph node metastases are present at presentation in approximately half of the cases, but distant metastases are relatively uncommon, probably less than 20%. With locally confined disease, radical surgery produces fairly good results and even in advanced cases, the prognosis is better than with other forms of HCC at a similar stage.

MRI Appearances

Imaging shows a well-defined tumor with lobulated or scalloped margins, more commonly in the left lobe than in the right. The lesions are typically solitary but in a minority of cases (10–20%) multiple nodules are present.

MRI typically shows a heterogeneous mass with mainly solid components, and in the majority of cases an extensive central "scar". On unenhanced T1w images, the lesions show varying degrees of hypointensity, sometimes with isointense areas. The central scar is always hypointense. On T2w images, the lesions show varying degrees of hyperintensity, often heterogeneously, and again sometimes with areas of isointensity. The central scar is typically hypointense on T2w images. Patchy calcification within the central scar is a well-recognized feature on CT, but may be quite subtle on MRI. Calcification is suggested by clusters of small, well-defined foci showing very low signal intensity on both T1w and T2w imaging. Enhancement with gadolinium is typically heterogeneous and may occur either in the arterial or portal phases, or both. The central scar is usually avascular and shows little or no enhancement, but occasionally some late enhancement will be seen in the scar. Uptake of mangafodipir into FLH lesions has been described. In our experience, these lesions do not take up SPIO contrast.

INFLAMMATORY PSEUDOTUMOR

Inflammatory pseudotumor is a rare focal liver lesion which may be problematic in differential diagnosis. The cause of this condition is unknown, but it has been suggested that chronic inflammatory disease of the biliary tract may be a predisposing factor in some cases. Pathology shows a mass of fibrous tissue with infiltration by chronic inflammatory cells, and areas of central coagulative necrosis may be present. There is no neoplasia, although isolated case reports have suggested the possibility of later malignant transformation. Although the lesions are histologically benign, they may pursue an aggressive course so surgical resection is the recommended treatment.

When the lesions are small, the patients may be asymptomatic, but in cases which present clinically, symptoms are usually of weight loss, fever, and upper abdominal pain. Liver function tests are usually normal unless the fibrotic mass encroaches on the porta hepatis.

In most cases, the patients are of middle age and there is a slight preponderance of males in the cases reported so far. Because of the relative rarity of this condition, the imaging findings described below must be regarded as a preliminary assessment only.

MRI Appearances

Most of the cases described have been solitary with exceptional cases showing two or three lesions. The masses are round, oval, lobulated or irregular in outline. One of the major characteristics of these lesions is they are ill-defined, particularly on unenhanced images. About two thirds of the lesions show hypointensity on unenhanced T1w images, the remainder have been isointense. On T2w imaging, the lesions are mildly hyperintense, or isointense. With gadolinium enhancement the lesions typically remain hypovascular in the arterial and portal phases, although an enhancing rim is often seen. Delayed images may show diffuse or nodular enhancement within the mass, and linear areas of late enhancement may produce a septated appearance. The margin of the lesion is usually more clearly defined after gadolinium, but it may still be infiltrative in character. In cases where SPIO contrast has been given, the margins of the lesion typically show uptake, indicating the presence of functioning Kupffer cells between the infiltrating sheets of inflammatory fibrosis, but in a few patients given gadobenate, no enhancement occurred. Although the lesions most commonly occur within the liver parenchyma, hilar location may present a difficult differential diagnosis. Segmental or lobar bile duct dilatation, and stenosis or occlusion of portal vein branches, accompanied by arterial hyperperfusion of the related liver segments, may produce an appearance which is virtually indistinguishable from that of hilar cholangiocarcinoma. Needle biopsy can be diagnostic, but surgery may be indicated irrespective of histology if the lesion is infiltrative, or affects the hilar structures, or both.

HEPATIC LYMPHOMA

Liver involvement in lymphoma occurs in 5–10% of patients with NHL and 10–20% of Hodgkin's disease patients. Splenic disease virtually always accompanies liver involvement, though the converse is not true. In over 90% of cases, lymphoma of the liver is manifest as diffuse infiltration which may cause hepatomegaly, but is otherwise unrecognizable on imaging. Focal lymphomatous masses are seen in under 10% of cases and are almost invariably accompanied by advanced abdominal lymph node disease, often with other extra nodal sites of involvement. Contrast- enhanced CT is used for staging of thoraco-abdominal lymphoma, so the characterization of lymphomatous masses in the liver is rarely a diagnostic problem, and MRI is seldom needed.

Patients who undergo organ transplantation followed by cyclosporin treatment for suppressing rejection have an increased risk of developing non-Hodgkin's lymphomas. Such lesions following liver transplantation usually present within a few months of transplantation with a soft tissue mass at the liver hilum which compresses—but does not completely obstruct—the bile ducts and portal veins.

Primary hepatic lymphoma is a very rare tumor usually presenting in middle-aged patients as a solitary intrahepatic mass, sometimes with enlarged nodes at the liver hilum.

MRI Appearances

Reported MR appearances of lymphomatous tumors in the liver are somewhat variable, but overlap almost completely with the appearance of metastatic tumors, so biopsy will usually be needed for diagnosis. The lesions may vary in size from sub-cm up to greater than 10 cm, and they are almost always well-defined. Primary lymphomas may be solitary or multiple, secondary lymphomas are usually multiple. Post-transplant lymphomas are solitary and typically hilar in position. On unenhanced T1w images, lymphoma in all of these categories most commonly shows hypointensity with a minority being isointense and occasional hyperintense cases have been described. Appearances on T2w images are also variable— most commonly the lesions are hyperintense, but cases of iso- and hypointensity have also been recorded. It has been suggested that the signal intensity on T2 relates to the degree of co-existing inflammatory infiltration within the mass, and this variation is paralleled by the post-gadolinium enhancement characteristics. Those tumors which have fairly high signal on T2w images tend to show quite marked early enhancement after Gadolinium, while those which are only slightly hyper- or isointense on T2w imaging show little or no enhancement, although these lesion often have a hypervascular enhancing rim.

MISCELLANEOUS TUMORS

Occasional instances of numerous different mesenchymal and epithelial primary liver tumors have been described. Experience with most of them is limited to a few case reports, so the imaging appearances are insufficiently established to provide a reliable guide to diagnosis. However, a few consistent observations have been made.

In primary angiosarcoma of the liver, formerly associated with occupational exposure to vinyl chloride, the lesions are single or multiple, heterogeneously hypointense on T1 and hyperintense on T2w imaging. Enhancement with gadolinium is patchy and progressive, giving an appearance reminiscent of giant hemangiomas. However, the lesions are fairly rapidly progressive and patients are usually ill at the time of presentation. Epithelioid heamangio-endothelioma (EHE) is marginally more common in women than men, and presents as a nodular, confluent or diffusely infiltrating tumor. The lesions typically show a high fluid content with areas of coagulative necrosis producing a target appearance with rings of hypo- and hyperintensity on T2w imaging. These tumors are characteristically peripheral within the liver, and local invasion with retraction of the adjacent liver capsule is a characteristic feature. The lesions show enhancement around the periphery on post-Gd T1w imaging.

Other primary mesenchymal lesions include leiomyosarcoma, malignant fibrous histiocytoma, adenofibroma, plasmacytoma, and primary neurendocrine tumors including carcinoid, pheochromoctyoma, and ganglioneuroma. Heterogeneous structure, hypointensity on T1w and hyperintensity on T2w imaging are described with all of these lesions, but the features are non-specific and histology is required for pathologic diagnosis.

ILLUSTRATIVE FIGURES

Typical FNH—Figures 1–4
Telangiectatic FNH—Figures 5–7
Large, multiple, lobulated FNH—Figures 8–13
FNH with enlarged vessels—Figures 14–16
FNH and fatty change—Figures 17–19
FNH containing fat—Figure 20
FNH with hemangioma—Figures 21–22
FNH in cirrhosis—Figure 23
Evolution of FNH—Figures 24–25
FNH versus metastasis—Figure 26
FNH with specific contrast agents—Figure 27
Typical adenoma—Figure 28
Adenoma with hemorrhage—Figures 29–30
Multiple adenomas—Figures 31–34
Co-existing adenoma and FNH—Figure 35
Typical hemangiomas—Figures 36–38
Angiographic correlation—Figures 39–40
Giant hemangioma—Figures 41–44
Atypical hemangiomas, THIDs—Figures 45–47
Hemangiomas and cysts—Figures 48–49
Hemangiomas in fatty liver—Figures 50–51
Hemangiomas in haemochromatosis—Figures 52–53
Hemangioma with SPIO T1 enhancement—Figure 54
Hemangioma with FNH—Figure 55
Growing hemangiomas—Figures 56–57
Differentials—hemangioma-like lesions—Figures 58–60
Angiomyolipomas—Figures 61–62
Peripheral cholangiocarcinomas—Figures 63–69
HCC in non-cirrhotic liver—Figures 70–77
Fibrolamellar HCC—Figures 78–82
Inflammatory pseudotumor—Figures 83–86
Hepatic lymphoma—Figures 87–89
Miscellaneous tumors—Figures 90–94

REFERENCES

1. Mortele KJ, Praet M, Van Vlierberghe H, et al. CT and MR imaging findings of focal nodular hyperplasia of the liver: radiologic-pathologic correlation. Am J Roentgenol 2000; 175:687–692.
2. Attal P, Vilgrain V, Brancatelli G, et al. Telangiectatic focal nodular hyperplasia: US, CT, and MR imaging findings with histopathologic correlation in 13 cases. Radiology 2003; 228:465–472.
3. Ba-Ssalamah A, Schima W, Schmook MT, et al. Atypical focal nodular hyperplasia of the liver: imaging features of non-specific and liver-specific contrast agents. Am J Roentgenol 2002; 179:1447–1456.
4. Chung KY, Mayo-Smith WW, Saini S, et al. Hepatocellular adenoma: MR imaging features with pathologic correlation. Am J Roentgenol 1995; 165:303–308.
5. Paulson EK, McClennan JS, Washington K, et al. Hepatic adenoma: MR characteristics and correlation with pathologic findings. Am J Roentgenol 1994; 163:113–116.
6. Semelka RC, Sofka CM. Hepatic hemangiomas. Magn Reson Imaging Clin N Am 1997; 5:241–253.

7. Vilgrain V, Boulos L, Vullierme M-P, et al. Imaging of atypical hemangiomas of the liver with pathologic correlation. Radiographics 2000; 20:379–397.

8. Coumbaras M, Wendum D, Monnier-Cholley L, et al. CT and MR imaging features of pathologically proven atypical giant hemangiomas of the liver. Am J Roentgenol 2002; 179:1457–1463.

9. Hogemann D, Flemming P, Kreipe H, et al. Correlation of MRI and CT findings with histopathology in hepatic angiomyolipoma. Eur Radiol 2001; 11:1389–1395.

10. Ichikawa T, Federle MP, Grazioli L, et al. Fibrolamellar carcinoma: imaging and pathologic findings in 31 recent cases. Radiology 1999; 213:352–361.

11. Yan FH, Zhou KR, Jiang YP, et al. Inflammatory pseudotumor of the liver: 13 cases of MRI findings. World J Gastroenterol 2001; 7:422–424.

12. Kelekis NL, Semelka RC, Siegelman ES, et al. Focal hepatic lymphoma: magnetic resonance demonstration using current techniques including gadolinium enhancement. Magn Reson Imaging 1997; 15:625–636.

13. Van Beers B, Roche A, Mathieu D, et al. Epithelioid hemangioendothelioma of the liver: MR and CT findings. J Comput Assist Tomogr 1992; 16:420–424.

14. Powers C, Ros PR, Stoupis C, et al. Primary liver neoplasms: MR imaging with pathologic correlation. Radiographics 1994; 14:459–482.

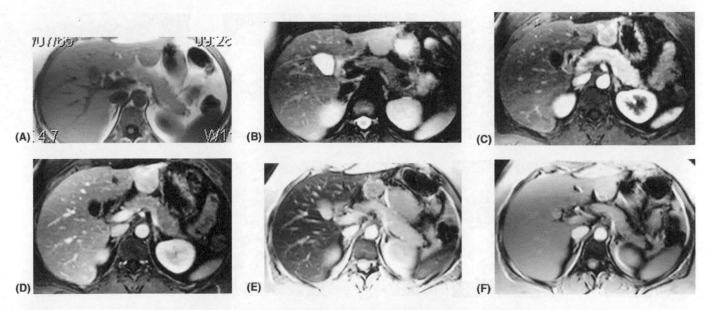

Figure 1. *Typical FNH:* A 3 cm-mass in the left lobe was detected incidentally on sonography. The lesion was isointense with adjacent liver on unenhanced T1w (**A**) and T2w (**B**) images. Post-Gd arterial phase T1w image (**C**) showed an intense blush which faded considerably by the venous phase (**D**), although remaining hyperintense. On post-SPIO T2w images, the lesion was hyperintense to surrounding liver (**E**); in order to find the degree of uptake of SPIO by the lesion, measurements of signal intensity loss in liver and lesion were made using an identical GRE sequence before (**F**) and after SPIO (**E**). The signal of liver fell by 82% while the signal of the lesion fell by 75%, confirming its benign hepatocellular nature.

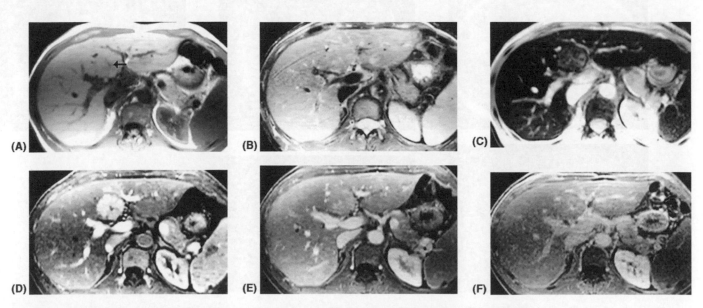

Figure 2. *Typical FNH:* A 3.5-cm lesion in segment 4 was isointense with liver on T1w and T2w images (**A**, **B**) with a faintly visible small central scar[arrow in (**A**)]. The lesion took up almost as much SPIO (PSIL of 48%) as the adjacent liver, becoming only mildly hyperintense on the post-SPIO T2w image (**C**). Post-Gd arterial phase, venous phase and delayed T1w images (**D**, **E**, **F**) showed typical intense transient enhancement in the arterial phase, the lesion becoming isointense later. The central scar remained unenhanced in the arterial phase, but became hyperintense compared with the rest of the lesion on the delayed image.

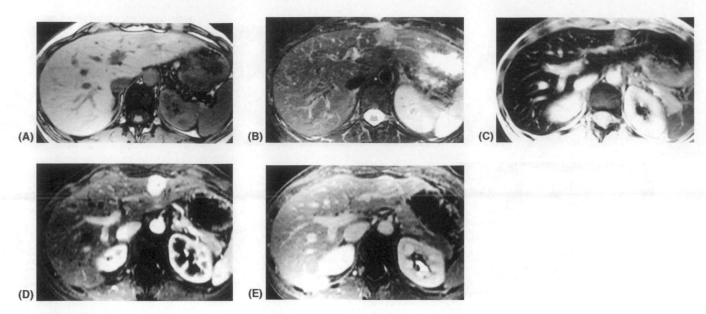

Figure 3. *Typical FNH:* A 2-cm lesion on the anterior aspect of the left lobe was minimally hypointense on T1w (**A**) and mildly hyperintense on T2w images (**B**). The lesion showed over 30% signal loss after SPIO (**C**). Post-Gd arterial and delayed T1w images (**D, E**) showed intense transient enhancement. A tiny central scar was visible (**C, D**).

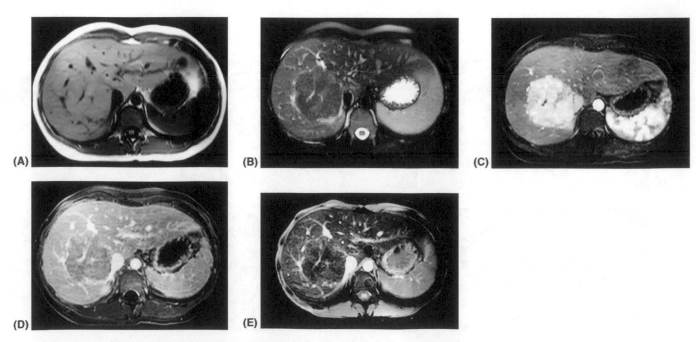

Figure 4. *Typical FNH:* Unenhanced T1w and HASTE images (**A, B**) showed a mass in the right lobe which was largely isointense with adjacent liver but contained a central linear scar which was hyperintense on T2w and hypointense on T1w images. Post-Gd T1w images in arterial and delayed phases (**C, D**) showed intense but heterogeneous arterial enhancement with prominent vessels around the periphery of the mass, and late enhancement of the central scar. Post-SPIO T2w imaging (**E**) showed the lesion to remain isointense with liver, with prominence of the unenhanced central scar.

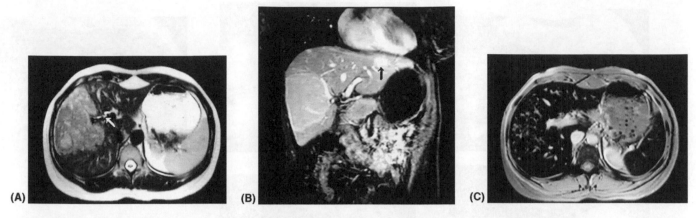

Figure 5. *FNH with telangiectatic histology:* T2w imaging (**A**) showed a large mass with heterogeneous hyperintensity. Post-Gd T1w coronal image (**B**) showed the lesion to be hypervascular; note a second hypervascular lesion in segment 2 (arrow). The post-SPIO T2w image (**C**) showed marked contrast uptake by the lesion but also a nodular heterogeneity within it. A prominent feeding artery was also visible [arrow in (**A**)].

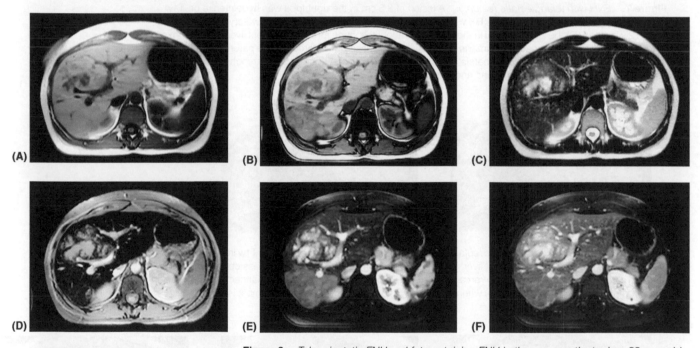

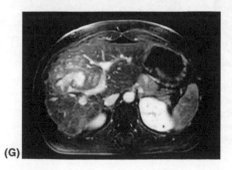

Figure 6. *Telangiectatic FNH and fat-containing FNH in the same patient:* In a 33-year-old female patient with a history of oral contraceptive usage, in-phase T1w imaging (**A**) showed an isointense lesion replacing the posterior aspect of the right lobe, with a second heterogeneous lesion centered in segment 4. The opposed-phase T1w image (**B**) showed both lesions to be hypointense compared with surrounding liver indicating the presence of fat within them. The posterior lesion was isointense on FSE T2w imaging (**C**), while the segment 4 lesion showed mixed hyperintensity. Post-SPIO T2w images (**D**) showed uniform contrast uptake in the posterior lesion, patchy uptake in the segment 4 lesion. Post-Gd T1w images in arterial, venous and delayed phases (**E**, **F**, **G**) showed the posterior lesion to be hyperintense only during the arterial phase, becoming isointense in the later phases. The segment 4 lesion showed more marked early enhancement in the areas which were hyperintense on T2w images, and this intensity persisted in the delayed images, in keeping with the vascular components of the lesion. The peripheral part of the segment 4 lesion showed similar transient hypointense enhancement to that of the more posterior lesion. Diagnosis: (1) a fat-containing but otherwise typical FNH in segment 6, (2) a telangiectatic FNH centered in segment 4; both confirmed on histology of the resected specimen.

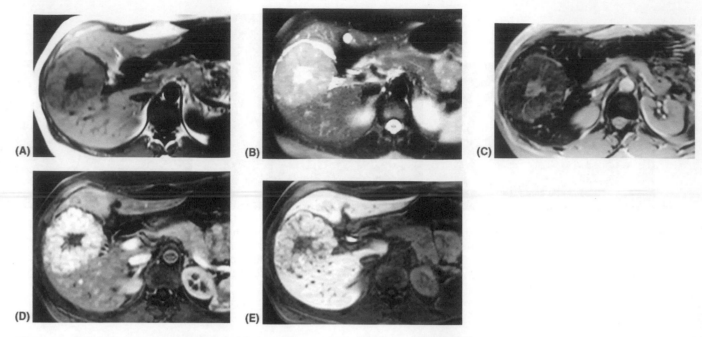

Figure 7. *FNH with telangiectatic features:* A lesion of 8.5 cm in the right lobe was hypointense on T1w (**A**) and hyperintense on T2w images (**B**), with internal septation and a central area of watery signal. On post-SPIO T2w images (**C**) the loss of signal in the lesion was about the same as in the adjacent liver. After gadoxetic acid contrast, the arterial phase T1w image (**D**) showed an intense but heterogeneous parenchymal blush, while the delayed image (**E**) showed persistent retention of the contrast agent in the parenchyma of the lesion and in the adjacent liver. The septations and central area never enhanced.

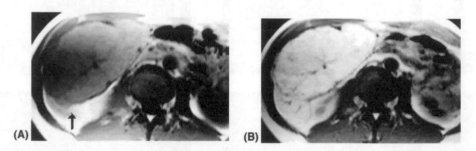

Figure 8. *Large FNH:* A 9-cm mass replaced the inferior part of the right lobe and on T1w images was mildly hypointense to the remaining adjacent liver, just visible posteriorly [arrow in (**A**)]. The mass contained a central scar with a few irregular septa. These remained visible within diffuse parenchymal enhancement in the lesion on post-mangafodipir T1w images (**B**) when both lesion and adjacent liver became almost isointense with adjacent fat.

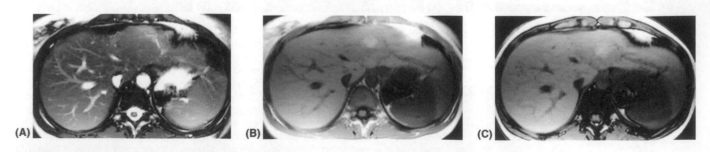

Figure 9. *Multiple FNH:* A 6-cm lesion in the left lobe was isointense with adjacent liver on true FISP (**A**), in-phase and opposed-phase T1w (**B**, **C**) and T2w (**D**) images, but was detectable by its mass effect. The lesion showed considerable uptake of SPIO, although less than adjacent liver (**E**). On the arterial phase post-Gd T1w images (**F**) the lesion showed intense, fairly homogeneous enhancement with a hint of a central scar and a second lesion of about 1 cm was shown in the lateral aspect of the left lobe (arrow). Both lesions became isointense with liver on venous phase T1w images (**G**). (*Continued*)

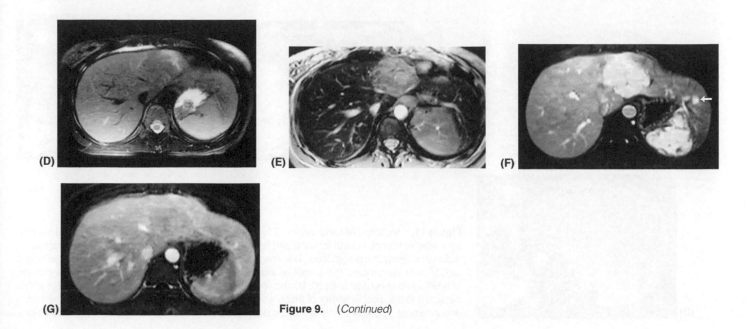

Figure 9.   (*Continued*)

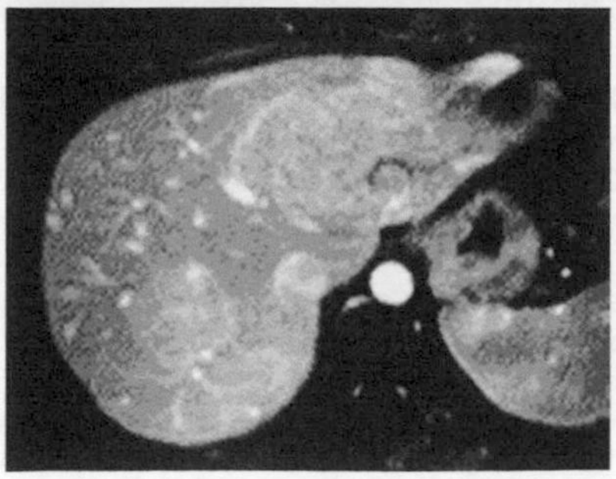

Figure 10.   *Multiple FNH:*   A 7-cm mass in the left lobe and a 4 cm mass in the right lobe were mildly hypointense on T1w (**A**) and hyperintense on T2w (**B**) images. Both lesions showed considerable uptake of SPIO contrast, although remaining hyperintense to adjacent liver (**C**). Both lesions showed heterogeneous but intense enhancement in the post-Gd arterial phase T1w images (**D**) which faded rapidly to become isointense in the venous phase (**E**).

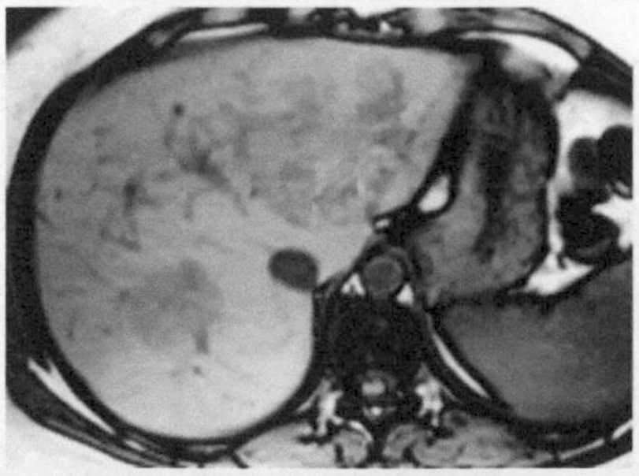

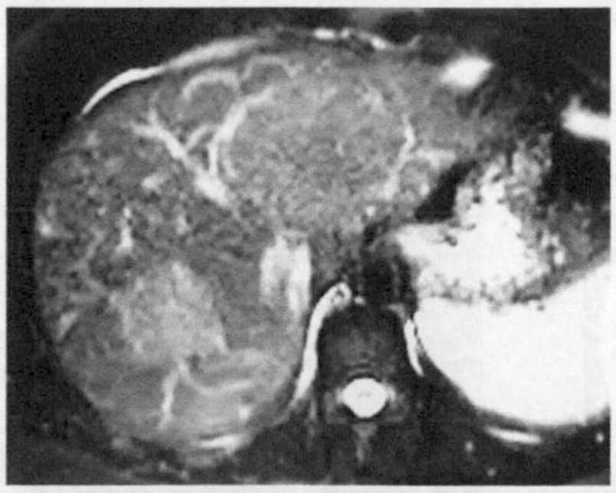

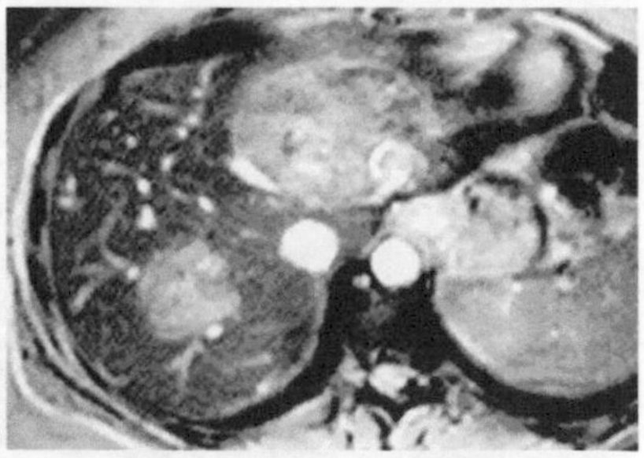

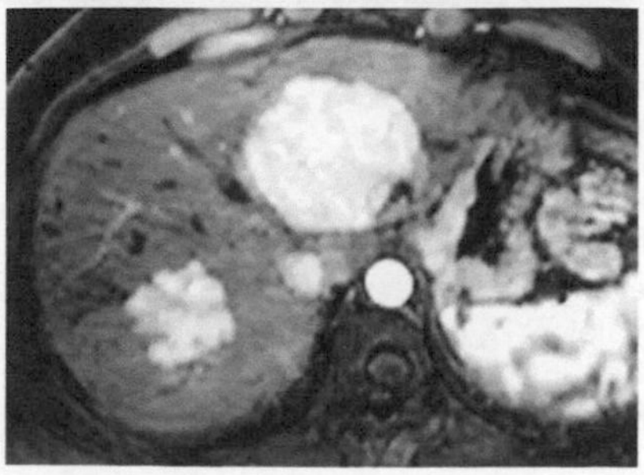

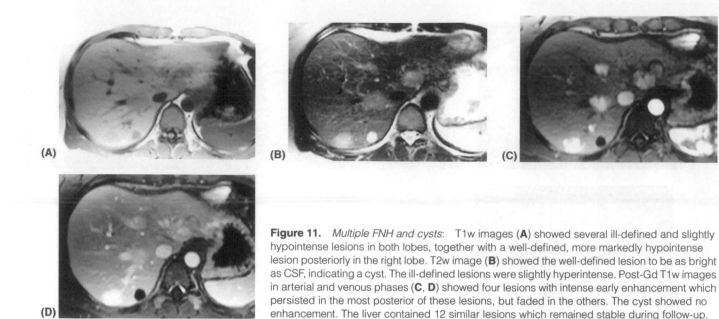

Figure 11.   *Multiple FNH and cysts:*   T1w images (**A**) showed several ill-defined and slightly hypointense lesions in both lobes, together with a well-defined, more markedly hypointense lesion posteriorly in the right lobe. T2w image (**B**) showed the well-defined lesion to be as bright as CSF, indicating a cyst. The ill-defined lesions were slightly hyperintense. Post-Gd T1w images in arterial and venous phases (**C**, **D**) showed four lesions with intense early enhancement which persisted in the most posterior of these lesions, but faded in the others. The cyst showed no enhancement. The liver contained 12 similar lesions which remained stable during follow-up.

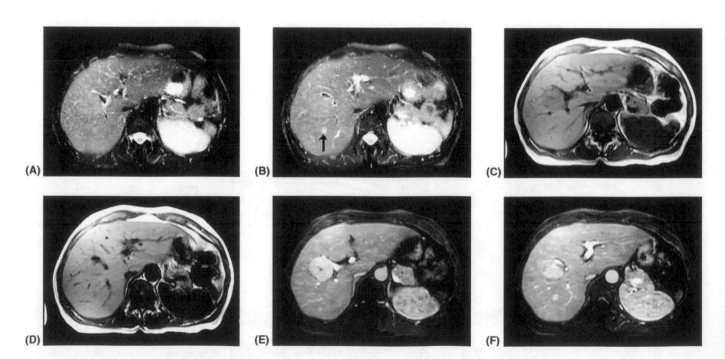

Figure 12.   *Multiple FNH with varying signal characteristics:*   Heavily T2w images (**A**, **B**) showed a moderately hyperintense 1 cm lesion in segment 7 (arrow), together with a 4 cm lesion close to the porta hepatis which was only faintly visible (**A**, **B**). On T1w images (**C**, **D**) the lesions were both marginally hypointense. Post-Gd T1w images showed a vivid arterial enhancement in both lesions (**E**, **F**) fading on delayed images (**G**, **H**) which also showed enhancement in the central scar of the larger lesion. On subsequent post-SPIO T2w images (**I**, **J**) the smaller lesion (arrow) demonstrated a signal intensity loss greater than background liver. The larger lesion showed a PSIL of over 30% but became more conspicuous due to a greater PSIL of approximately 80% in the background liver. For reasons which are not clear, small FNHs often have a particular avidity for SPIO accumulation. The appearance of the smaller lesion in this patient could not be characterized without post-SPIO imaging. (*Continued*)

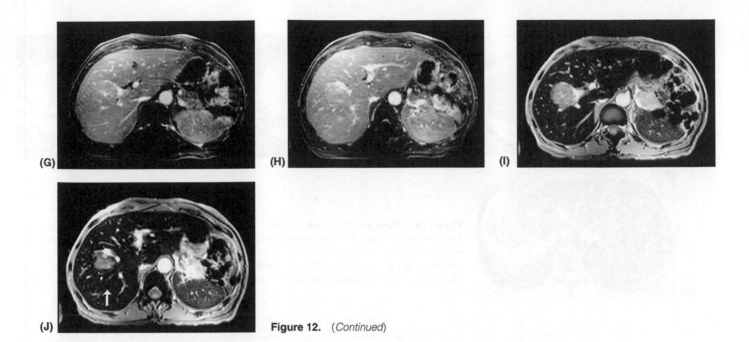

Figure 12. (*Continued*)

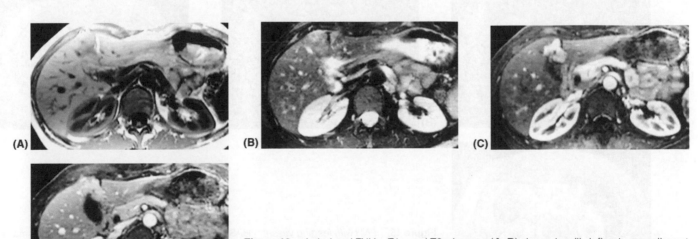

Figure 13. *Lobulated FNH:* T1w and T2w images (**A**, **B**) showed an ill-defined area adjacent to the falciform ligament which was slightly hypointense on T1w and hyperintense on T2w imaging. Post-Gd T1w images showed an intense arterial blush (**C**) and a central non-enhancing scar, with only minimal hyperintensity on the venous phase (**D**).

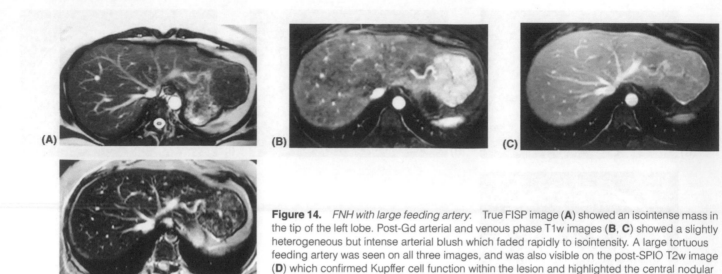

Figure 14. *FNH with large feeding artery:* True FISP image (**A**) showed an isointense mass in the tip of the left lobe. Post-Gd arterial and venous phase T1w images (**B**, **C**) showed a slightly heterogeneous but intense arterial blush which faded rapidly to isointensity. A large tortuous feeding artery was seen on all three images, and was also visible on the post-SPIO T2w image (**D**) which confirmed Kupffer cell function within the lesion and highlighted the central nodular scar.

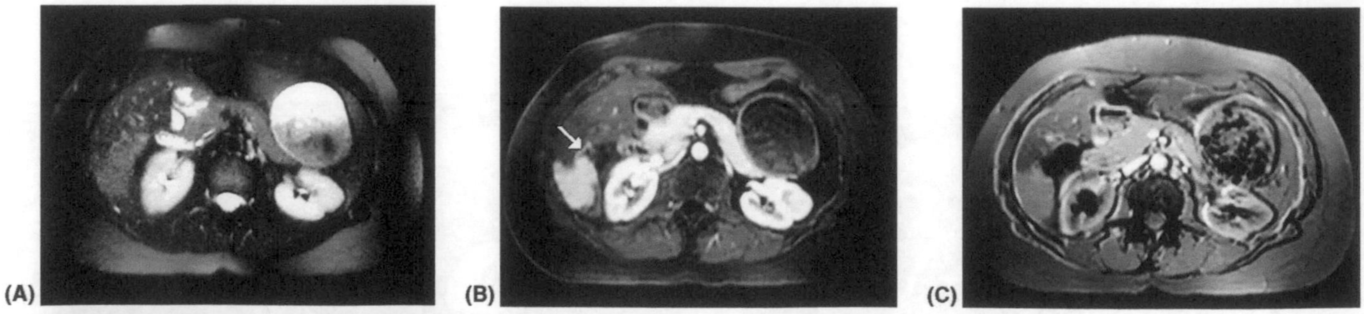

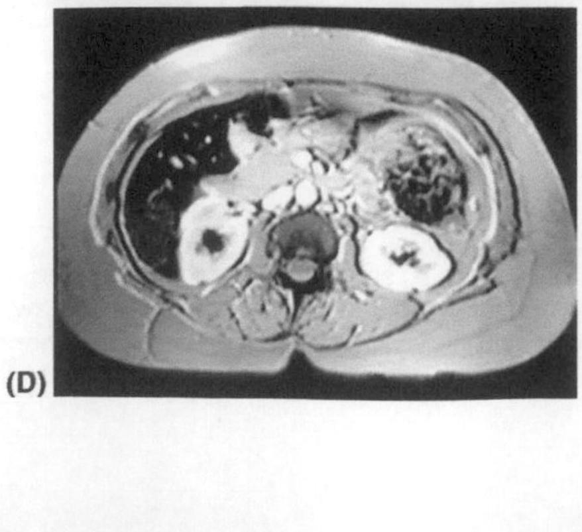

Figure 15. *FNH with feeding vessel:* HASTE image (**A**) showed an almost isointense mass in the posterior aspect of the right lobe. Post-Gd arterial phase T1w image (**B**) showed the mass to be hypervascular with a dominant feeding artery (arrow). From the pre- and post-SPIO T2w images (**C**, **D**) it was apparent the lesion took up as much SPIO contrast as the adjacent liver parenchyma.

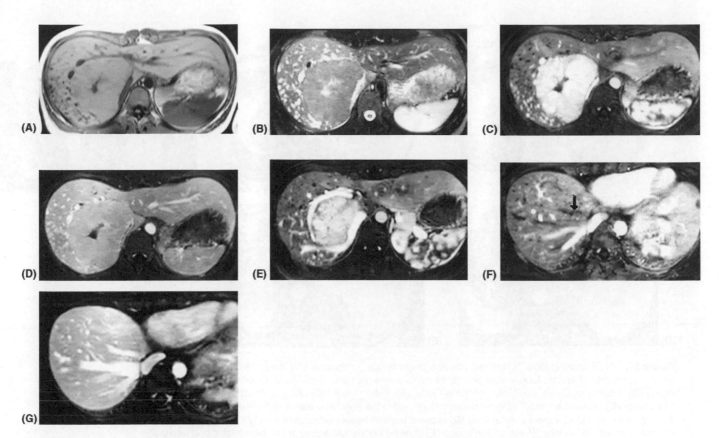

Figure 16. *FNH with arterio-venous shunting*:   Unenhanced T1w and T2w images (**A**, **B**) showed a large lesion which remained isointense with adjacent liver parenchyma but contained a well-defined central scar, hypointense on T1w and hyperintense on T2w images. Large vessels were visibly stretched around the periphery of the lesion. Arterial and venous post-Gd T1w images (**C**, **D**) showed an intense parenchymal blush in the arterial phase, fading rapidly to isointensity, but no enhancement of the central scar. Arterial phase image at a more caudal position (**E**) showed early filling of large veins around the periphery of the lesion. Arterial phase image (**F**) at a more cranial level than (**C**) and (**D**) showed early contrast enhancement of the right hepatic vein at a time when the middle hepatic vein (arrow) remained unenhanced. A venous phase image (**G**) immediately cranial to (**F**) showed a distended right hepatic vein. While the arterial supply of FNH is typically through a central vessel, venous drainage is less well-established, but abnormally large veins are sometimes visible at the periphery of the lesion.

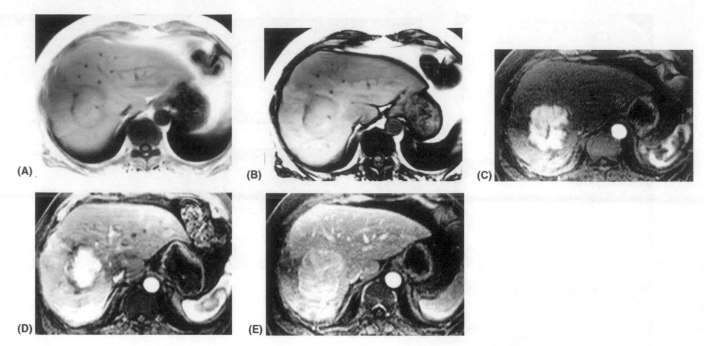

Figure 17. *FNH causing lobar hypo-perfusion and fatty change*: In-phase T1w image (**A**) showed an isointense lesion in the right lobe visible only by its hypointense rim (pseudocapsule). Opposed-phase T1w image (**B**) showed relative hypointensity of the left lobe suggesting lobar fatty change. Arterial phase post-Gd T1w image (**C**) showed a typical intense vascular blush within the FNH, and also a well-defined central scar. Arterial phase image at a more caudal level (**D**) showed marked hyper-perfusion of the right lobe with normal arterialization of the left lobe. Portal phase image (**E**) showed normal enhancement of the left lobe and rather patchy residual enhancement of the periphery of the right lobe. Appearances are explained by compression of the right main portal vein branch by the FNH causing increased arterialization of the right lobe. Because of its reduced portal flow, the right lobe was protected from the fatty infiltration which has occurred in the left lobe. The central scar enhancement (**E**) is typical of FNH, but the capsular enhancement (**E**) is an unusual feature. Biopsy showed the presence of portal tracts, confirming FNH rather than adenoma.

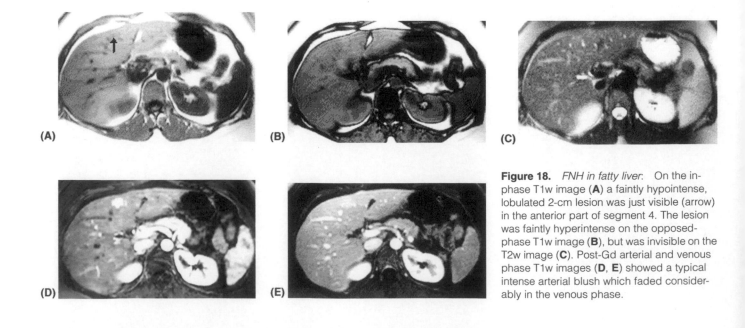

Figure 18. *FNH in fatty liver*: On the in-phase T1w image (**A**) a faintly hypointense, lobulated 2-cm lesion was just visible (arrow) in the anterior part of segment 4. The lesion was faintly hyperintense on the opposed-phase T1w image (**B**), but was invisible on the T2w image (**C**). Post-Gd arterial and venous phase T1w images (**D, E**) showed a typical intense arterial blush which faded considerably in the venous phase.

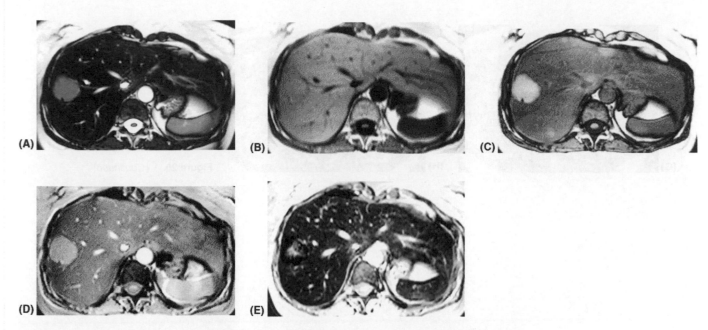

Figure 19. *FNH in fatty liver:* The true FISP image (**A**) showed a rounded 3-cm mass in the lateral part of the right lobe which was hyperintense to the adjacent liver. The liver signal intensity was less than normal owing to diffuse fatty change. On the in-phase T1w image (**B**), the lesion was isointense with the liver but it appeared markedly hyperintense on the opposed-phase T1w image (**C**) which also showed several other areas of relative hyperintensity, indicating focal fatty sparing. GRE T2w image (**D**) again showed the lesion to be hyperintense, but the same sequence obtained after SPIO (**E**) showed the lesion had taken up even more contrast than the normal liver parenchyma so the periphery of the lesion then appeared blacker than the adjacent liver. The central scar in the lesion only became visible after SPIO.

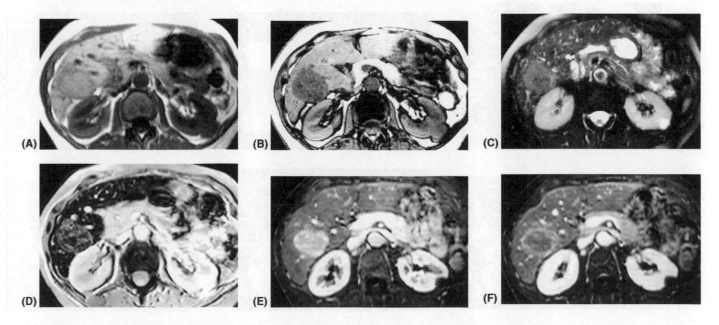

Figure 20. *Evolution of FNH containing fat:* On the in-phase T1w image (**A**) a lesion in segment 5 was almost isointense with adjacent liver. On the opposed-phase T1w image (**B**), the lesion was markedly hypointense, even though the liver signal was diffusely reduced by fatty change to be almost isointense with the renal parenchyma. On the T2w image (**C**), the lesion was slightly hyperintense to liver and on the post-SPIO T2w image (**D**) both lesion and liver showed an equal diminution of signal. Post-Gd T1w images showed a well-defined arterial blush (**E**), fading rapidly to isointensity in the venous phase (**F**). Note the low signal intensity of the liver parenchyma in the post-Gd T1w images, resulting from severe fatty change—the TE of the dynamic sequence approximates to opposed-phase. Further in-phase and opposed-phase images (**G**, **H**) obtained six months later show that the fatty change within both liver and lesion had resolved, and the lesion then appeared minimally hypointense on both in-phase and opposed-phase T1w images. (*Continued*)

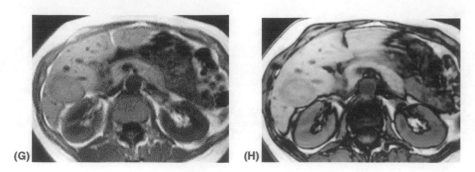

Figure 20. (*Continued*)

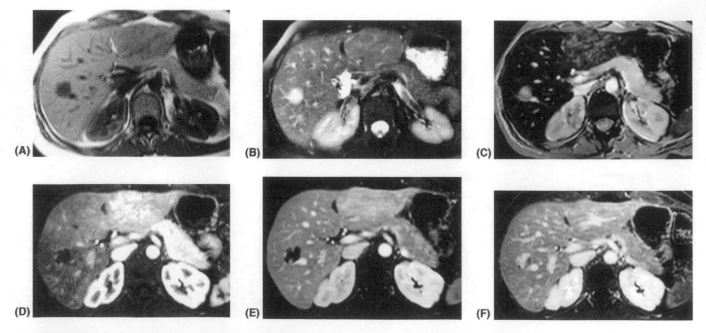

Figure 21. *FNH and hemangioma*: The unenhanced T1w image (**A**) showed a well-defined and markedly hypointense lesion in the right lobe, and the impression of an isointense mass expanding the lateral segments of the left lobe. The T2w image (**B**) showed the right lobe lesion to be markedly hyperintense, while the mass in the left lobe was isointense. On post-SPIO T2w images (**C**), the left lobe lesion showed considerable contrast uptake, although a little less than the adjacent liver. The right lobe lesion remained hyperintense. Arterial phase and venous phase post-Gd T1w images (**D**, **E**) showed a heterogeneous arterial blush in the left lobe lesion, while the right lobe lesion showed a little nodular enhancement around the periphery. A delayed image (**F**) showed substantial infilling of the right lobe lesion giving the typical appearance of a benign hemangioma. The left lobe lesion was then again isointense apart from a well-defined central scar which showed increased enhancement.

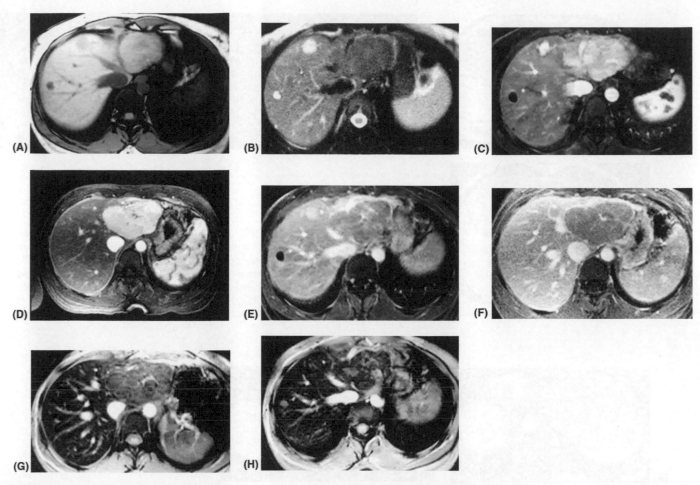

Figure 22.   *Multiple FNH with other benign lesions*:   The unenhanced T1w images (**A**) showed a markedly hypointense lesion of 1.5 cm in the lateral aspect of the right lobe, a 2.5 cm lesion lying anteriorly in segment 4 which was less hypointense, and a 6x8 cm isointense mass replacing segments 2 and 3. The T2w images (**B**) showed the right lobe lesion to be isointense with CSF, the segment 4 lesion to be just a little less hyperintense, and the large left lobe mass to be isointense. Arterial phase post-Gd T1w imaging (**C**) showed no enhancement in the right lobe lesion with an intense blush in the segment 4 lesion and also diffusely increased arterialization of the larger left lobe lesion. A slightly more caudal slice in the arterial phase (**D**) showed more uniform enhancement of the left lobe mass with a non-enhancing central scar, typical of FNH. Venous phase and delayed phase images (**E**, **F**) confirmed no enhancement in the right lobe lesion (cyst), partial washout of the segment 4 lesion (small FNH), and marginal hypointensity of the left lobe lesion apart from increased delayed enhancement of the central scar (large FNH). Post-SPIO T2w images (**G**, **H**) showed contrast uptake in both FNH lesions. The liver contained several further foci of FNH, cysts and hemangiomas at other levels. Follow-up imaging showed no progression in any of the lesions.

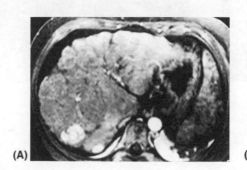

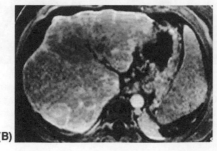

Figure 23.   *FNH in cirrhosis*:   On arterial and venous phase post-Gd T1w images (**A**, **B**) two hypervascular nodules were seen posteriorly in the right lobe of a cirrhotic liver showing macro-nodular change in a 9-year-old boy with cirrhosis following neonatal hepatitis. Biopsies were suggestive of focal nodular hyperplasia and at liver transplantation one year later, the ex-plant showed no evidence of malignancy.

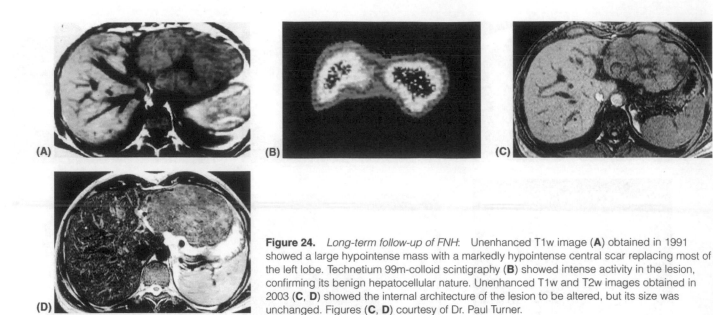

Figure 24. *Long-term follow-up of FNH:* Unenhanced T1w image (**A**) obtained in 1991 showed a large hypointense mass with a markedly hypointense central scar replacing most of the left lobe. Technetium 99m-colloid scintigraphy (**B**) showed intense activity in the lesion, confirming its benign hepatocellular nature. Unenhanced T1w and T2w images obtained in 2003 (**C**, **D**) showed the internal architecture of the lesion to be altered, but its size was unchanged. Figures (**C**, **D**) courtesy of Dr. Paul Turner.

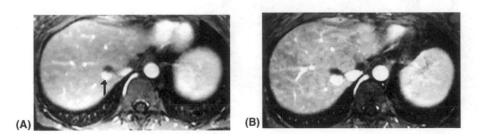

Figure 25. *Enlarging FNH:* In a patient with a history of previous liver resection of FNH, a post-Gd arterial phase T1w image (**A**) showed a 12 mm lesion (arrow) immediately posterior to the right hepatic vein and lateral to the IVC. The same sequence repeated 17 months later (**B**) shows the lesion has enlarged, measuring 17 mm. Several new sub-cm lesions also appeared during the period of surveillance. Only a small minority of FNH lesions enlarge over time—a few regress but most lesions remain unchanged.

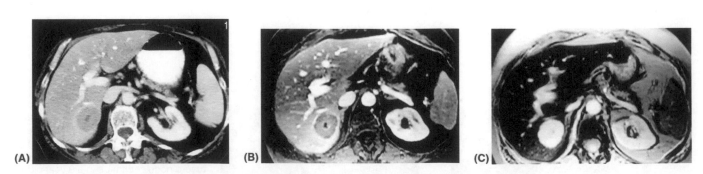

Figure 26. *FNH vs. metastasis:* Venous phase CT (**A**) showed a lesion which was almost iso-attenuating, with a hypo-attenuating central scar. Post-Gd early venous phase T1w image (**B**) showed the lesion to be hypoenhancing, with a vascular rim and a non-enhancing central scar. Post-SPIO T2w image (**C**) showed the lesion to have no uptake of contrast, indicating its non-hepatocellular nature. Histology—neuroendocrine metastasis.

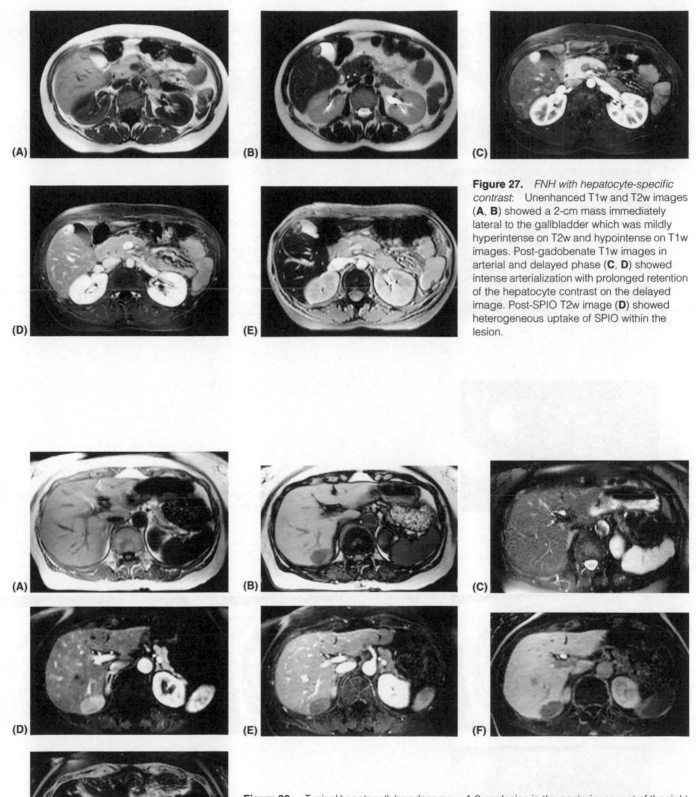

Figure 27. *FNH with hepatocyte-specific contrast*: Unenhanced T1w and T2w images (**A**, **B**) showed a 2-cm mass immediately lateral to the gallbladder which was mildly hyperintense on T2w and hypointense on T1w images. Post-gadobenate T1w images in arterial and delayed phase (**C**, **D**) showed intense arterialization with prolonged retention of the hepatocyte contrast on the delayed image. Post-SPIO T2w image (**D**) showed heterogeneous uptake of SPIO within the lesion.

Figure 28. *Typical hepatocellular adenoma*: A 3-cm lesion in the posterior aspect of the right lobe was almost invisible on the in-phase T1w image (**A**) but owing to its fat content, the lesion was hypointense on the opposed-phase T1w image (**B**). The lesion was isointense on HASTE T2w imaging (**C**). Post-gadobenate T1w images showed an early arterial blush (**D**) which faded rapidly in the venous phase (**E**). The lesion remained hypointense on the 60-minute delayed T1w image (**F**) but the post-SPIO T2w image (**G**) showed uptake of contrast in the lesion, confirming its hepatocellular nature.

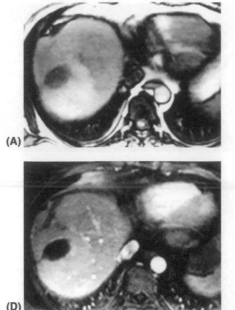

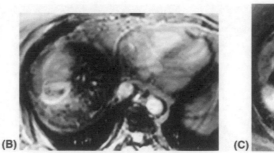

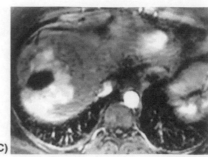

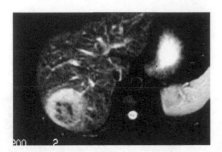

Figure 29. *Adenoma with hemorrhage:* In a female patient aged 40, a 9-cm lesion in the right lobe showed a lobulated outline and was hyperintense on the T1w image (**A**) with a central area of marked hypointensity corresponding to previous hemorrhage. On the T2w image (**B**), the lesion was mildly hyperintense with the haemorrhagic area showing a rim of marked hyperintensity fluid surrounding a central isointense solid hematoma. Post-Gd arterial and venous phase T1w images (**C**, **D**) showed marked arterial enhancement which faded to become isointense in the venous phase. The hematoma showed no enhancement. Note also a small area of sub-capsular hematoma over the surface of segment 8. On post-SPIO T2w images (not illustrated) the lesion showed some signal loss, but less than normal liver.

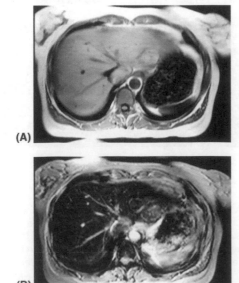

Figure 30. *Adenoma with recent hemorrhage:* T2w imaging showed a hyperintense lesion with nodular hypointensity resulting from hemorrhage into an adenoma.

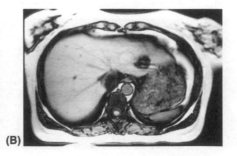

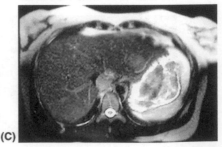

Figure 31. *Multiple adenomas:* Two lesions each of about 3 cm size were faintly visible in segments 1 and 2 on the in-phase T1w image (**A**) but were markedly hypointense on the opposed phase T1w image (**B**) indicating considerable fat content. The lesions were only faintly hyperintense on T2w images (**C**) but showed considerable uptake of SPIO contrast (**D**). Post-Gd T1w images (**E**, **F**) showed a heterogeneous arterial phase blush in both lesions which faded fairly rapidly so the lesions became hypointense in the venous phase. (*Continued*)

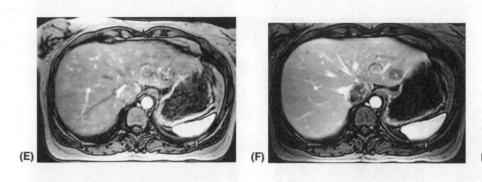

(E)   (F)   **Figure 31.**   (*Continued*)

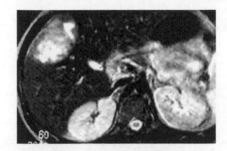

Figure 32.   *Multiple adenomas in glycogen storage disease*:   T2w imaging showed a heterogeneous hyperintense lesion subsequently confirmed as adenoma with hemorrhage. At other levels, smaller non-haemorrhagic lesions were present.

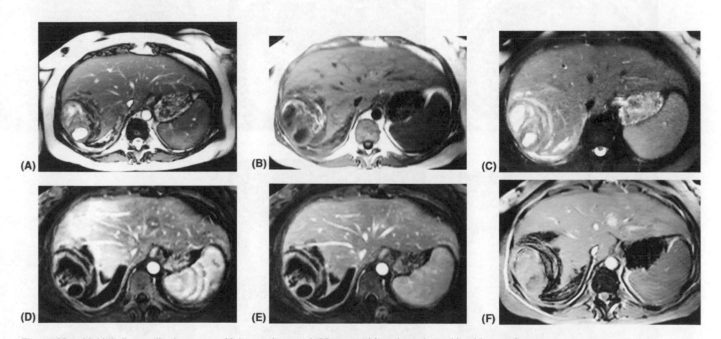

(A)   (B)   (C)

(D)   (E)   (F)

Figure 33.   *Multiple liver cell adenomas with hemorrhage*:   A 30-year-old female patient with a history of oral contraceptive usage presented with signs of acute intra-abdominal bleeding and right upper quadrant pain. True FISP imaging (**A**) showed a heterogeneous 8 cm mass posteriorly in the right lobe. On T1w and T2w images, (**B**, **C**), areas of liquefaction were shown together with elements of solid tissue which were almost isointense with liver, and areas of fresh hemorrhage indicated by hyperintensity on T1w images. Post-Gd T1w images showed marked arterial phase enhancement (**D**) in the residual solid components of the lesion, but also showed areas of arterial blush in the medial part of segment 7, and in segments 8 and 4, all of which were isointense on the unenhanced images. The venous phase image (**E**) showed the enhancement had faded to isointensity. GRE T2w images before and after SPIO (**F**, **G**) showed the lesions in segment 4 and 8 had taken up as much contrast as the normal left lobe. RAO coronal post-Gd T1w image (**H**) showed the extensive sub-hepatic and intraperitoneal hemorrhage arising from capsular rupture adjacent to the right lobe lesion. Note also the flask-shaped common bile duct, with an asymptomatic type 1 choledochal cyst. Resection histology showed numerous adenomas, the largest in segment 7, with extensive hemorrhage. (*Continued*)

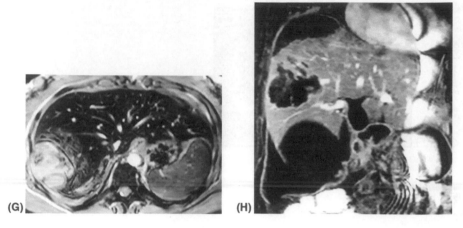

(G)   (H)   **Figure 33.**   (*Continued*)

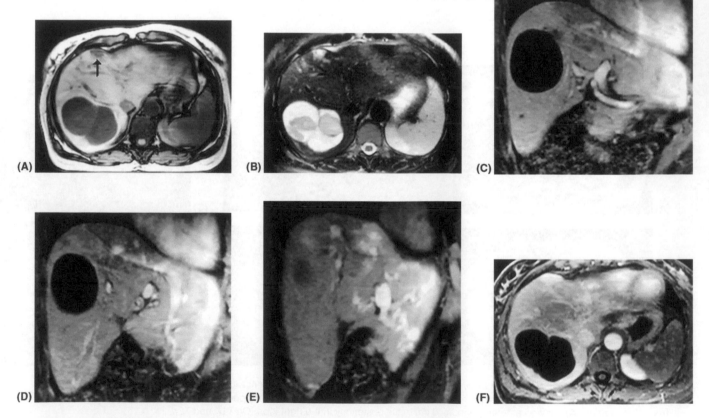

(A)   (B)   (C)

(D)   (E)   (F)

Figure 34.   *Liver adenomatosis with cystic degeneration*:   A female patient aged 48 presented with a cystic mass in the liver 5 years after an acute episode of right upper quadrant pain. The T1w image (**A**) showed a bi-loculated cystic area in segment 7, a small hypointense lesion on the anterior aspect of segment 4, and several prominent vascular channels. The T2w image (**B**) showed the bi-locular cyst containing solid elements in segment 7, the segment 4 lesion was hyperintense and the remainder of the liver slightly heterogeneous. Coronal post-Gd T1w images in the arterial phase (**C**, **D**, **E**) showed that although the cystic lesion was avascular, there were several small nodular areas of bright arterial enhancement elsewhere in the liver, together with enlarged and tortuous vascular channels involving both hepatic and portal veins. Axial venous phase image (**F**) showed persistent enhancement in the segment 4 lesion and around the periphery of the cystic area. Resection histology confirmed multiple adenomas with cystic degeneration.

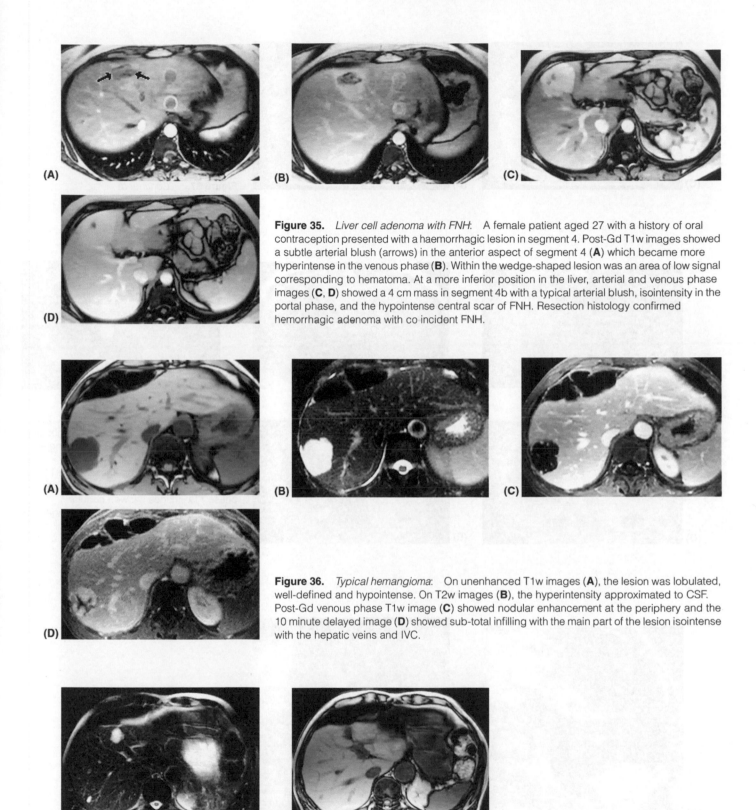

Figure 35.   *Liver cell adenoma with FNH:*   A female patient aged 27 with a history of oral contraception presented with a haemorrhagic lesion in segment 4. Post-Gd T1w images showed a subtle arterial blush (arrows) in the anterior aspect of segment 4 (**A**) which became more hyperintense in the venous phase (**B**). Within the wedge-shaped lesion was an area of low signal corresponding to hematoma. At a more inferior position in the liver, arterial and venous phase images (**C**, **D**) showed a 4 cm mass in segment 4b with a typical arterial blush, isointensity in the portal phase, and the hypointense central scar of FNH. Resection histology confirmed hemorrhagic adenoma with co-incident FNH.

Figure 36.   *Typical hemangioma:*   On unenhanced T1w images (**A**), the lesion was lobulated, well-defined and hypointense. On T2w images (**B**), the hyperintensity approximated to CSF. Post-Gd venous phase T1w image (**C**) showed nodular enhancement at the periphery and the 10 minute delayed image (**D**) showed sub-total infilling with the main part of the lesion isointense with the hepatic veins and IVC.

Figure 37.   *Typical hemangiomas:*   T2w image (**A**) showed a 2 cm lesion lying anteriorly in segment 8, and a sub-cm lesion in segment 7 with similar hyperintensity. On unenhanced T1w images (**B**) both lesions showed similar hypointensity. Arterial phase image post-Gd T1w images (**C**) showed peripheral nodular enhancement in both lesions while the delayed image (**D**) showed complete homogeneous enhancement of both lesions. (*Continued*)

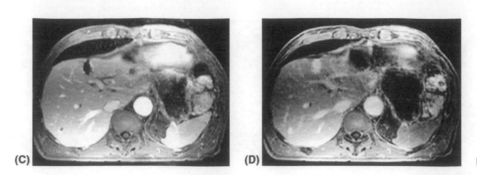

Figure 37.   (*Continued*)

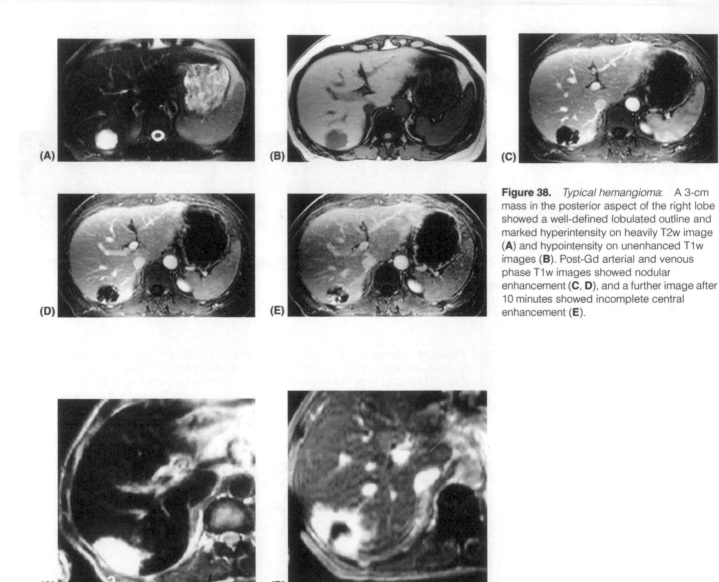

Figure 38.   *Typical hemangioma*:   A 3-cm mass in the posterior aspect of the right lobe showed a well-defined lobulated outline and marked hyperintensity on heavily T2w image (**A**) and hypointensity on unenhanced T1w images (**B**). Post-Gd arterial and venous phase T1w images showed nodular enhancement (**C**, **D**), and a further image after 10 minutes showed incomplete central enhancement (**E**).

Figure 39.   *Typical hemangioma with angiographic correlation*:   Heavily T2w image (**A**) showed a markedly hyperintense lesion in the posterior aspect of the right lobe. Delayed post-Gd T1w image (**B**) showed homogeneous enhancement of most of the lesion with a central unenhanced area. Arterial phase and venous phase angiography (**C**, **D**) showed the characteristic perfusion pattern with prominent tortuous arteries supplying the hypervascular periphery of the lesion which showed a persistent parenchymal blush after contrast had cleared from the adjacent liver parenchyma. (*Continued*)

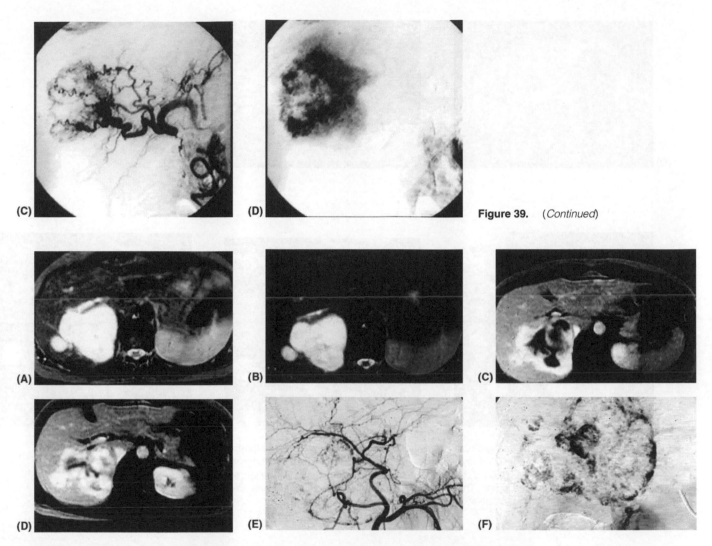

Figure 40. *Hemangioma with angiographic correlation:* The lobulated lesion in the right lobe showed high signal on T2w imaging with TE of 90m sec (**A**) which was only slightly less when the TE was increased to 180m sec (**B**). Post-Gd T1w images in venous and delayed phases (**C, D**) showed centripetal enhancement. Arterial and venous phase angiograms (**E, F**) showed typical nodular malformed vessels around the periphery of the lesion with a discontinuous blush in the venous phase.

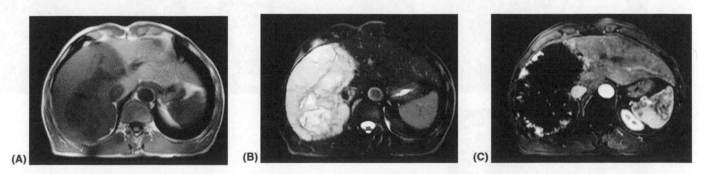

Figure 41. *Giant hemangioma:* Unenhanced T1w (**A**) and heavily T2w (**B**) images showed a well-defined, heterogeneous lesion with complex internal structure replacing most of the right lobe, and with the usual characteristics of hypointensity on T1w and marked hyperintensity on T2w imaging. Post-Gd T1w images in arterial, venous and delayed phases (**C, D, E**) showed typical peripheral nodular enhancement, progressing centripetally. The central area which showed particular hyperintensity on T2w and hypointensity on unenhanced T1w images remained unenhanced at 10 minutes after injection. (*Continued*)

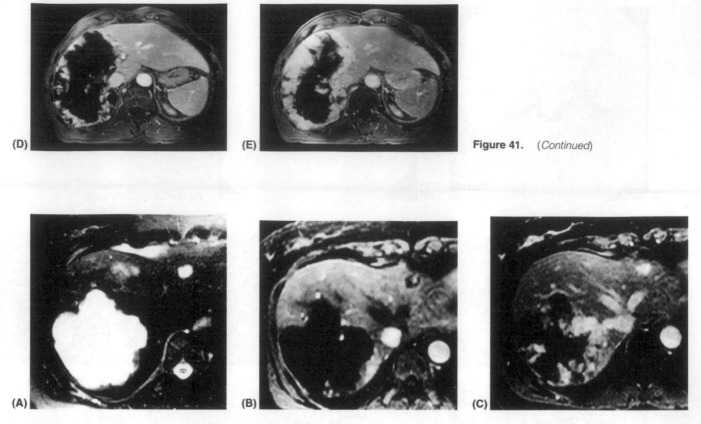

(D)   (E)   **Figure 41.** *(Continued)*

(A)   (B)   (C)

Figure 42. *Giant and typical hemangiomas:* Heavily T2w image (**A**) showed a large lobulated lesion replacing most of segment 7 and a 2-cm hyperintense lesion in the anterior aspect of segment 2. Post-Gd arterial and delayed T1w images (**B, C**) showed peripheral nodular enhancement in the large lesion with some centripetal infilling on the delayed image. The small lesion showed eccentric nodular enhancement on the early image, but filled in completely on the delayed image.

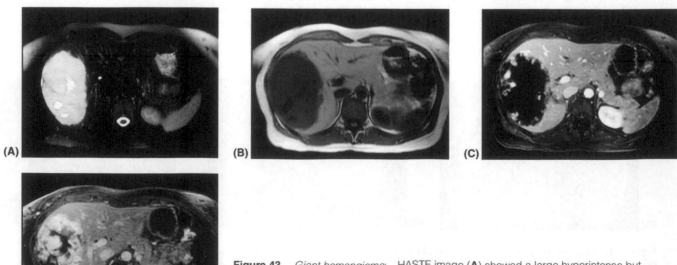

(A)   (B)   (C)

(D)

Figure 43. *Giant hemangioma:* HASTE image (**A**) showed a large hyperintense but heterogeneous lesion occupying much of the right lobe. Unenhanced T1w image (**B**) showed similar heterogeneity within the hypointense lesion. Post-Gd T1w images in venous and delayed phases (**C, D**) showed typical peripheral nodular and discontinuous enhancement followed by centripetal infilling with residual unenhanced scar tissue in the center of the lesion.

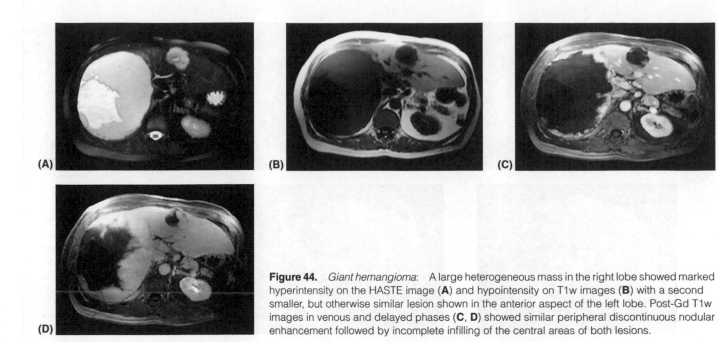

Figure 44. *Giant hemangioma:* A large heterogeneous mass in the right lobe showed marked hyperintensity on the HASTE image (**A**) and hypointensity on T1w images (**B**) with a second smaller, but otherwise similar lesion shown in the anterior aspect of the left lobe. Post-Gd T1w images in venous and delayed phases (**C**, **D**) showed similar peripheral discontinuous nodular enhancement followed by incomplete infilling of the central areas of both lesions.

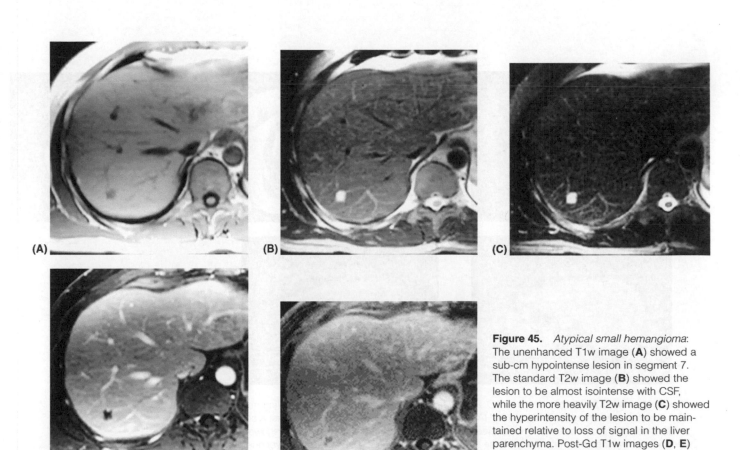

Figure 45. *Atypical small hemangioma:* The unenhanced T1w image (**A**) showed a sub-cm hypointense lesion in segment 7. The standard T2w image (**B**) showed the lesion to be almost isointense with CSF, while the more heavily T2w image (**C**) showed the hyperintensity of the lesion to be maintained relative to loss of signal in the liver parenchyma. Post-Gd T1w images (**D**, **E**) showed peripheral nodular enhancement at first, but no delayed infilling.

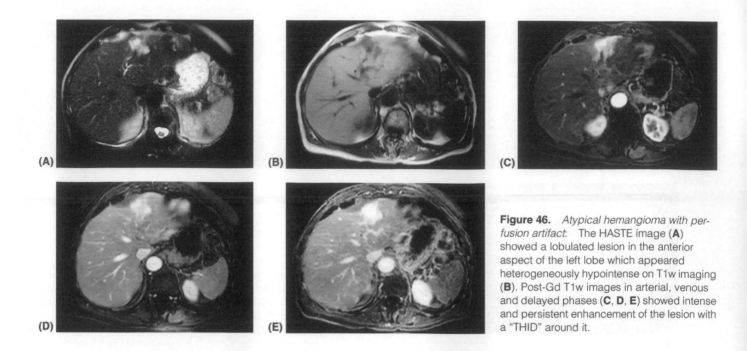

Figure 46. *Atypical hemangioma with perfusion artifact:* The HASTE image (**A**) showed a lobulated lesion in the anterior aspect of the left lobe which appeared heterogeneously hypointense on T1w imaging (**B**). Post-Gd T1w images in arterial, venous and delayed phases (**C**, **D**, **E**) showed intense and persistent enhancement of the lesion with a "THID" around it.

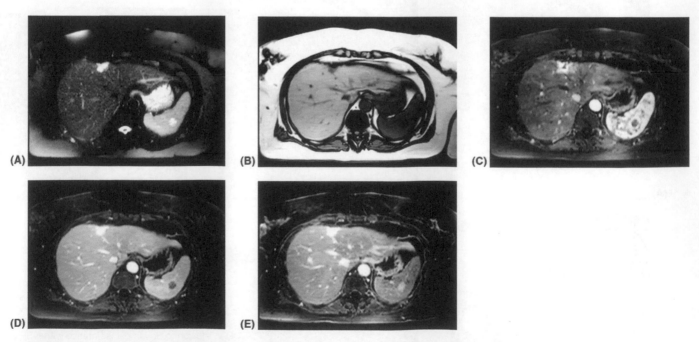

Figure 47. *Small hemangioma with THID and splenic hemangioma:* A small lesion lying anteriorly in the left lobe appeared markedly hyperintense on HASTE (**A**) and hypointense on T1w (**B**) images. A second lesion with similar characteristics was shown in the spleen. On post-Gd T1w images, the liver lesion showed typical nodular peripheral enhancement in the early phase (**C**) with persistent infilling of the lesion on venous phase and delayed images (**D**, **E**). The splenic lesion showed only a faint nodular peripheral enhancement in the venous phase (**D**) with delayed enhancement of the center of the lesion on the final image (**E**).

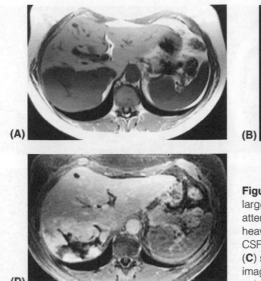 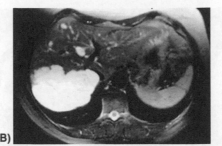 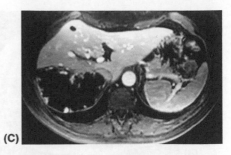

Figure 48. *Large hemangioma and small cyst:* The unenhanced T1w image (**A**) showed a large, well-defined but irregularly-shaped lesion occupying most of segment 7. Note the lower attenuation "scar" centrally, and also the small round lesion in the anterior part of segment 4. A heavily T2w image (**B**) showed both lesions were very hyperintense, approaching the signal of CSF, but the larger lesion showed internal architecture. Early venous phase post-Gd T1w image (**C**) showed nodular peripheral enhancement in the larger lesion and the 10 minute delayed image (**D**) showed incomplete central enhancement. The small segment 4 cyst showed no enhancement.

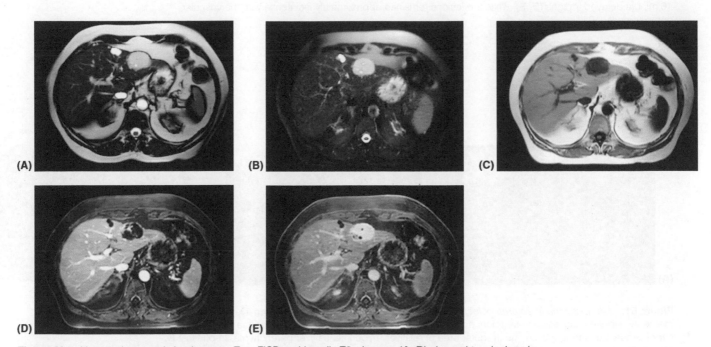

Figure 49. *Hemangioma and simple cyst:* True FISP and heavily T2w images (**A**, **B**) showed two lesions in the anterior aspect of the left lobe; the smaller lesion appeared isointense with CSF, the larger lesion was less hyperintense, with several small foci of higher intensity within it. Both lesions showed hypointensity on unenhanced T1 (**C**). Post-Gd venous phase and delayed phase T1w images (**D**, **E**) showed the smaller lesion does not enhance, while the larger lesion shows nodular enhancement which was mostly peripheral at first, with almost total infilling later. Note that the small internal foci which were particularly hyperintense on T2w imaging failed to enhance, suggesting areas of hyalinization within the lesion.

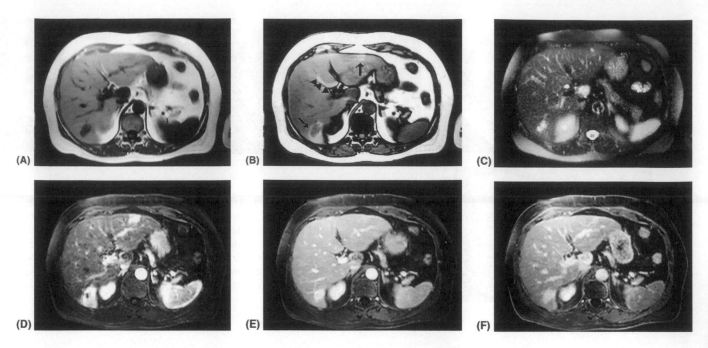

Figure 50. *Fatty liver with two hemangiomas each associated with a THID and focal fatty sparing:* In-phase (**A**) and opposed-phase (**B**) T1w images showed diffuse fatty change with a small linear area of focal sparing on the posterior aspect of segment 4 (arrowheads). There was also a 2 cm lesion in segment 6 (arrow) and a sub-cm lesion in the anterior surface of segment 3 (arrow). Both of these lesions were surrounded by a wedge-shaped area of focal fatty sparing, visible in (**B**). T2w image (**C**) showed fairly well-defined lesions with hyperintense signal, not quite as intense as CSF. Post-Gd arterial phase T1w image (**D**) showed that both of the small lesions were associated with "THIDs"—areas of increased arterial perfusion surrounding the lesions and extending to the liver surface—which faded to isointensity with the liver parenchyma on venous phase and 10 minute delayed images (**E**, **F**), while the lesions remained approximately isointense with the vascular compartment.

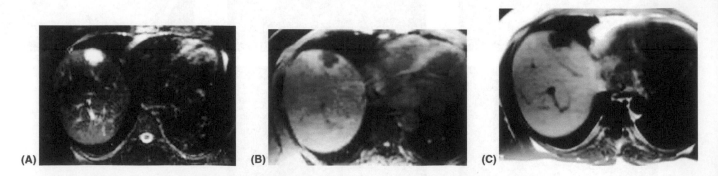

Figure 51. *Hemangioma in an area of focal fatty sparing:* T2w image showed uniform liver signal with a markedly hyperintense lesion in segment 4 (**A**). Opposed-phase T1w image (**B**) showed the lesion to be hypointense, but surrounded by an irregular area of relatively hyperintense liver parenchyma. In-phase T1w image (**C**) showed the hypointense lesion with isointense signal from the adjacent liver parenchyma, confirming that the parenchymal abnormality on the opposed-phase image was caused by focal fatty sparing. Arterial and venous phase post-Gd T1w images (**D**, **E**) showed heterogeneous early enhancement of the lesion with a persistent homogeneous blush on the delayed image (**E**). Note the relatively increased perfusion in the area of focal fatty sparing around the lesion compared with the rest of the liver, which remained relatively hypointense after Gd because the sequence used for dynamic acquisition (VIBE) has a TE which is close to opposed-phase. (*Continued*)

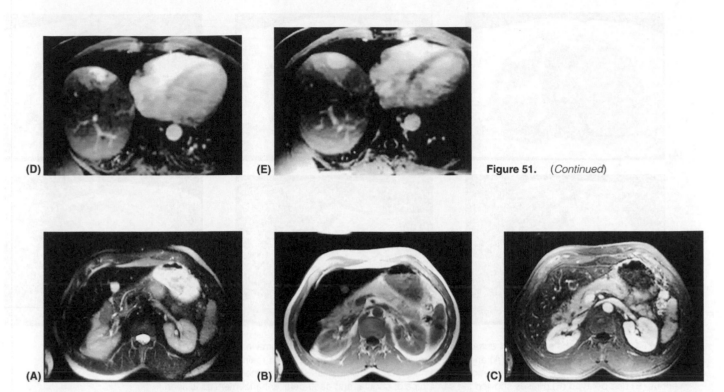

Figure 51. (*Continued*)

Figure 52. *Hemangioma in hemochromatosis*: A T2w image (**A**) showed a well-defined, brightly hyperintense lesion in the posterior aspect of the left lobe. The unenhanced T1w image (**B**) showed the liver parenchyma was severely hypointense compared to normal, so the lesion appears hyperintense. Post-Gd venous phase T1w image (**C**) showed nodular discontinuous enhancement around the periphery of the lesion.

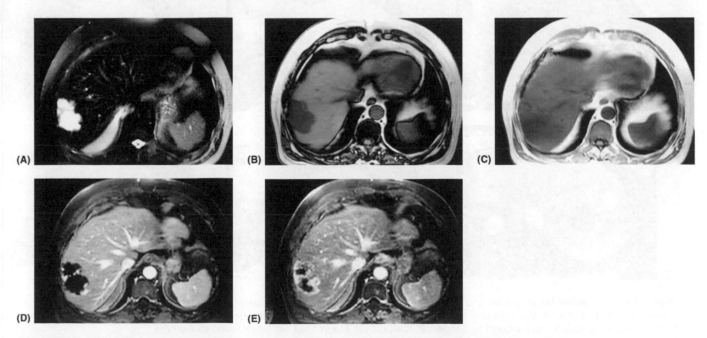

Figure 53. *Hemangioma in hemochromatosis*: The HASTE image (**A**) showed a lobulated hyperintense hemangioma in segment 7 which appeared typically hypointense on opposed-phase T1w images (**B**). However, the lesion was almost invisible on the in-phase T1w image (**C**) because the background liver signal was reduced due to iron deposition. Post-Gd T1w images (**D**, **E**) showed typical peripheral nodular enhancement with subsequent partial infilling of the center of the lesion.

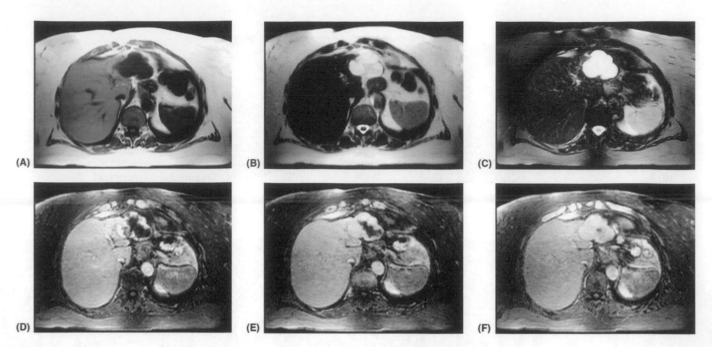

Figure 54.   *Hemangioma showing T1 enhancement with SPIO contrast*:   A hemangioma in the left lobe showed typical hypointensity on T1w (**A**) and hyperintensity on HASTE (**B**) images, and maintained marked hyperintensity on T2w images with TE extended to 180msec (**C**). Dynamic post-SPIO T1w images in arterial (**D**) venous (**E**) and delayed (**F**) phases showed the same type of nodular and centripetal enhancement as is seen with post-Gd imaging.

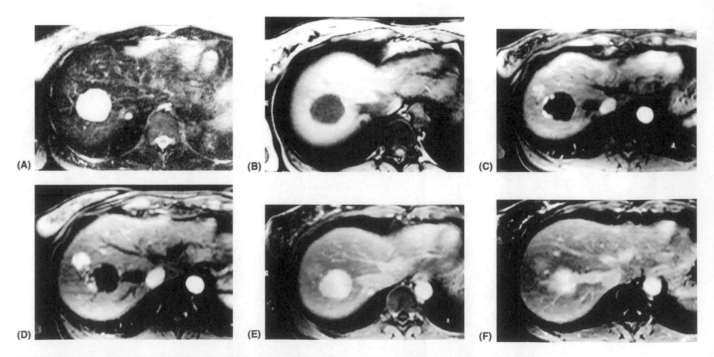

Figure 55.   *Co-existent hemangiomas and FNH*:   In a patient with known colorectal cancer, T2w images (**A**) showed two lesions of 5 cm and 1 cm size, both well-defined and markedly hyperintense. Both lesions were uniformly hypointense on unenhanced T1w images (**B**). On post-Gd T1w images, the larger lesion showed the typical discontinuous, nodular, peripheral enhancement of hemangioma, while the smaller lesion showed no early enhancement (**C**). However, a third hypervascular lesion was seen just antero-lateral to the larger hemangioma, and was better appreciated on the adjacent slice (**D**). Delayed images (**E**, **F**) showed complete uniform enhancement of both hemangiomas, while the more vascular lesion faded almost to isointensity, suggesting FNH. Post-SPIO T2w imaging (not illustrated) confirmed FNH.

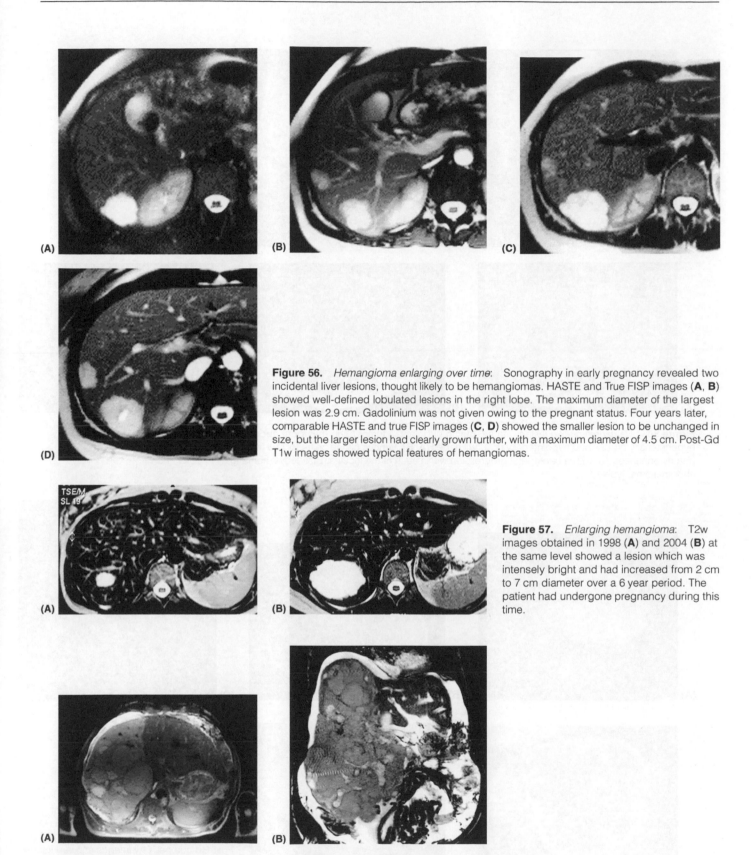

Figure 56. *Hemangioma enlarging over time*: Sonography in early pregnancy revealed two incidental liver lesions, thought likely to be hemangiomas. HASTE and True FISP images (**A**, **B**) showed well-defined lobulated lesions in the right lobe. The maximum diameter of the largest lesion was 2.9 cm. Gadolinium was not given owing to the pregnant status. Four years later, comparable HASTE and true FISP images (**C**, **D**) showed the smaller lesion to be unchanged in size, but the larger lesion had clearly grown further, with a maximum diameter of 4.5 cm. Post-Gd T1w images showed typical features of hemangiomas.

Figure 57. *Enlarging hemangioma*: T2w images obtained in 1998 (**A**) and 2004 (**B**) at the same level showed a lesion which was intensely bright and had increased from 2 cm to 7 cm diameter over a 6 year period. The patient had undergone pregnancy during this time.

Figure 58. *Hemangioma-like lesion*: In a 79-year-old male patient, a huge heterogeneous mass replaced the right lobe of the liver. Axial and coronal true FISP images (**A**, **B**) showed the full extent of the mass, also a considerable amount of ascites. Coronal post-Gd T1w images showed patchy nodular enhancement in the portal phase (**C**) with considerable infilling of the tumor mass on delayed images (**D**). Histology—hemangiosarcoma. (*Continued*)

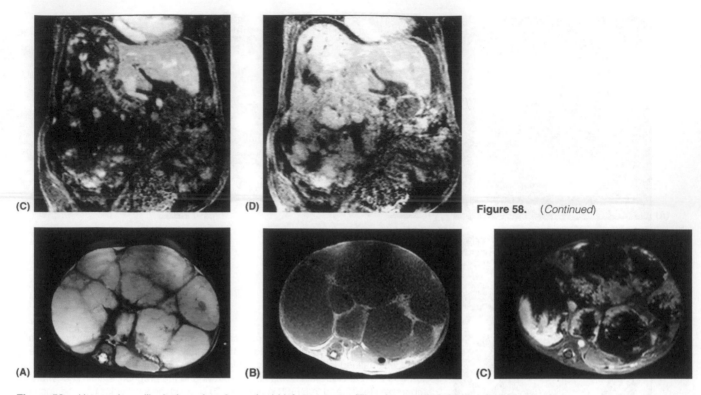

(C)   (D)   **Figure 58.** (*Continued*)

(A)   (B)   (C)

Figure 59. *Hemangioma-like lesion*:   In a 6-month-old infant, a tumor filling the upper abdomen showed hyperintensity on T2w and hypointensity on T1w images (**A**, **B**). Venous phase post-Gd T1w image (**C**) showed patchy enhancement with a centripetal progression within each of the locules. Histology—hemangio-endothelioma, type 1.

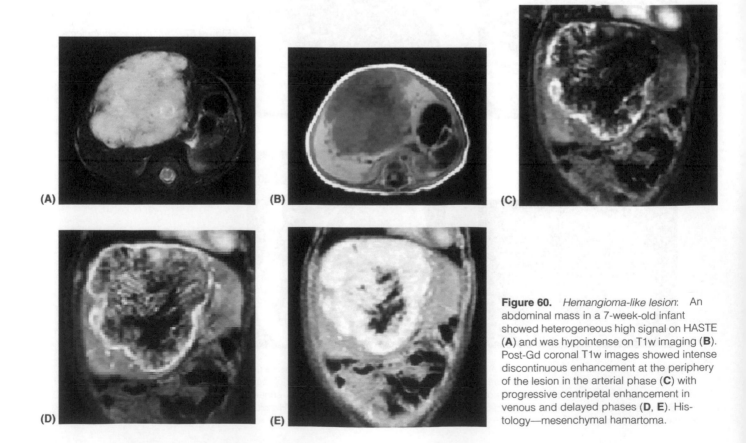

(A)   (B)   (C)

(D)   (E)   **Figure 60.** *Hemangioma-like lesion*:   An abdominal mass in a 7-week-old infant showed heterogeneous high signal on HASTE (**A**) and was hypointense on T1w imaging (**B**). Post-Gd coronal T1w images showed intense discontinuous enhancement at the periphery of the lesion in the arterial phase (**C**) with progressive centripetal enhancement in venous and delayed phases (**D**, **E**). Histology—mesenchymal hamartoma.

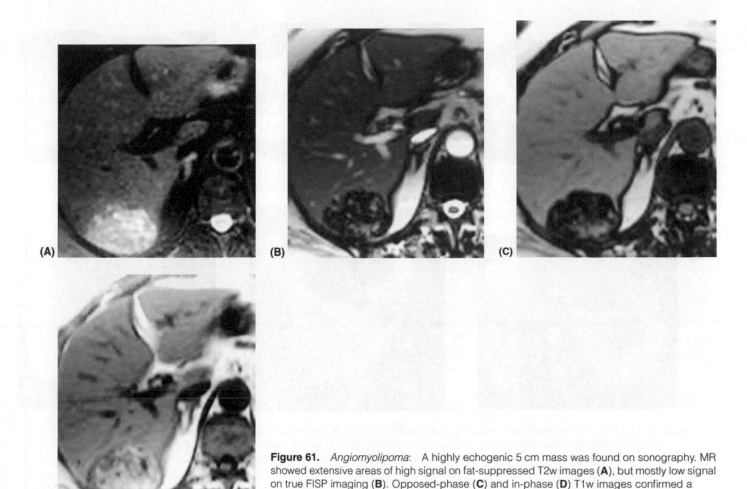

Figure 61. *Angiomyolipoma*:   A highly echogenic 5 cm mass was found on sonography. MR showed extensive areas of high signal on fat-suppressed T2w images (**A**), but mostly low signal on true FISP imaging (**B**). Opposed-phase (**C**) and in-phase (**D**) T1w images confirmed a considerable fat component producing lower signal on (**C**) and high signal on (**D**).

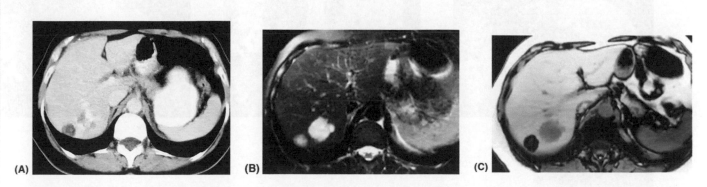

Figure 62. *Angiomyolipoma and hemangioma*:   In a patient with previous breast carcinoma, surveillance sonography showed echogenic lesions in the right lobe. Portal phase CT (**A**) showed patchy enhancement in one of the lesions, the second being relatively avascular. T2w images (**B**) showed both lesions to be hyperintense. One of the lesions was hypointense on opposed-phase (**C**) and hyperintense on in-phase (**D**) T1w images confirming a high fat content. The second lesion was hypointense on both in- and opposed-phase, but post-Gd T1w arterial phase (**E**) and delayed phase (**F**) images showed the characteristic enhancement pattern of a benign hemangioma. The fat-containing lesion showed no enhancement. (*Continued*)

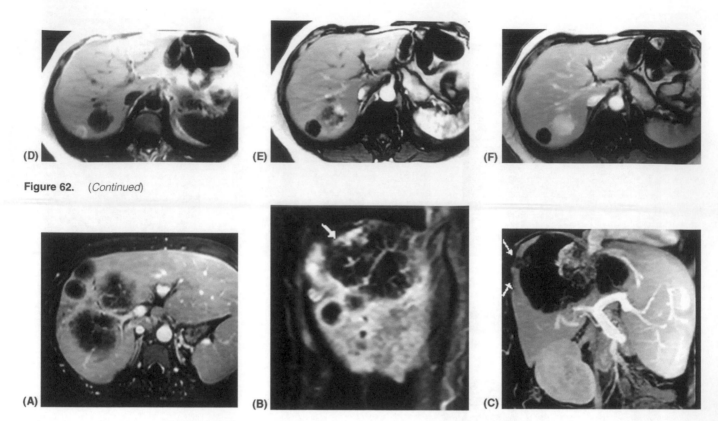

Figure 62. (*Continued*)

Figure 63. *Intrahepatic cholangiocarcinoma*: Axial (**A**) and RAO coronal (**B, C**) post-Gd T1w images showed a lobulated tumor with several satellite lesions. The peripheral enhancing rim is typically seen on early images, while more central enhancement is often seen on delayed images (**C**). Note also small areas of capsular retraction (arrows) in (**B**) and (**C**).

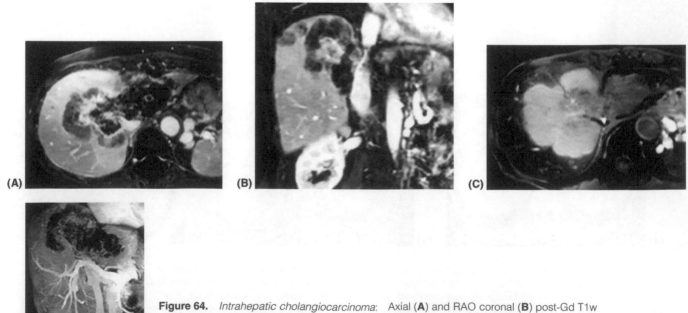

Figure 64. *Intrahepatic cholangiocarcinoma*: Axial (**A**) and RAO coronal (**B**) post-Gd T1w venous phase images showed lobulated tumor with satellite lesions and some central enhancement. The full intrahepatic extent of the mass was best shown on post-SPIO T2w images (**C**). Coronal MIP image (**D**) showed occlusion of the left main portal vein branch.

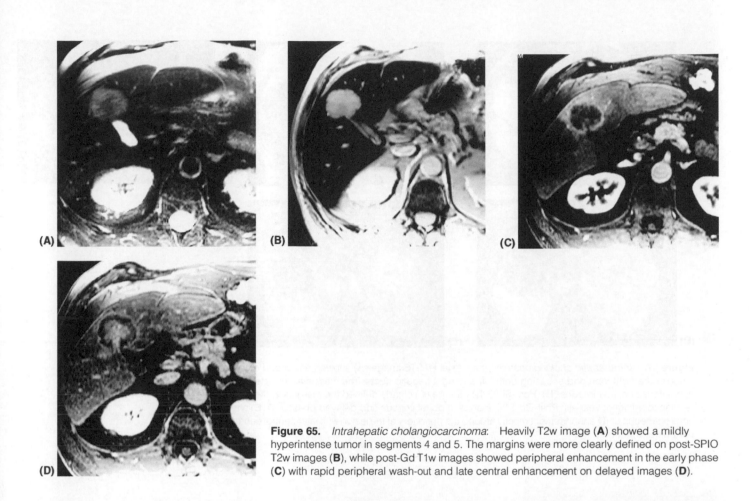

Figure 65. *Intrahepatic cholangiocarcinoma*:   Heavily T2w image (**A**) showed a mildly hyperintense tumor in segments 4 and 5. The margins were more clearly defined on post-SPIO T2w images (**B**), while post-Gd T1w images showed peripheral enhancement in the early phase (**C**) with rapid peripheral wash-out and late central enhancement on delayed images (**D**).

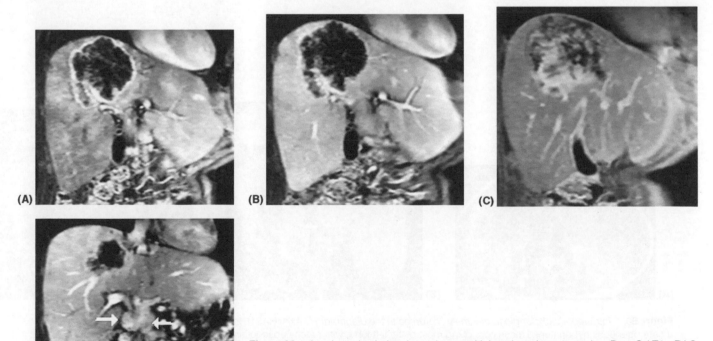

Figure 66. *Intrahepatic cholangiocarcinoma with lymph node metastasis*:   Post-Gd T1w RAO coronal images showed a tumor with a brightly enhancing rim in the arterial phase (**A**) which faded considerably by the venous phase (**B**). Delayed images (**C**) showed patchy central enhancement and large hilar lymph nodes (arrows) were shown on a more posterior slice (**D**).

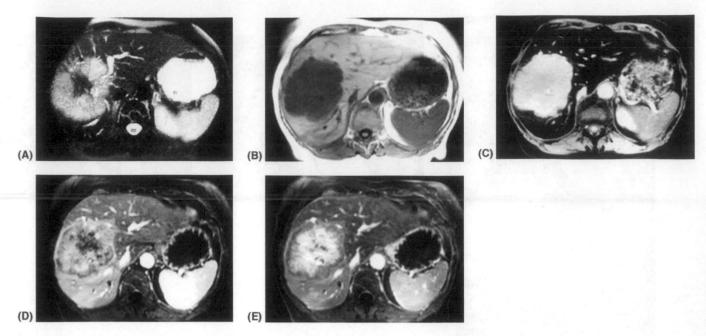

Figure 67. *Intrahepatic cholangiocarcinoma*: Axial HASTE image (**A**) showed a rounded mass occupying much of the right lobe and encasing both left and right hepatic ducts. The mass was well-defined and hypointense on T1w images (**B**). Post-SPIO T2w image (**C**) clearly defined the margins of the mass and its relation to adjacent vessels. Post-Gd T1w images in portal venous and delayed phases (**D**, **E**) showed typical heterogeneous early enhancement mostly around the periphery of the lesion with later central enhancement and peripheral wash-out.

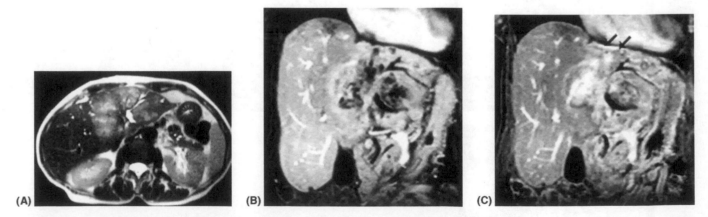

Figure 68. *Intrahepatic cholangiocarcinoma with spread to the diaphragm*: Axial HASTE image (**A**) showed a heterogeneous hyperintense mass occupying most of the left lobe, with patchy obstruction of intrahepatic ducts. Coronal post-Gd venous phase T1w image (**B**) showed heterogeneous hypo-intensity with patchy enhancement and multiple duct obstructions. Delayed post-Gd coronal T1w image (**C**) showed enhancement along the diaphragmatic surface of segment 2 (arrows). Laparoscopic biopsy confirmed peritoneal and diaphragmatic involvement.

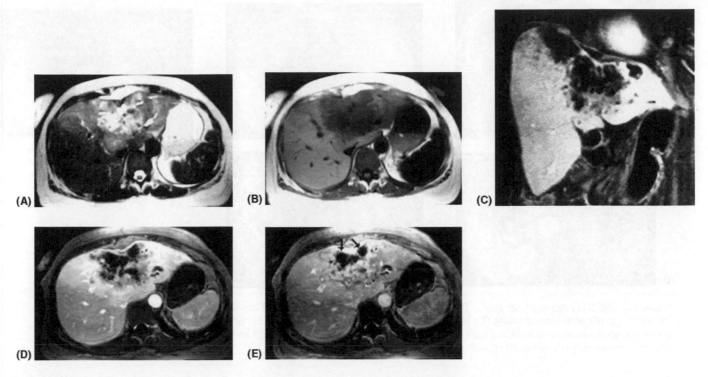

Figure 69. *Intrahepatic cholangiocarcinoma with capsular indrawing:* Unenhanced images showed a heterogeneous tumor lying centrally within the left lobe and causing indrawing of the anterior liver surface seen on T2w (**A**) and T1w (**B**) images. Post-Gd venous phase coronal T1w image (**C**) also showed capsular retraction on the superior surface of the left lobe. Note also several satellite lesions around the irregular margins of the tumor. Abnormal capsular enhancement was shown in the axial post-Gd venous phase T1w image (**D**), but the intense enhancement of the surface disease was best seen (arrows) after a 10 minute delay (**E**).

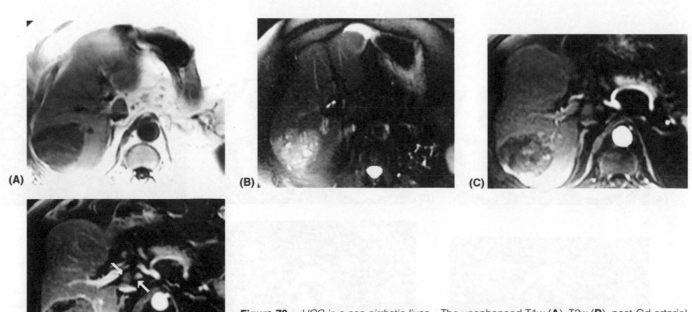

Figure 70. *HCC in a non-cirrhotic liver:* The unenhanced T1w (**A**), T2w (**B**), post-Gd arterial phase (**C**) and venous phase (**D**) T1w images showed a heterogeneous tumor with rim enhancement lying within a morphologically normal liver. HCC was confirmed on histology. Note the enlarged porto-caval nodes [arrows in (**D**)].

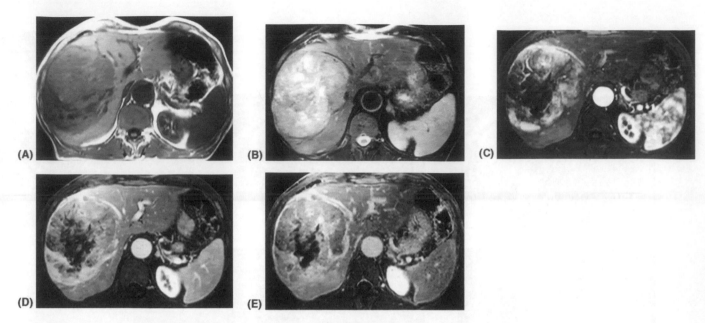

Figure 71. *HCC in a non-cirrhotic liver.* The unenhanced T1w (**A**), T2w (**B**), post-Gd arterial phase (**C**), venous phase (**D**) and delayed phase (**E**) T1w images showed a large heterogeneous tumor with patchy peripheral enhancement and a central area which remained unenhanced on the delayed image. Histology showed a moderately differentiated HCC in a non-cirrhotic liver.

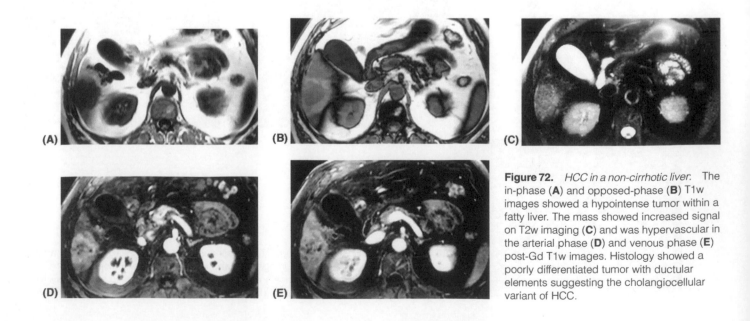

Figure 72. *HCC in a non-cirrhotic liver.* The in-phase (**A**) and opposed-phase (**B**) T1w images showed a hypointense tumor within a fatty liver. The mass showed increased signal on T2w imaging (**C**) and was hypervascular in the arterial phase (**D**) and venous phase (**E**) post-Gd T1w images. Histology showed a poorly differentiated tumor with ductular elements suggesting the cholangiocellular variant of HCC.

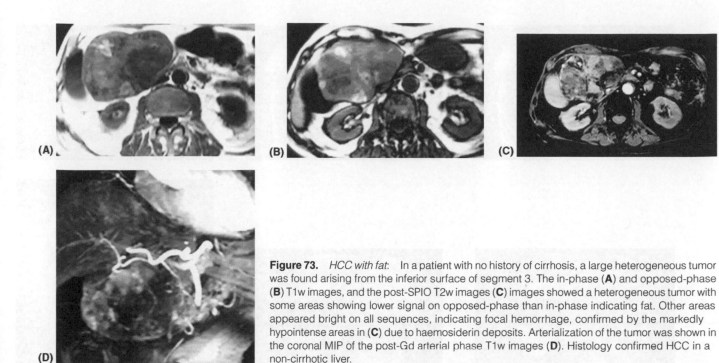

Figure 73. *HCC with fat:* In a patient with no history of cirrhosis, a large heterogeneous tumor was found arising from the inferior surface of segment 3. The in-phase (**A**) and opposed-phase (**B**) T1w images, and the post-SPIO T2w images (**C**) images showed a heterogeneous tumor with some areas showing lower signal on opposed-phase than in-phase indicating fat. Other areas appeared bright on all sequences, indicating focal hemorrhage, confirmed by the markedly hypointense areas in (**C**) due to haemosiderin deposits. Arterialization of the tumor was shown in the coronal MIP of the post-Gd arterial phase T1w images (**D**). Histology confirmed HCC in a non-cirrhotic liver.

Figure 74. *HCC in non-cirrhotic liver:* A 67-year-old man presented with a 15-cm mass in the right lobe. Unenhanced T1w images showed a heterogeneous mass with foci of hyperintensity on both in-phase (**A**) and opposed-phase (**B**) images. Note the more marked hypointensity of the main tumor mass on the opposed-phase imaging, indicating fat content. The lesion was hyperintense on HASTE imaging (**C**) and showed no uptake of SPIO contrast (**D**). Post-Gd T1w images showed arterial phase hypervascularity (**E**) with a central non-enhancing area, but marked capsular enhancement on delayed images (**F**).

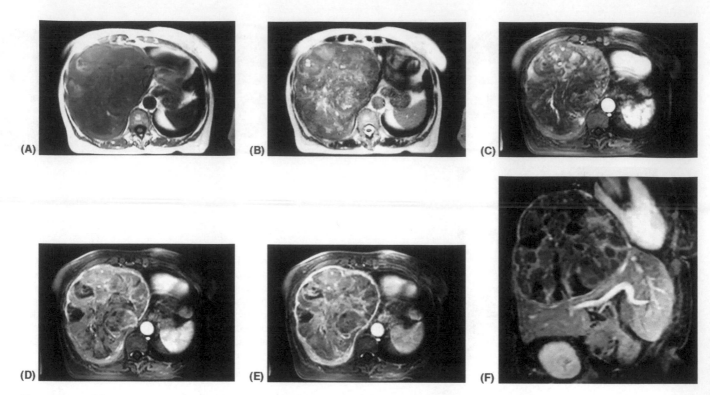

Figure 75. *HCC in non-cirrhotic liver.* This female patient aged 67 presented with a 13-cm right lobe mass. Unenhanced T1w (**A**) and HASTE (**B**) images showed a heterogeneous tumor with foci of high signal indicating local hemorrhage. Post-Gd T1w imaging in arterial, venous and delayed phases (**C**, **D**, **E**) showed typical heterogeneous arterial hypervascularity with most of the tumor mass being hypovascular compared with liver parenchyma and capsular enhancement being notable in the delayed image. On the RAO coronal MIP image (**F**), the tumor appeared clear of the portal branches and the left hepatic vein, so resection was undertaken.

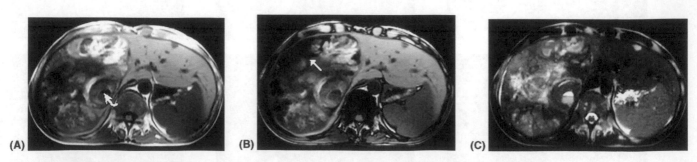

Figure 76. *HCC and hemangioma in non-cirrhotic liver.* A man aged 41 presented with a 15-cm mass in the right lobe. Unenhanced in-phase (**A**) and opposed-phase (**B**) T1w images showed the large markedly heterogeneous tumor. Note the areas of marked signal drop out (arrow) in the opposed-phase image indicating local fat deposition within the tumor. A central nodule adjacent to the cava contained a blood-filled cavity within which a fluid-fluid level was visible [curved arrow in (**A**)]. The fluid level was also visible on HASTE (**C**) and post-SPIO T2w imaging (**D**). Histology confirmed HCC in non-cirrhotic liver with local hemorrhage into the tumor adjacent to the cava, causing the fluid level. Also note the 2 cm lesion on the anterior surface of segment 3 visible on all sequences, which showed the enhancement characteristics of a benign hemangioma, also confirmed at resection. The coronal post-Gd T1w MIP image (**E**) showed the left portal vein and left hepatic vein to be uninvolved and successful resection was performed. (*Continued*)

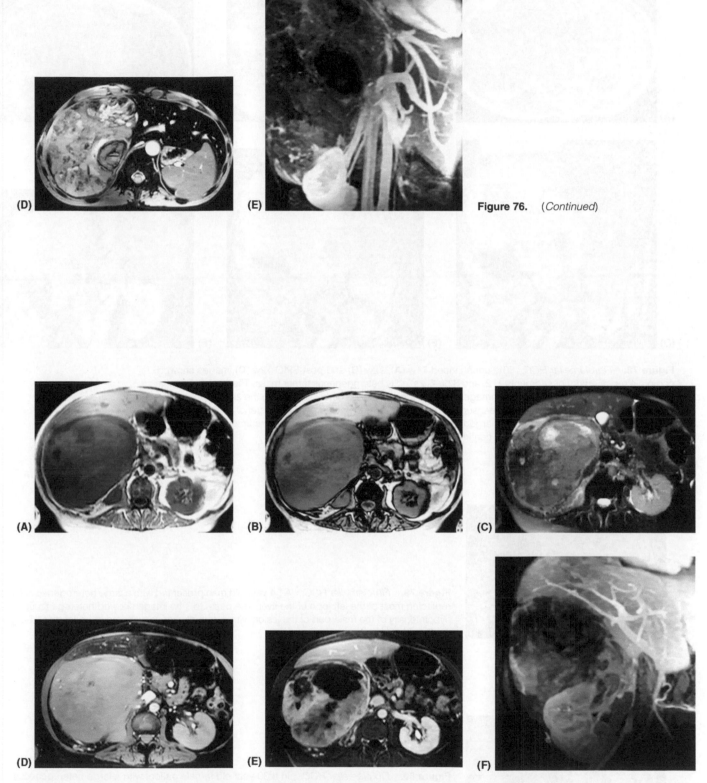

Figure 76.   (*Continued*)

Figure 77.   *Differential diagnosis of HCC:*   In a non-cirrhotic patient, exophytic HCC was suspected when a large heterogeneous tumor showed low signal intensity on both in-phase and opposed-phase T1w images (**A**, **B**) and heterogeneous hyperintensity on HASTE images (**C**). The lesion took up no SPIO contrast (**D**) and showed marked heterogeneous enhancement on post-Gd T1w images (**E**). Coronal MIP image (**F**) showed the intimate relationship of the tumor to the right lobe of liver and right kidney. Histology—liposarcoma.

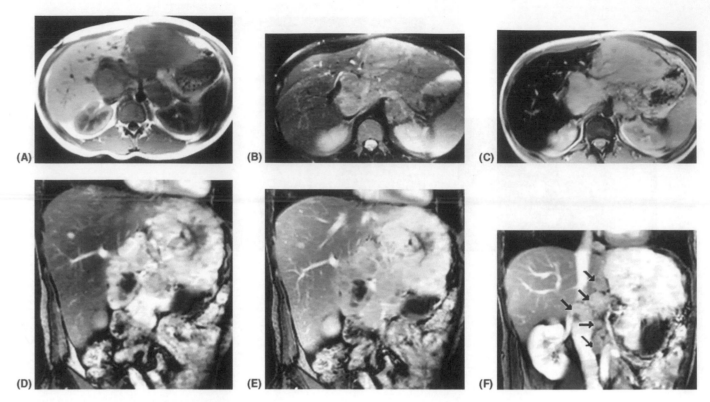

Figure 78. *Fibrolamellar HCC:* The unenhanced T1w (**A**), T2w (**B**) and post-SPIO T2w (**C**) images showed complete replacement of segments 1, 2, and 3 by the slightly heterogeneous tumor mass. The post-Gd arterial phase (**D**) and venous phase (**E**) T1w images showed the mass to be highly vascular in the arterial phase with some central areas of non-enhancement suggesting fibrotic scar elements. A more posterior slice from the venous phase (**F**) showed multiple enlarged nodes in the porta hepatis, right cardiophrenic angle, and the aorto-caval space (arrows). Histology confirmed fibrolamellar HCC.

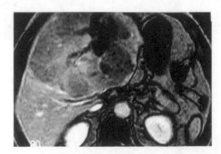

Figure 79. *Fibrolamellar HCC:* A 54-year-old man presented with a large heterogeneous tumor replacing most of the left lobe of the liver. The post-Gd T1w image showed heterogeneous hypointensity of the main part of the lesion with a central scar showing no enhancement. Surgery confirmed FLH.

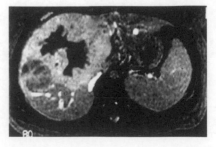

Figure 80. *Fibrolamellar HCC:* In a 30-year-old female patient with a large heterogeneous tumor centred in segment 4 but extending into the right lobe, post-Gd T1w images showed a large non-enhancing central scar within a hypervascular lesion, with persistent parenchymal enhancement in the portal phase. A separate nodule of tumor adjacent to the lateral margin of the right lobe showed less specific features. Histology of the resection specimen confirmed FLH with a separate nodule of moderately differentiated tumor.

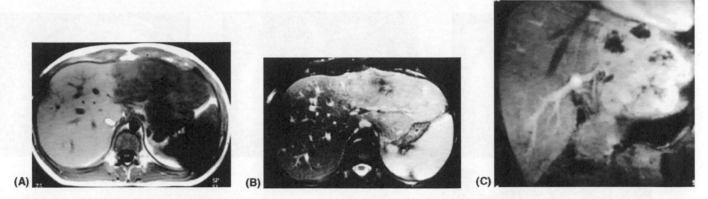

Figure 81. *Fibrolamellar HCC:* In a 16-year-old boy, an extensive tumor replacing the left lobe of the liver showed patchy hypointensity on T1w (**A**) and hyperintensity on T2w imaging (**B**). The central scar was represented by an ill-defined low signal area on T2w images, but post-Gd T1w imaging in the late arterial phase (**C**) showed more well-defined areas of non-enhancement within a diffusely enhancing tumor mass. Resection histology confirmed HCC with fibrolamellar components.

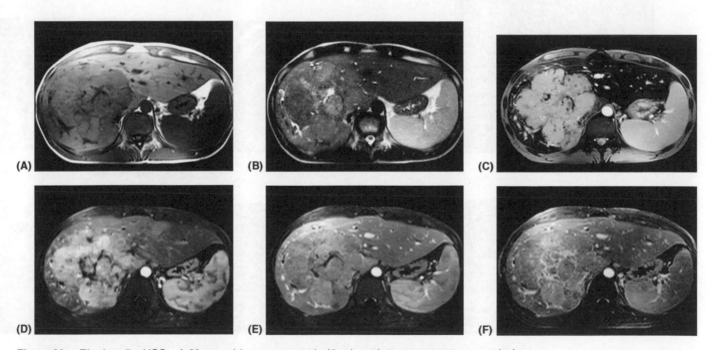

Figure 82. *Fibrolamellar HCC:* A 20-year-old man presented with a large heterogeneous tumor replacing most of the right lobe. The lesion showed heterogeneous hypointensity on T1w imaging (**A**) and mild hyperintensity on T2w images (**B**). The lesion showed no uptake of SPIO contrast (**C**). The foci of low signal within the lesion represent areas of calcification, previously shown on CT. Post-Gd T1w imaging in arterial (**D**) and venous (**E**) phases showed a marked arterial enhancement in most of the lesion which faded to isointensity by the venous phase. The central scar was best seen on the post-Gd images and remained hypointense up to the portal phase. However, further T1w imaging after 10 minutes delay (**F**) showed considerable enhancement of the central scar which then appeared hyperintense. Resection histology confirmed FLH.

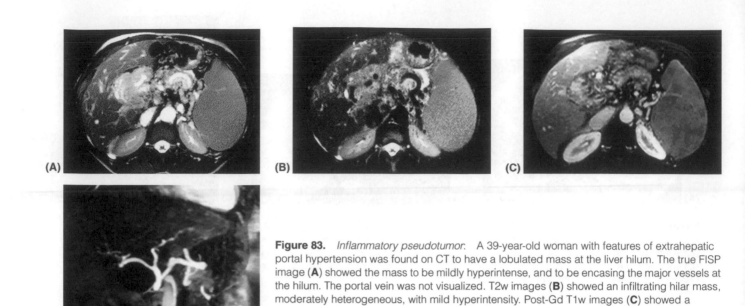

Figure 83. *Inflammatory pseudotumor.* A 39-year-old woman with features of extrahepatic portal hypertension was found on CT to have a lobulated mass at the liver hilum. The true FISP image (**A**) showed the mass to be mildly hyperintense, and to be encasing the major vessels at the hilum. The portal vein was not visualized. T2w images (**B**) showed an infiltrating hilar mass, moderately heterogeneous, with mild hyperintensity. Post-Gd T1w images (**C**) showed a moderate degree of heterogeneous enhancement within the lesion, and the arterial phase MIP image (**D**) showed no evidence of arterial encasement, even though the mass was clearly surrounding the arteries on cross-sectional images. The lack of vascular invasion favored the diagnosis of lymphoma, but histology was that of inflammatory pseudotumor.

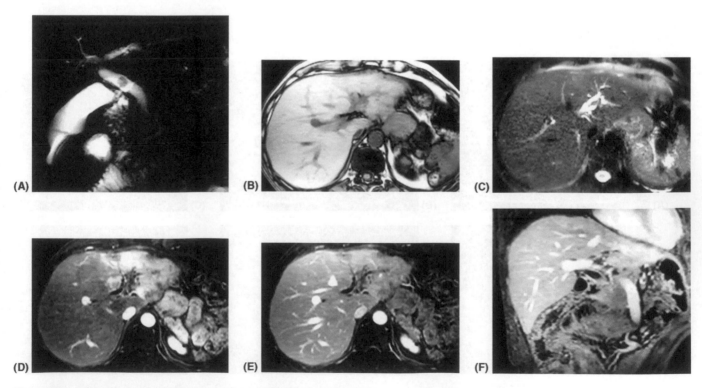

Figure 84. *Inflammatory pseudotumor.* A 59-year-old man presented with a stone in the common bile duct, but MRCP (**A**) also showed segmental obstruction of the left lobe ducts at the liver hilum. On T1w images (**B**) subtle heterogeneity was visible in segments 2 and 3, and HASTE images (**C**) showed dilatation of the left lobe ducts but no parenchymal lesion. Post-Gd T1w images showed heterogeneous arterial enhancement in most of the left lobe (**D**) with several peripheral areas of lesser perfusion and an ill-defined perihilar mass. The peripheral hypointense areas persisted in the venous phase (**E**) and the impression of a hilar mass was confirmed on the venous phase MIP (**F**) which also showed occlusion of the left portal branch. Biopsy histology revealed inflammatory pseudotumor, and the appearances remained stable during 12 months follow-up with no surgery.

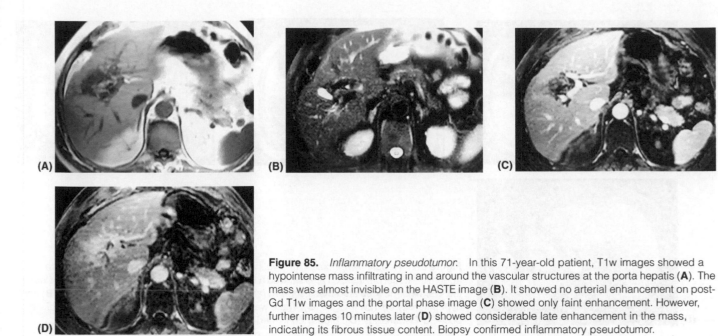

Figure 85. *Inflammatory pseudotumor.* In this 71-year-old patient, T1w images showed a hypointense mass infiltrating in and around the vascular structures at the porta hepatis (**A**). The mass was almost invisible on the HASTE image (**B**). It showed no arterial enhancement on post-Gd T1w images and the portal phase image (**C**) showed only faint enhancement. However, further images 10 minutes later (**D**) showed considerable late enhancement in the mass, indicating its fibrous tissue content. Biopsy confirmed inflammatory pseudotumor.

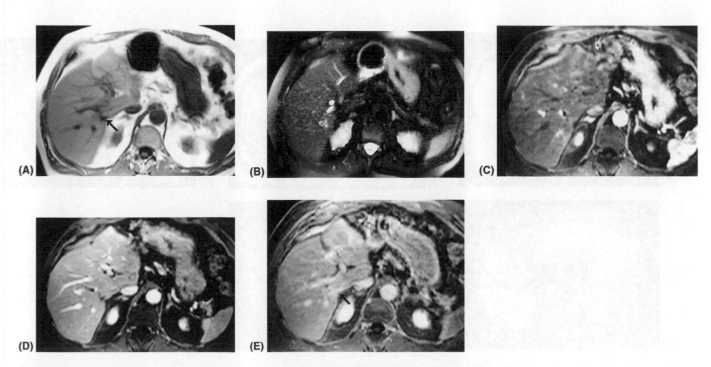

Figure 86. *Post-infective scarring.* An elderly patient with a suspected liver abscess in segment 6 was treated conservatively before being sent for MRI. On T1w images (**A**), the lesion was manifest only as a small area of hypointensity (arrow) associated with indrawing of the liver capsule. The lesion was invisible on HASTE images (**B**). The abnormality was hypointense on post-Gd T1w images in arterial and portal venous phases (**C, D**) and was best seen 10 minutes later (**E**) when the fibrotic component showed considerably more enhancement than the adjacent liver (arrow).

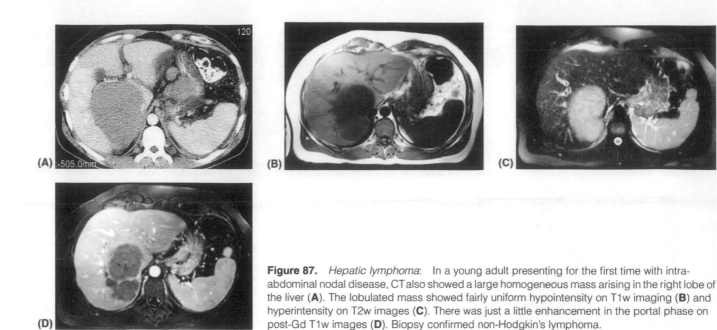

Figure 87. *Hepatic lymphoma:* In a young adult presenting for the first time with intra-abdominal nodal disease, CT also showed a large homogeneous mass arising in the right lobe of the liver (**A**). The lobulated mass showed fairly uniform hypointensity on T1w imaging (**B**) and hyperintensity on T2w images (**C**). There was just a little enhancement in the portal phase on post-Gd T1w images (**D**). Biopsy confirmed non-Hodgkin's lymphoma.

Figure 88. *Porta hepatis lymphoma:* Four months after successful liver transplantation, this patient presented with a mass at the liver hilum which was hypoattenuating on CT with rim enhancement (**A**). The lesion showed uniform hypointensity on T1w imaging (**B**) and heterogeneous hyperintensity on T2w images (**C**). Post-Gd T1w images showed an enhancing rim in the arterial phase (**D**) with no enhancement of the central part of the lesion in the portal phase (**E**). Diagnosis—post-transplant non-Hodgkin's lymphoma (confirmed on biopsy).

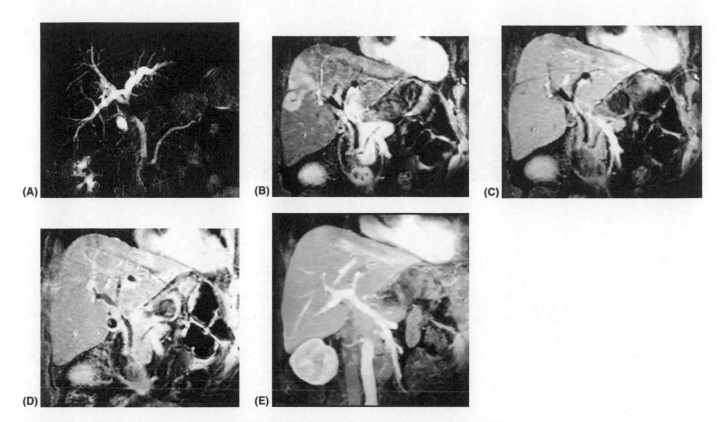

Figure 89. *Hepatic hilar lymphoma*:   A man aged 73 with jaundice was shown on CT to have a hilar obstruction and a combined endoscopic/percutaneous stent procedure was performed. Subsequent MRCP (**A**) showed a smooth stricture of the common hepatic duct with upstream dilatation of the biliary tree. Arterial phase post-Gd T1w imaging (**B**) showed an intensely enhancing mass encasing the common hepatic duct and extending into segment 3 along the line of the main left hepatic duct. The patchy perfusion abnormality shown adjacent to the lateral margin of the right lobe is related to previous percutaneous transhepatic catheterization. Enhancement in the obstructing mass faded in the portal phase (**C**) and images 10 minutes later (**D**) showed only a little persisting enhancement in the abnormal tissue. However, the venous MIP image (**E**) showed narrowing of the left branch of the portal vein corresponding with the site of intrahepatic extension of the mass. Histology revealed non-Hodgkin's lymphoma.

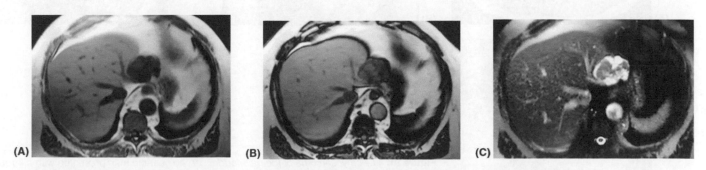

Figure 90. *Biliary adenofibroma*:   A non-cirrhotic patient presented with a complex 6 cm mass arising close to the tip of the left lobe of the liver. In-phase and opposed-phase T1w images (**A**, **B**) showed the mass to be heterogeneously hypointense, with no visible fat content. The lesion showed heterogeneous hyperintensity on T2w imaging (**C**) and no uptake of SPIO contrast (**D**). Post-Gd T1w imaging (**E**) showed quite marked, but patchy, portal phase enhancement. The pre-operative imaging diagnosis was of either sporadic HCC or a mixed mesenchymal tumor. Resection histology showed biliary adenofibroma. (*Continued*)

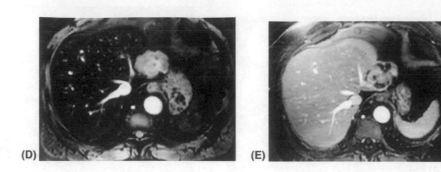

(D)   (E)   **Figure 90.**   (*Continued*)

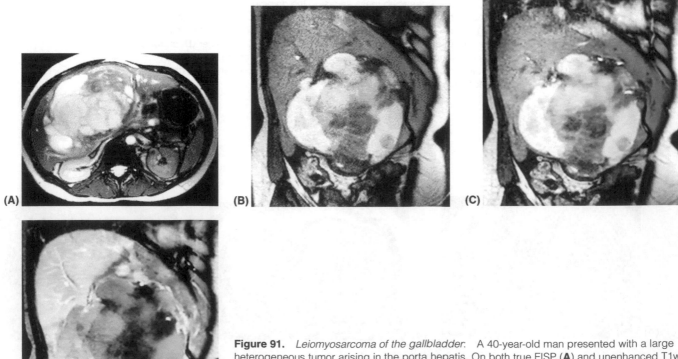

(A)   (B)   (C)

(D)   **Figure 91.**   *Leiomyosarcoma of the gallbladder.*   A 40-year-old man presented with a large heterogeneous tumor arising in the porta hepatis. On both true FISP (**A**) and unenhanced T1w imaging (**B**), the lesion showed a complex structure with numerous areas of hyperintensity and internal septation. Post-Gd T1w coronal images in arterial (**C**) and venous (**D**) phases showed very little enhancement within the mass. Grossly abnormal architecture suggested a malignant mesenchymal tumor. Resection histology confirmed leiomyosarcoma, probably arising in the gallbladder.

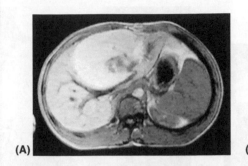
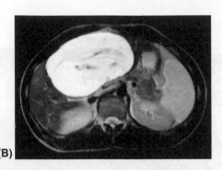
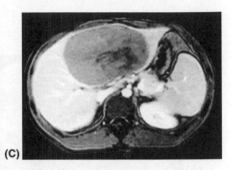

Figure 92. *Malignant mesenchymal tumor.* In a 23-year-old man, unenhanced T1w imaging (**A**) showed a cystic tumor arising in the left lobe of the liver. The mass contained solid components within the lumen, and the hyperintensity of the fluid within the lesion suggested a mucin-secreting tumor. On T2w imaging (**B**), the fluid component was brightly hyperintense, but again hypointense solid areas were shown within the lesion. Post-Gd T1w imaging (**C**) showed no enhancement in the lesion in either arterial or portal phases. Pre-operative diagnosis was of biliary cystadenoma with mesenchymal stroma. Resection histology showed a cystic tumor with a wall composed of undifferentiated small malignant cells.

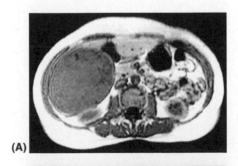
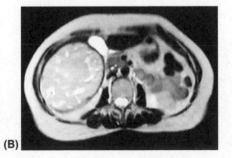
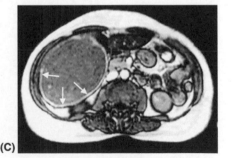
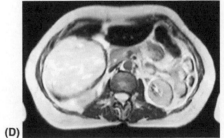

Figure 93. *Malignant mesenchymal tumor.* A 64-year-old woman presented with a large mass arising in the right lobe of the liver. The mass appeared well-defined, heterogeneous and hypointense on T1w images (**A**). On T2w imaging (**B**), the mass again showed a peripheral rim or capsule of hypointense signal, surrounding a hyperintense mass with numerous ill-defined areas of more marked hyperintensity suggesting areas of necrosis or possibly dilated pathologic vessels. Post-Gd T1w image (**C**) showed late enhancement in the capsule (arrows) with relatively mild and fairly uniform enhancement within the tumor mass. The lesion did not take up SPIO contrast (**D**). Pre-operative diagnosis was of a malignant mesenchymal tumor; resection histology showed leiomyosarcoma.

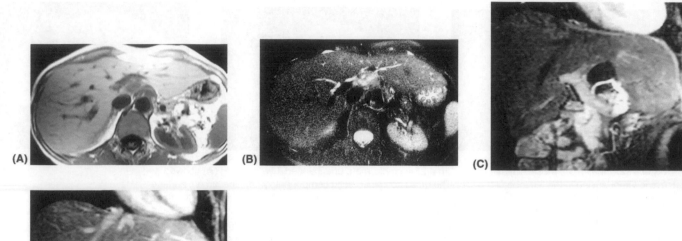

Figure 94. *Benign mesenchymal tumor.* In a 40-year-old woman presenting with post-cholecystectomy pain, CT showed a mass arising in the porta hepatis or caudate lobe of the liver. The lesion was hypointense on T1w imaging (**A**) and showed heterogeneous hyperintensity on HASTE imaging (**B**). Though no enhancement was seen on initial T1w images after gadolinium (**C**), some enhancement was visible (arrow) on delayed images (**D**). Imaging features suggested a mesenchymal tumor with a substantial fibrous component. Resection histology showed ganglioneuroma.

CHAPTER 7

Fat and the Liver

THE IMPORTANCE OF FAT IN LIVER DISEASE

Although the liver is a major site of lipid metabolism, little fat is normally stored there. The abnormal accumulation of fat in the liver is manifest microscopically as visible globules of intracellular lipid, and macroscopically by changes in the visual appearance of the liver. These are also detectable by imaging using sonography, CT or MRI.

Abnormal deposition of fat in the liver may mimic disease, may complicate existing disease, and may disguise or conceal disease. The presence of fat within focal liver lesions is a pointer towards specific pathologies.

CAUSES OF FATTY LIVER

Fatty infiltration of the liver is a common manifestation of alcoholic liver disease, and is reversible with abstinence. Lipid deposition is also common in uncomplicated obesity, in diabetic patients, and in those with severe malnutrition. These and other less common aetiologies are grouped together as 'non-alcoholic fatty liver disease'. A combination of fat deposition, fibrosis, and inflammatory change forms the basis for the diagnosis of non-alcoholic steatohepatitis (NASH) which is also most commonly found in diabetic patients. The mechanism for the relationship between obesity, adult onset diabetes, and NASH remains unclear, but about 20% of patients with NASH progress to cirrhosis within 5 years of diagnosis. Lipid deposition is also associated with hypertriglyceridaemia from any cause, and is fairly common in patients undergoing chemotherapy for malignant disease. The character of the fat deposition in all these conditions is rather similar, and areas of the liver affected by fatty change associated with any of these conditions produce the same appearance on imaging. Lipid deposits in acute fatty liver of pregnancy and Reye's syndrome are of a different character—the microvesicular deposits of fat are much smaller and the total amount of fat deposited is much less—so changes on imaging are less characteristic with these rare conditions.

IMAGING THE FATTY LIVER

Intracellular fat globules produce interfaces which reflect sound waves, so the characteristic appearance of fatty liver at sonography is of increased echogenicity. Since fat contains only carbon, hydrogen, and a little oxygen, its average atomic number (about 6.3) is less than that of other soft tissues (about 7.4) which contain more oxygen and also nitrogen, sulphur, and phosphorus. Because of this, significant fatty change in the liver leads to reduced attenuation on CT which is best appreciated on unenhanced images. Attempts have been made to quantitate the amount of fat in the liver at CT and sonography by correlating the changes in attenuation and echogenicity with pathologic estimates of fat content based on biopsy specimens. With both sonography and CT, there is little difficulty in recognizing cases of gross fatty change, but the quantitative methods require careful calibration and have not been shown to be accurate with minor degrees of fatty change.

CHEMICAL SHIFT MRI

When placed in a magnetic field, protons in fatty tissues resonate at a slightly lower frequency than those in watery tissues. These frequencies are sufficiently similar for both sets of protons to be excited by the same RF impulse, and sufficiently different for the peaks and troughs of their interference pattern to be detectable separately. Imaging with an echo time (TE) which coincides with one of the peaks of the interference pattern is described as in-phase imaging, while acquiring data at a TE coinciding with one of the troughs in the pattern is described as opposed-phase imaging (Fig. 1). Where fat and water protons are mixed in the same image voxel, in-phase, and opposed-phase images will show a distinct difference in signal intensity. This is seen normally in vertebral bone marrow but not in the normal liver which does not contain enough fat to demonstrate this effect. With the T1-weighted gradient echo sequences used for chemical shift acquisitions, the signal intensity from fat protons is considerably greater than that from water protons. In vitro work has indicated that the proportion of fat content which would produce approximately equal signal intensities from fat and water protons mixed in the same voxel is in the region of 15–20%. In vivo, the relationship is more complex due to interactions with proteins and other large molecules, but it is clear that small degrees of lipid deposition produce visible differences between in-phase and opposed-phase images, and larger amounts of fatty infiltration produce a severe loss of liver signal on the opposed-phase images. With extremely fatty livers, the signal from fat may considerably outweigh the water signal, so the loss of signal on opposed-phase images is less marked, but in such cases the additive effect of the fat signal renders the liver distinctly brighter than normal on in-phase images. With severe degrees of fatty infiltration, phase cancellation artifact may be visible along the margins of the intrahepatic veins on opposed-phase sequences, perhaps best seen on True FISP images.

GEOGRAPHIC DISTRIBUTION OF FATTY CHANGE

Fatty infiltration is commonly diffuse but may be patchy or focal. Diffuse fatty change results in uniform changes in signal intensity across the liver, as described above. The normal lobar architecture of the liver is maintained, but enlarged nodes may develop at the porta hepatis. Occasionally fatty change may affect one lobe only, the demarcation being distinctly in line with anatomic landmarks. This phenomenon could be explained by laminar flow in the portal vein—fat from the intestine entering the right lobe via the superior mesenteric vein, while the left lobe receives fat-free blood from the stomach, spleen, and pancreas—but this supposition has not been proven. However, both focal fatty change and focal sparing within a diffusely fatty liver may be seen at specific sites in the liver which are known to be associated with non-portal venous inflow. These include the anterior surface of segment 4 adjacent to the falciform ligament, the posterior surface of segments 2,3 and 4 close to the porta hepatis, and the surface of segment 5 adjacent to the gallbladder fossa. In these areas, the portal inflow which occurs in the rest of the liver may be displaced by blood flowing into the liver parenchyma from the parabiliary venous plexus, the cholecystic veins, the inferior vein of Sappey and the para-umbilical veins. These observations suggest that the distribution of focal fatty change, or focal sparing within a fatty liver, is related to the intrahepatic distribution of portal blood flow.

Less easy to explain is the occasional finding of nodules of fat scattered through an otherwise normal liver or the converse appearance—nodules of focal sparing within a diffusely fatty liver. Nodular fatty change associated with areas of intervening fibrosis is a feature of alcoholic hepatitis and early cirrhosis and similar appearances may be seen in NASH.

TUMORS IN THE FATTY LIVER

The increased echogenicity of the fatty liver at sonography may make echogenic tumors more difficult to detect, and because most tumors are hypo-attenuating relative to normal liver on CT, the presence of fatty change may disguise or conceal them. Focal areas of fatty change or fatty sparing may be indistinguishable on both sonography and CT from metastases or other significant mass lesions. In such cases, chemical shift MRI will highlight the fatty tissues within which focal lesions are clearly visualized on the in-phase images. Focal areas of fatty change show reduced signal on opposed-phase images, while being similar to normal liver on in-phase images. With focal fatty sparing, the normal areas of liver tissue show similar signal on in-phase and opposed-phase images, while the rest of the liver shows reduced signal on the opposed-phase. Not infrequently, the presence of a mass lesion in a diffusely fatty liver may be signalled on the opposed-phase image (as on CT) by a halo of apparently normal liver tissue surrounding the lesion. It is postulated that this rim of preserved normal liver occurs as a result of compression of the portal inflow around the mass, or possibly as a result of arterio-portal shunting in the peri-lesional liver tissue. This 'halo' phenomenon may be seen with either benign or malignant lesions and is not specific for any particular pathology.

FAT IN LIVER TUMORS

A further application of chemical shift imaging is to seek the presence of fat within mass lesions since fat deposits are associated with only a few types of liver tumor. Fat is a fairly frequent component of hepatocellular carcinomas and the discovery of fat within a cirrhotic nodule should raise suspicion of malignant change since regenerative and dysplastic nodules rarely contain enough fat to be visible on imaging. Fat is also a fairly common constituent of hepatic adenomas and has occasionally been seen in focal nodular hyperplasia. In all of these hepatocellular lesions, the proportion of fat is usually small and its distribution heterogeneous. More extensive fat deposition is typical of angiomyolipomas in the liver. Lipomas and liposarcomas contain little else but fat, although metastases from liposarcomas contain soft tissue elements which increase in proportion to the aggressiveness of the malignancy. Fat is rarely seen in other metastases but has been described in deposits from renal cell primaries. Where radio-frequency ablation has been carried out on tumors within a fatty liver, fat components may be released from the surrounding liver into the cavity produced by ablation. Finally, gallbladder carcinoma may contain areas of fat which are demonstrable on chemical shift imaging, possibly as a result of the stone formation which commonly precedes malignant change in the gallbladder wall.

ILLUSTRATIVE FIGURES

Effect of varying TE on signal intensity from a fat and water mixture—Figure 1
Diffuse fatty change—Figures 2,3
Focal or lobar fatty change—Figures 4–7
Focal sparing in diffusely fatty liver—Figures 8–9
Differentials—focal fatty change or metastasis?—Figures 10–13 and Figures 27–28
Fatty change with fibrosis—Figures 14–17
Nodular fatty change—Figure 18
Nodular sparing in fatty liver—Figure 19
Neoplasms containing fat—Figures 20–22
Mass lesions within diffusely fatty liver—Figures 23–26 and Figures 33–34
Halo sign of focal lesion within fatty liver—Figures 29–32
Effect of RF ablation in fatty liver—Figure 35

See also:

Fat in cirrhotic nodules and HCC—Chapter 9
Fat in other focal liver lesions—Chapter 6

REFERENCES

1. Prasad SR, Wang H, Rosas H, et al. Fat-containing lesions of the liver: radiologic-pathologic correlation. Radiographics 2005; 25:321–331.
2. Basaran C, Karcaaltincaba M, Akata D, et al. Fat-containing lesions of the liver: cross-sectional imaging findings with emphasis on MRI. AJR Am J Roentgenol 2005; 184:1103–1110.
3. Kroncke TJ, Taupitz M, Kivelitz D, et al. Multifocal nodular fatty infiltration of the liver mimicking metastatic disease on CT: imaging findings and diagnosis using MR imaging. Eur Radiol 2000; 10:1095–1100.
4. Venkataraman S, Braga L, Semelka RC. Imaging the fatty liver. Magn Reson Imaging Clin N Am 2002; 10:93–103.
5. Chung JJ, Kim MJ, Kim JH, et al. Fat sparing of surrounding liver from metastasis in patients with fatty liver: MR imaging with histopathologic correlation. Am J Roentgenol 2003; 180:1347–1350.
6. Rinella ME, McCarthy R, Thakrar K, et al. Dual-echo, chemical shift gradient-echo magnetic resonance imaging to quantify hepatic steatosis: implications for living liver donation. Liver Transpl 2003; 9:851–856.

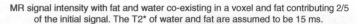

MR signal intensity with fat and water co-existing in a voxel and fat contributing 2/5 of the initial signal. The T2* of water and fat are assumed to be 15 ms.

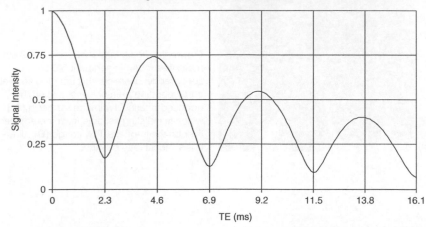

Figure 1. Influence of TE on signal intensity from mixed fat/water tissues at 1.5 T.

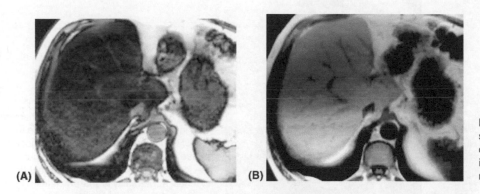

Figure 2. *Diffuse fatty infiltration*: The signal intensity in the liver was much less on opposed-phased (**A**) than on in-phase T1w images (**B**). Signal intensity from fat and from muscle was unchanged.

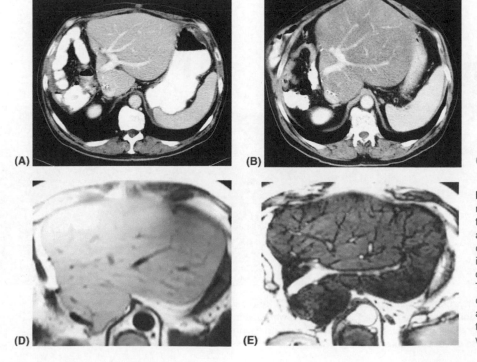

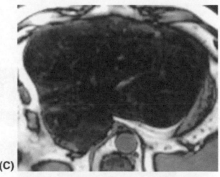

Figure 3. *Diffuse fatty infiltration*: Following right hemi-hepatectomy for colorectal metastases, CT images before (**A**) and two years after the start of chemotherapy (**B**) showed the development of fatty change. Chemical shift imaging showed a gross reduction in signal in opposed-phase (**C**) compared with in-phase T1w images (**D**). Because of the severe degree of fatty change, phase cancellation artifact (a black line between vessels and liver tissue) is visible on the True FISP sequence (**E**) which is an opposed-phase acquisition.

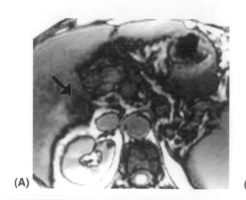

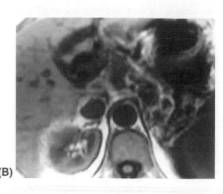

(A) **(B)**

Figure 4. *Focal fatty infiltration*: A 2-cm mass was found in segment 5/6 by sonography; chemical shift imaging showed a corresponding area of low signal on the opposed-phase T1w image [arrow in (**A**)] which is indistinguishable from the adjacent liver on the in-phase T1w image (**B**): diagnosis—focal fatty change.

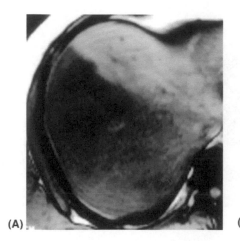

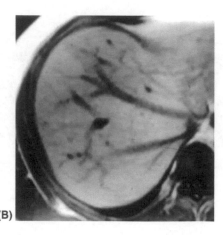

(A) **(B)**

Figure 5. *Lobar fatty infiltration*: Chemical shift imaging showed diffuse reduction in signal within the right lobe on the opposed-phase T1w image (**A**) with normal signal on the in-phase T1w image (**B**). Note that the extent of abnormality is sharply defined by the position of the middle hepatic vein.

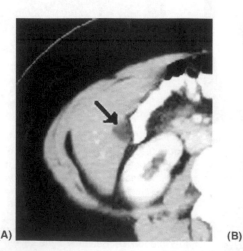

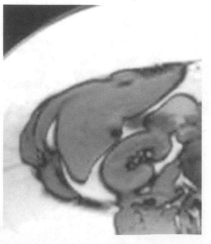

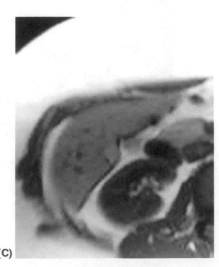

(A) **(B)** **(C)**

Figure 6. *Focal fatty infiltration*: A 2-cm hypo-attenuating nodule was shown on CT [arrow in (**A**)]. Chemical shift imaging showed low signal in the lesion on opposed-phase T1w image (**B**), while the in-phase T1w images (**C**) showed the lesion to have slightly higher signal than the adjacent liver indicating a very high fat content within this area. Note the thickness of subcutaneous fat in this patient.

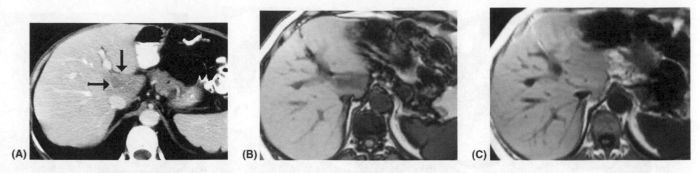

Figure 7. *Focal fatty change:* An ill-defined lesion shown in segment 1 on CT [arrows in (**A**)] showed low signal on the opposed-phase T1w image (**B**) and was iso-intense on the in-phase T1w image (**C**).

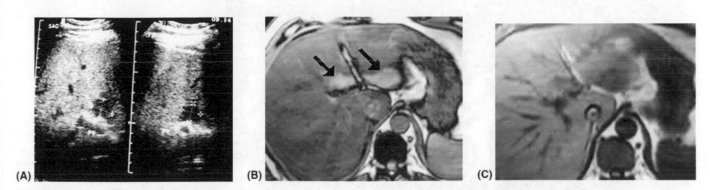

Figure 8. *Focal sparing within a severely fatty liver:* A 2-cm echo-poor lesion found on sonography within a fatty liver (**A**) was hyperintense to surrounding liver on the opposed-phase T1w image [arrows in (**B**)], but hypointense on in-phase T1w imaging (**C**).

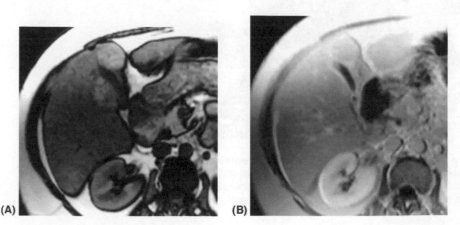

Figure 9. *Focal sparing within a fatty liver:* Sonography showed two areas of reduced echogenicity adjacent to the gallbladder fossa. These appeared hyperintense on opposed-phase (**A**) and iso-intense on in-phase T1w imaging (**B**).

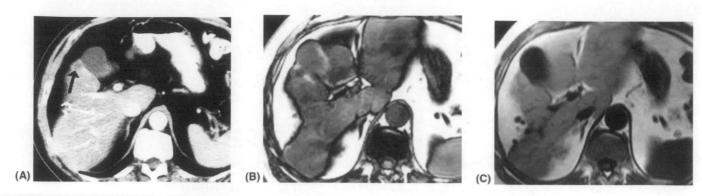

Figure 10.   *Focal fat or metastasis?*   Following partial hepatectomy and local metastatectomy for colorectal liver deposits, CT showed a 1-cm low attenuation area adjacent to the gallbladder [arrow in (**A**)]. The lesion showed low signal on opposed-phase (**B**) and isointensity on in-phase T1w imaging (**C**) confirming focal fatty change.

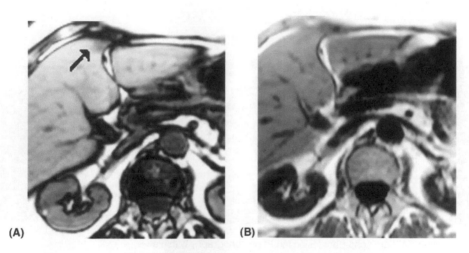

Figure 11.   *Focal fat or metastasis?*   In a patient with previous colorectal malignancy, CT showed a focal area of low attenuation adjacent to the falciform ligament [arrow in (**A**)], which was hypointense on opposed-phase (**A**) and hyperintense on in-phase T1w imaging (**B**). Diagnosis—focal fat deposition.

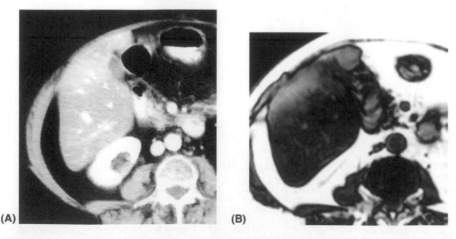

Figure 12.   *Focal fat or metastasis?*   In a patient with previous hepatic resection for colorectal metastases, a subtle perfusion alteration adjacent to the cut surface of the residual liver was observed on CT (**A**). Opposed-phase (**B**) and in-phase (**C**) T1w images showed diffuse fatty change in the liver remnant, and a focal lesion which was markedly hypointense on the in-phase image. Post-SPIO T2*w imaging (**D**) confirmed this was a further metastatic deposit. (*Continued*)

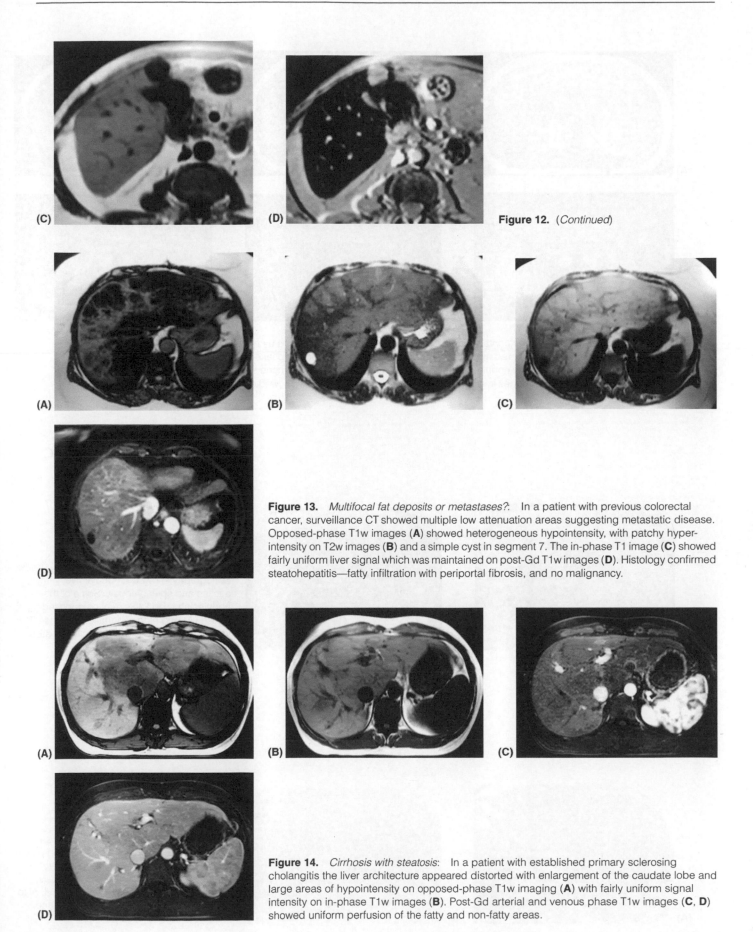

Figure 12. (*Continued*)

Figure 13. *Multifocal fat deposits or metastases?*: In a patient with previous colorectal cancer, surveillance CT showed multiple low attenuation areas suggesting metastatic disease. Opposed-phase T1w images (**A**) showed heterogeneous hypointensity, with patchy hyper-intensity on T2w images (**B**) and a simple cyst in segment 7. The in-phase T1 image (**C**) showed fairly uniform liver signal which was maintained on post-Gd T1w images (**D**). Histology confirmed steatohepatitis—fatty infiltration with periportal fibrosis, and no malignancy.

Figure 14. *Cirrhosis with steatosis*: In a patient with established primary sclerosing cholangitis the liver architecture appeared distorted with enlargement of the caudate lobe and large areas of hypointensity on opposed-phase T1w imaging (**A**) with fairly uniform signal intensity on in-phase T1w images (**B**). Post-Gd arterial and venous phase T1w images (**C**, **D**) showed uniform perfusion of the fatty and non-fatty areas.

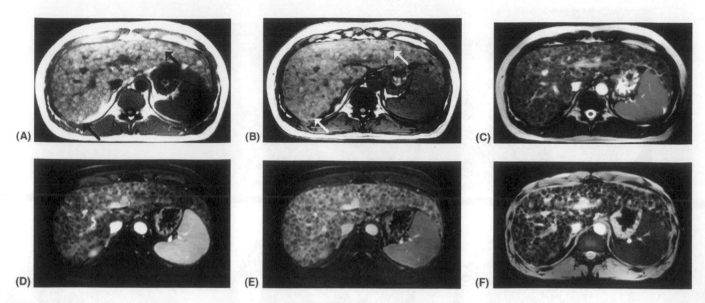

Figure 15. *Benign cirrhotic nodules containing fat*: In a patient with cirrhosis caused by hepatitis B chronicity, some of the nodules appeared more intense on in-phase (**A**) than opposed-phase T1w images (**B**) indicating fat content (arrows). All the nodules were isointense on HASTE images (**C**), none showed hypervascularity on post-Gd T1w images in arterial and venous phases (**D, E**) and all showed normal uptake of SPIO (**F**).

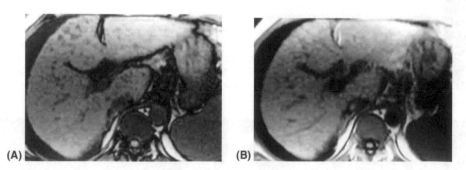

Figure 16. *Alcohol-induced steatohepatitis*: Sonography showed a nodular liver with ascites and splenomegaly. Some of the nodules showed low signal on opposed-phase (**A**) and higher signal on in-phase T1w images (**B**). Diagnosis—alcoholic hepatitis with cirrhosis.

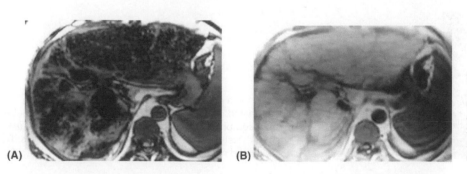

Figure 17. *Alcohol-induced steatosis with cirrhosis*: Opposed-phase (**A**) and in-phase (**B**) T1w images showed extensive fatty change with intervening areas of fibrosis. Similar appearances are seen in NASH. Also note relative enlargement of left lobe and moderate splenomegaly.

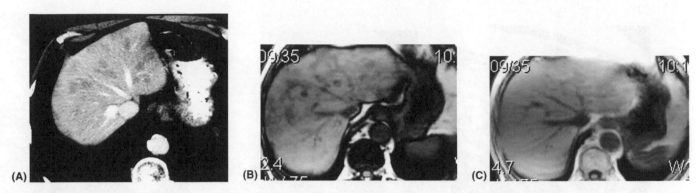

Figure 18. *Nodular fat deposition:* CT (**A**) showed multiple low attenuation nodules in the liver of a man with no history or clinical evidence of malignancy. The nodules were visible on opposed-phase (**B**), but not on in-phase T1w images (**C**).

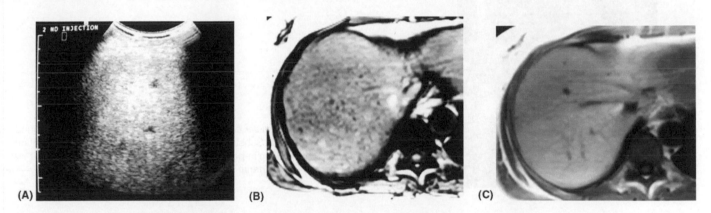

Figure 19. *Fatty infiltration with multiple small nodules of focal sparing:* Multiple echo-poor foci were found in a fatty liver at sonography (**A**). Liver architecture appeared nodular on opposed-phase (**B**) but homogeneous on in-phase T1w images (**C**).

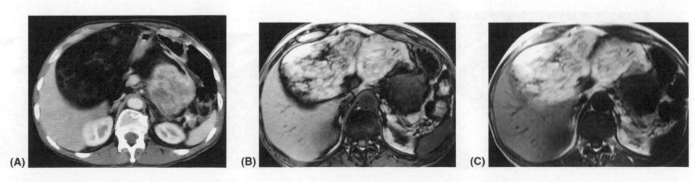

Figure 20. *Liposarcoma:* A large fat-containing tumor replaced the left lobe of liver on CT (**A**). Opposed-phase (**B**) and in-phase (**C**) T1w images showed the tumor was almost entirely fat, with phase cancellation artifact in (**B**) at the interface between liver tissue and tumor.

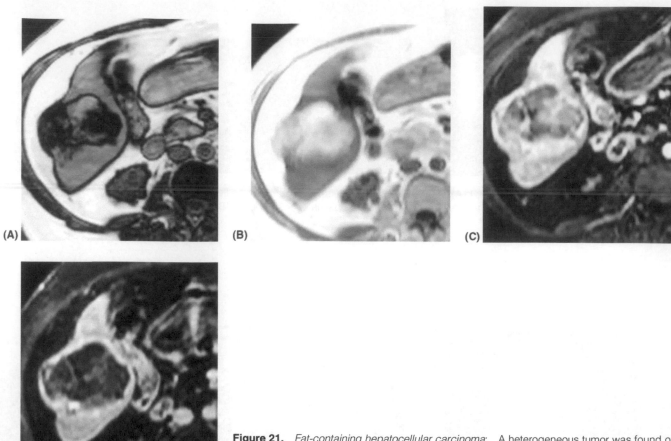

Figure 21. *Fat-containing hepatocellular carcinoma*: A heterogeneous tumor was found on sonography in a non-cirrhotic patient. Substantial areas of the tumor showed low signal on opposed-phase (**A**) and high signal on in-phase (**B**) T1w images. Patchy enhancement with gadolinium was more marked in the arterial (**C**) than in the venous phase (**D**). Histology—well-differentiated HCC.

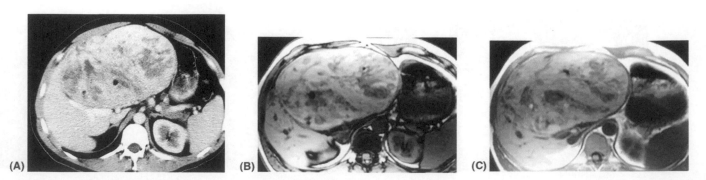

Figure 22. *Fat-containing hepatocellular carcinoma*: A large heterogeneous tumor contained small foci of very low attenuation on CT (**A**). Some of these areas were shown to be hypointense on opposed-phase (**B**) and hyperintense on in-phase T1w images (**C**). Histology—well-differentiated HCC.

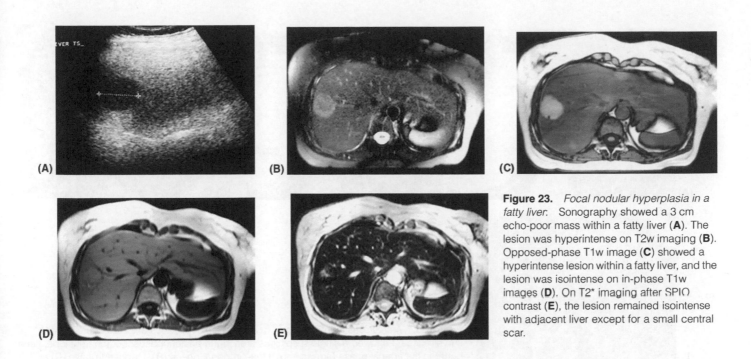

Figure 23. *Focal nodular hyperplasia in a fatty liver.* Sonography showed a 3 cm echo-poor mass within a fatty liver (**A**). The lesion was hyperintense on T2w imaging (**B**). Opposed-phase T1w image (**C**) showed a hyperintense lesion within a fatty liver, and the lesion was isointense on in-phase T1w images (**D**). On T2* imaging after SPIO contrast (**E**), the lesion remained isointense with adjacent liver except for a small central scar.

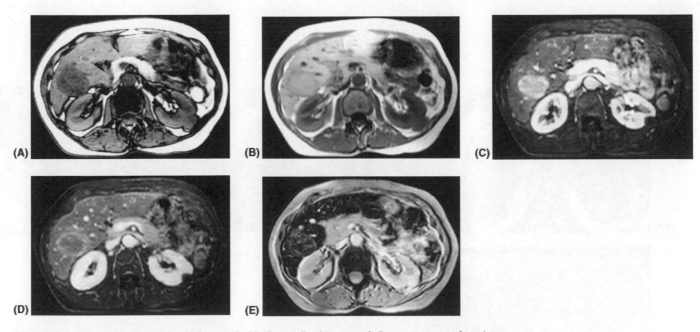

Figure 24. *Benign hepatocellular lesion, probably liver cell adenoma:* A 5-cm mass was found on sonography, within a diffusely fatty liver. Opposed-phase (**A**) and in-phase (**B**) T1w imaging confirmed diffuse fatty change in the liver, but also showed that the lesion contained more fat than the surrounding liver. After gadolinium the lesion showed marked arterial enhancement (**C**) which faded rapidly in the venous phase (**D**). With SPIO contrast (**E**) the lesion showed a degree of iron uptake almost equal to that of the surrounding liver.

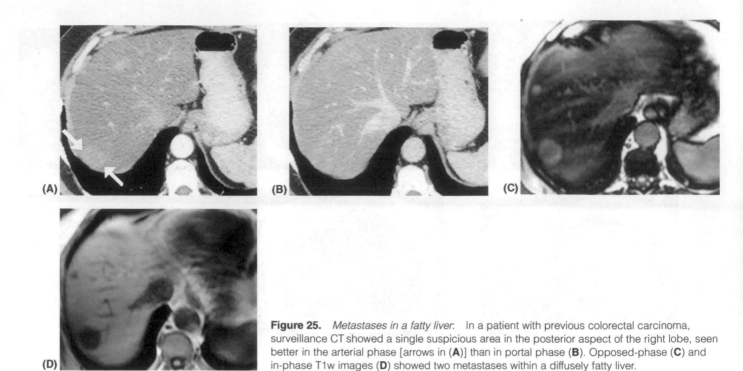

(A)

(B)

(C)

(D)

Figure 25. *Metastases in a fatty liver.* In a patient with previous colorectal carcinoma, surveillance CT showed a single suspicious area in the posterior aspect of the right lobe, seen better in the arterial phase [arrows in (**A**)] than in portal phase (**B**). Opposed-phase (**C**) and in-phase T1w images (**D**) showed two metastases within a diffusely fatty liver.

(A)

(B)

(C)

(D)

Figure 26. *Hemangioma in a fatty liver.* In a patient with a previous history of breast carcinoma, re-staging sonography showed focal lesions within a diffusely abnormal liver. Opposed-phase (**A**) and in-phase T1w images (**B**) showed a diffusely fatty liver with a 3-cm mass at the posterior aspect of the right lobe. Arterial (**C**) and delayed T1w images (**D**) after gadolinium showed typical enhancement pattern of a benign hemangioma in the right lobe, also a small area of focal nodular hyperplasia in the anterior aspect of segment 2 [arrow in (**C**)].

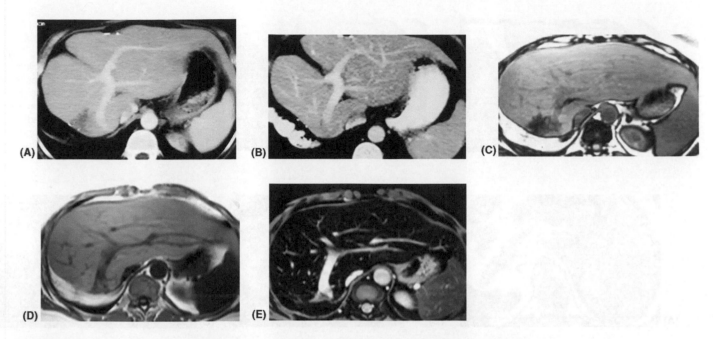

Figure 27. *Focal fat or metastasis?*: Surveillance CT one year after liver resection for colorectal metastases showed an ill-defined area of low attenuation adjacent to the cut surface of the liver (**A**) which was not visible on the immediate post-operative CT (**B**) of a year before. Opposed-phase (**C**) and in-phase T1w images (**D**) showed the abnormality to be a patch of focal fatty change. SPIO contrast was given to seek any other possible lesions—the suspicious area showed normal uptake of SPIO (**E**), confirming its benignity.

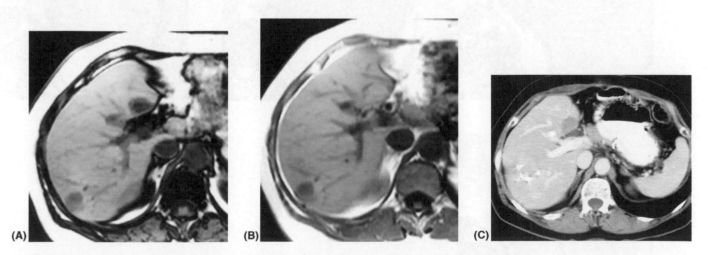

Figure 28. *Focal fat or metastasis?*: Liver CT in a patient with previous colorectal carcinoma showed a low attenuation lesion in the posterior aspect of the right lobe and a second lesion at segment 4 just anterior to the porta hepatis. Opposed-phase (**A**) and in-phase T1w images (**B**) confirmed the right lobe metastasis, but showed the segment 4 lesion to be an area of focal fatty change. Right lobe metastatectomy was performed, and further CT obtained one year later showed the segment 4 abnormality to be unchanged (**C**).

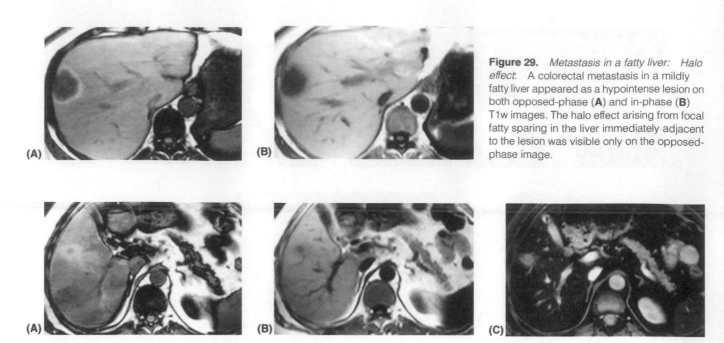

Figure 29. *Metastasis in a fatty liver: Halo effect.*   A colorectal metastasis in a mildly fatty liver appeared as a hypointense lesion on both opposed-phase (**A**) and in-phase (**B**) T1w images. The halo effect arising from focal fatty sparing in the liver immediately adjacent to the lesion was visible only on the opposed-phase image.

Figure 30.   *Metastasis in a fatty liver: Halo effect.*   Colorectal metastasis in a more severely fatty liver appeared as an isointense lesion surrounded by a halo of increased signal on the opposed-phase T1w image (**A**). The lesion was hypointense on the in-phase T1w image (**B**) where the halo was invisible. The true size of the lesion was confirmed on the post-SPIO T2*w image (**C**).

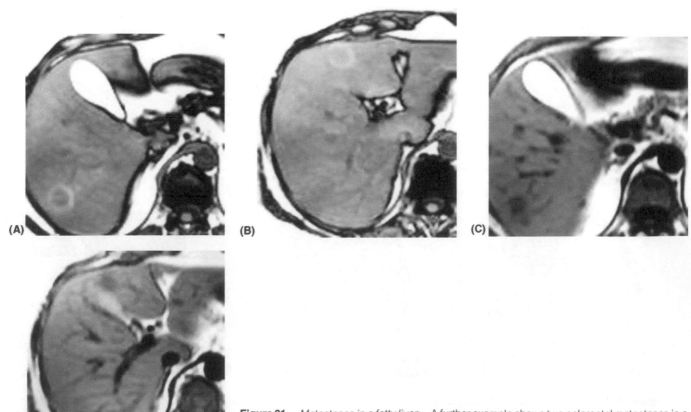

Figure 31.   *Metastases in a fatty liver.*   A further example shows two colorectal metastases in a fatty liver, each of which was surrounded by a halo of normal liver tissue highlighted on the opposed-phase T1w images (**A**, **B**). The in-phase T1w images (**C**, **D**) showed the lesions to be hypointense without the halo.

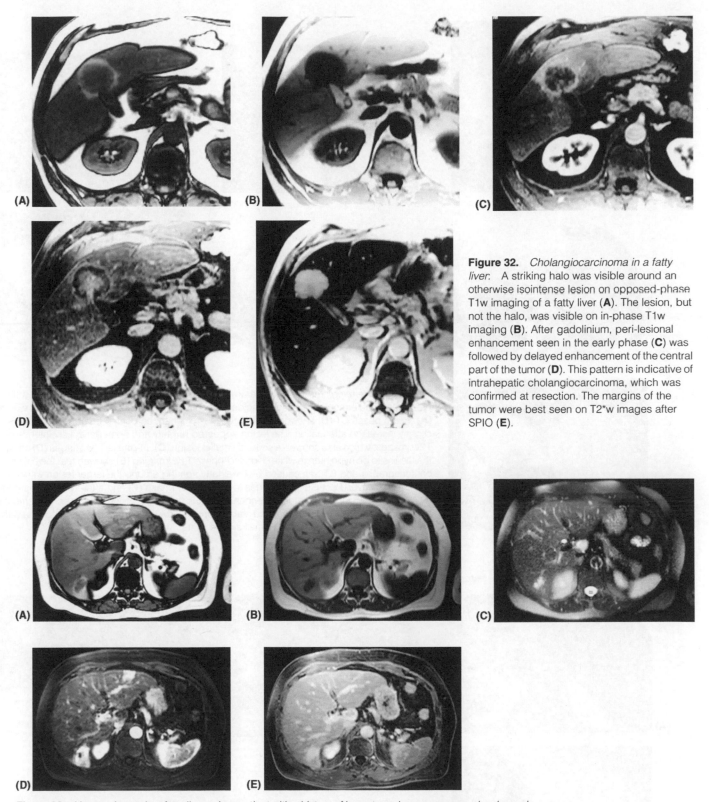

Figure 32. *Cholangiocarcinoma in a fatty liver.* A striking halo was visible around an otherwise isointense lesion on opposed-phase T1w imaging of a fatty liver (**A**). The lesion, but not the halo, was visible on in-phase T1w imaging (**B**). After gadolinium, peri-lesional enhancement seen in the early phase (**C**) was followed by delayed enhancement of the central part of the tumor (**D**). This pattern is indicative of intrahepatic cholangiocarcinoma, which was confirmed at resection. The margins of the tumor were best seen on T2*w images after SPIO (**E**).

Figure 33 *Hemangiomas in a fatty liver.* In a patient with a history of breast carcinoma, sonography showed several focal lesions within a fatty liver. Opposed-phase T1w images showed diffuse fatty infiltration plus multiple isointense lesions each surrounded by a halo of normal liver tissue (**A**). In-phase T1w images showed a liver of uniform signal containing hypointense lesions (**B**). The lesions all appeared bright on T2w images (**C**); arterial phase and delayed T1w images obtained after gadolinium (**D, E**) showed typical enhancement patterns of benign hemangiomata. Note that the 'THADs' surrounding the hemangiomas exactly correspond to the areas of focal fatty sparing shown in (**A**).

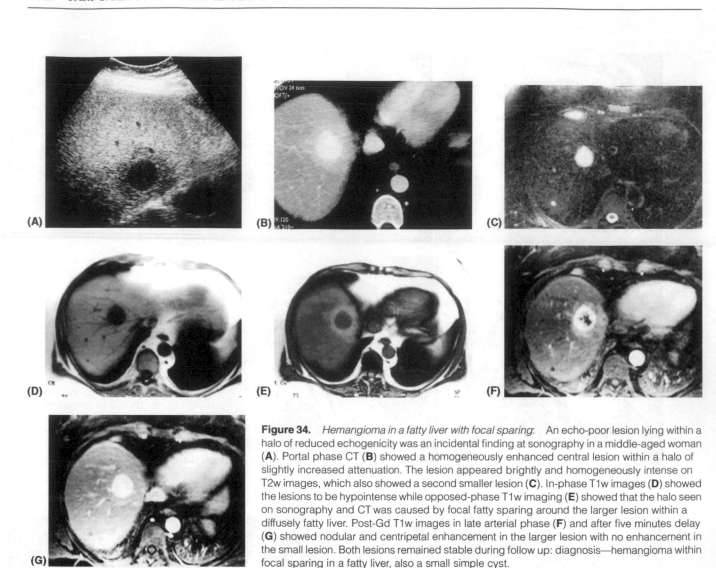

Figure 34. *Hemangioma in a fatty liver with focal sparing:* An echo-poor lesion lying within a halo of reduced echogenicity was an incidental finding at sonography in a middle-aged woman (**A**). Portal phase CT (**B**) showed a homogeneously enhanced central lesion within a halo of slightly increased attenuation. The lesion appeared brightly and homogeneously intense on T2w images, which also showed a second smaller lesion (**C**). In-phase T1w images (**D**) showed the lesions to be hypointense while opposed-phase T1w imaging (**E**) showed that the halo seen on sonography and CT was caused by focal fatty sparing around the larger lesion within a diffusely fatty liver. Post-Gd T1w images in late arterial phase (**F**) and after five minutes delay (**G**) showed nodular and centripetal enhancement in the larger lesion with no enhancement in the small lesion. Both lesions remained stable during follow up: diagnosis—hemangioma within focal sparing in a fatty liver, also a small simple cyst.

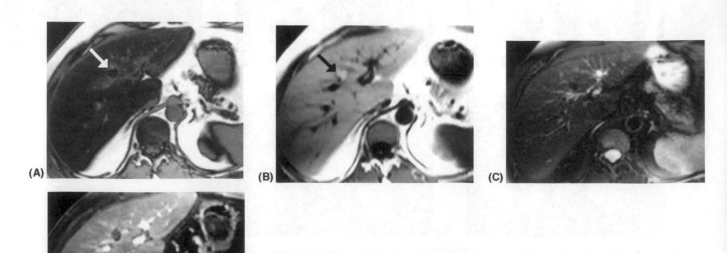

Figure 35. *Fat accumulation in RF ablation defect:* A patient underwent chemotherapy for colorectal liver metastases and then radio-frequency ablation was carried out on a residual lesion in segment 4. Post-RF opposed-phase (**A**) and in-phase T1w imaging (**B**) showed a diffusely fatty liver with an area of more marked fat accumulation at the site of ablation (arrows). The abnormality showed low signal on fat-suppressed T2w imaging (**C**) and no enhancement on T1w images after gadolinium (**D**).

CHAPTER 8

Structural and Vascular Changes in Diffuse Liver Disease

The main aim of imaging investigation is to identify the abnormal anatomy resulting from disease, so in the management of patients with diffuse liver disease imaging in general, and MRI in particular, has only a secondary role. With most forms of diffuse hepatic disorder, diagnosis is primarily based on thorough clinical assessment along with tests of liver function and immunologic screening, often supplemented by percutaneous needle biopsy of the liver. Imaging is required for the investigation of associated vascular abnormalities, particularly portal hypertension and obstructions or occlusions of hepatic veins or parts of the portal venous system. Imaging is also needed to seek evidence of other complications including local hemorrhage or infection, iron deposition, and malignant change. Finally, imaging is needed to assess the anatomic suitability of patients for liver resection or transplantation.

With this background, MR is mainly used to seek hepatocellular carcinoma (HCC) in cirrhotic patients, and to assess vascular anatomy in pre-operative cases. This chapter deals with structural and vascular changes in diffuse liver disease, while the subject of dysplasia and HCC developing in the cirrhotic liver is covered by chapter nine.

HEPATITIS AND LIVER FIBROSIS

The anatomic alterations in late stage cirrhosis are well established (see below), but the more subtle disturbances of early cirrhosis and of infective and toxic forms of hepatitis are less well established, although some studies have correlated MRI appearances with histology. However, in many cases liver involvement is heterogeneous both on imaging and at pathology, so although biopsy correlation is usually helpful and informative, it doesn't always allow the imaging findings to be explained and understood. Because of its unique magnetic properties, iron deposition is of particular interest and is discussed further below.

The pathologic processes associated with diffuse liver disease include inflammation, necrosis, regeneration, and healing by fibrosis. Edema frequently accompanies these changes and causes increased sinusoidal and venous pressures, leading to reduced portal flow and increased arterial flow. The type, severity, and chronicity of the infective or toxic agent which produces diffuse liver disease, and the possible combinations of different causative agents, produces a broad spectrum of manifestations in the patient's liver. Liver involvement is typically heterogeneous, and because liver tissue regenerates so rapidly, the appearance may change quite quickly over time.

MRI Appearances

Fibrosis produces hyperintensity on T2w and hypointensity on T1w images. Focal inflammation produces similar changes. However, post-Gd T1W images typically show that inflammatory tissue enhances rapidly in the first minute or so after injection, and the signal intensity fades thereafter. With fibrosis, enhancement is slower but persists for much longer, so the maximum contrast between fibrotic tissue and adjacent liver parenchyma is seen on delayed images, 10 minutes or more after contrast injection. Local necrosis and edema complicate matters by effectively reducing local perfusion, causing an overall diminution in tissue enhancement on post-Gd T1w images as well as local hypointensity on T1w and hyperintensity on T2w images. Fatty change is a frequent histological finding in diffuse liver disease of both acute and chronic type, but is often of minor degree and so unrecognizable on imaging. However, in some cases there are sufficient fat deposits to be detected by in-phase and opposed-phase T1w imaging. Liver fibrosis may be widespread and fairly diffuse, so producing, in combination with regenerative nodules, the honeycomb architectural pattern typical of cirrhosis, and detailed further below. Quite commonly, areas of fibrosis coalesce to form dense bands of tissue which may have a non-anatomical orientation in some patients, but in others fibrosis may be centered around the major vessels. With impairment of portal flow to one or other lobes of the liver, a unilateral fibrosis may be produced, and at segmental level, segment four is more often fibrotic or atrophied in advanced cirrhosis than other areas of the liver. Patchy fibrosis may develop as thick bands of dense fibrous tissue, or as a reticular pattern of thin plates of fibrosis. Near the liver surface, fibrosis may assume a wedge-shape, and indrawing of the liver capsule is sometimes a result.

Even when the liver parenchyma appears homogeneous on unenhanced T1w and T2w images, gadolinium enhancement often demonstrates abnormalities of perfusion. One characteristic pattern, usually associated with perivenular fibrosis on histology, shows marked peri-portal enhancement in the venous phase, producing a feathery pattern of signal intensity which highlights the unenhanced areas surrounding the main hepatic veins. This heterogeneity is generally lost on delayed images. In the hepatic venous phase, small but patent hepatic veins are visible, unlike the appearance typical of acute Budd-Chiari syndrome in which the affected hepatic veins do not fill with contrast.

Although the enhancement pattern seen typically in acute Budd-Chiari syndrome and in perivenular fibrosis appear to be specific for these pathologies, a more common manifestation of diffuse liver disease is heterogeneous arterial phase enhancement which may be widespread, focal or patchy. This pattern is non-specific and is seen in acute, sub-acute or chronic hepatitis, alcoholic liver disease, chronic Budd-Chiari, and in other forms of severe hepatic injury. In most cases the signal intensity becomes homogeneous in the venous phase but with severe inflammatory change or necrosis, heterogeneity may persist. Once extensive fibrosis has occurred, increased arterialization of the remaining parenchyma is inevitable, with the gradual obliteration of portal tracts causing diminished inflow of portal venous blood. Patients with chronic hepatic injury or hepatitis who have not yet developed established cirrhosis may still show a degree of heterogeneity of enhancement in the arterial phase, at a time when the liver is normal on unenhanced imaging, so the functional disturbance can only be detected by dynamic post-Gd T1w imaging.

IRON AND THE LIVER

Iron Metabolism

The body of the normal adult contains approximately 4 gms of iron, two thirds of which is incorporated in hemoglobin and myoglobin, and most of the other third is stored in the liver. The small remaining proportion is made up of transportable forms of iron in blood and tissues, and a small amount of iron bound within enzymes.

About 1–2 mg/day of dietary iron is normally absorbed from the intestine, and this is balanced by daily losses from skin and mucous membranes. In women during reproductive years, average daily losses and dietary absorption are both approximately doubled.

Iron is normally stored as ferritin, a molecule which comprises a protein shell enclosing a crystallised matrix of iron atoms complexed with phosphates and oxides. Iron in this form is fairly readily available for mobilization into the metabolic pool. When iron content exceeds the normal storage capacity, it is deposited as hemosiderin—an amorphous accumulation of iron oxides with protein fragments and lipids. In this form, the iron is less accessible for re-entry into the metabolic pool, so deposits of hemosiderin are less easily removed by chelation than ferritin, and may remain in tissues permanently.

Genetic Hemochromatosis

Genetic hemochromatosis (GH) is a metabolic disorder in which increased absorption of iron from the gut leads to excessive body iron stores. With advanced disease, total iron stores may rise to 40–60 gms. The defect has been linked to an abnormal gene in chromosome 6, and is transmitted as an autosomal recessive. The condition is relatively common, about one in 300 of the general population in Western countries. Although males and females are equally affected, clinical manifestations are more frequent in men because women are partly protected by normal menstrual losses. Clinical features are related to the deposition of iron in liver, pancreas, spleen, myocardium, and joints. The classic presentation is with adult onset diabetes, abnormal liver function, and increased skin pigmentation ("bronze diabetes") but this occurs in only a minority of cases. Some patients remain asymptomatic until the onset of cirrhosis and others may present for the first time with HCC.

Other Causes of Iron Overload

Iron from the breakdown of hemoglobin is normally recycled, so patients who receive transfusions for reasons other than blood loss are at risk of developing increased iron stores. The normal storage capacity of the body for iron is in the region of 10 gms, so the patients at risk are those who have received transfusions of 40–50 units of blood, or more. Iron deposition in GH is primarily in hepatocytes, but with more advanced disease the reticulo-endothelial cells of the liver, and spleen are also involved. With transfusional hemosiderosis, it is the reticulo-endothelial cells of the spleen, liver, and bone marrow which store the iron, although in the late stages iron deposition in hepatocytes and in other organs may eventually occur.

Even without transfusions, patients with some hemolytic anemias, particularly thalassaemia, also develop increased iron stores. As in GH, it is the hepatocytes which harbor most of the excess iron, since ferritin stored in the RE cells is preferentially mobilised for hemoglobin synthesis.

Excess iron deposition in hepatocytes is also a well-recognized feature of cirrhosis, particularly when resulting from alcoholic liver disease, or chronic hepatitis B or C infection. The degree of iron overload in these cases is generally much less than that typically seen with GH.

Siderotic Nodules

A second manifestation of iron deposition in the cirrhotic liver is the appearance of iron within regenerative nodules. The mechanism for this iron deposition is uncertain—it has been suggested that it could result from microscopic hemorrhages within areas of rapid parenchymal growth or possibly from the local up-regulation of transferrin receptors. Similar foci of iron deposition are not uncommon in the spleen of cirrhotic patients. The splenic foci, described as "Gamna-Gandy bodies," usually contain denser concentrations of iron than siderotic nodules in the liver, and are usually only a few mm in diameter.

Is Iron Carcinogenic?

Like other heavy metals, iron in its ionic form, particularly as $Fe3+$, has toxic effects. These appear to be related to its oxidative properties which mediate the production of free radicals. It is suggested that local toxicity produced by heavy deposition of iron in hepatocytes is responsible for stimulating periportal fibrosis leading to cirrhosis in patients with GH. HCC develops in about one third of patients with GH, but is rare in patients with other types of iron overload, unless associated with chronic hepatitis or alcoholic liver disease. There is some evidence that chronic inflammatory activity in patients with cirrhosis, particularly chronic infection with hepatitis B & C viruses, is associated with increased iron deposition in the liver and also with an increased risk of HCC, but whether it is the effect of inflammation or the iron itself which is carcinogenic is uncertain. Some clinical studies have suggested that the risk of HCC is greater in siderotic than in non-siderotic regenerative nodules, but careful explant correlations have shown only a marginal increase in the propensity to develop HCC in association with focal iron deposition.

MRI Appearances of Iron Deposition

Magnetic properties of iron vary a little according to the chemical form in which it is bound in tissues, but for practical purposes we may regard iron deposits as always being strongly paramagnetic—i.e., when placed in a strong magnetic field they become magnetized themselves—so producing local field inhomogeneities which result in loss of phase coherence in nearby protons. This effect is manifested in the images as shortening of both T1 and T2, but the T2 effects are strongly predominant. Because FSE sequences, particularly when a long echo train is used, involve repeated refocusing RF pulses, the de-phasing effects of iron deposits are minimized, so these sequences are insensitive for detecting iron deposition. Gradient echo sequences do not have these refocusing pulses, so are much more sensitive to the susceptibility effects of iron. De-phasing effects become more apparent as TE is lengthened, so a GRE T2w sequence with TE of 8–10 mSec or more is most effective for detecting iron in the liver. In order to minimize T1 effects, a flip angle of 10–30 degrees should be chosen.

Recent studies have shown good correlation between the liver-to-muscle signal intensity ratio and the histologic assessment of iron loading in liver biopsy specimens. However, because of variations in sequence parameters and differences in calibration factors between different MRI scanners, it is impossible to extrapolate specific measurements of this kind to general use. Currently, individual users still need to calibrate their own measurements with histologic results in order to predict reliably the degree of hepatic iron loading from MR measurements.

Patients with GH typically show diffuse loss of signal from the liver parenchyma, most apparent on GRE sequences with T2 weighting. With advanced disease, signal loss may also be apparent on T1w GRE sequences. A characteristic finding is that when in-phase and opposed-phase T1w GRE sequences are obtained, the liver parenchyma returns a lower signal on the in-phase image (because of its longer TE)—the opposite finding to that of fatty change. Iron deposition in the pancreas is also most apparent on T2w GRE sequences, but when severe it may also be apparent on T1w GRE images. In early stages of GH the spleen may be normal, but with more advanced disease iron deposition occurs in the spleen, and cirrhosis with portal hypertension may result in splenomegaly. Signal loss in the myocardium should be recognized as an indicator of iron deposition here, which may herald cardiac problems in patients who are candidates for liver resection or transplantation.

A similar effect of diffuse loss of signal from the liver parenchyma on T1w GRE sequences may also occur in patients with cirrhosis or in those with thalassaemia major, but in these instances the severity of the effect is relatively mild. Patients with transfusional hemosiderosis typically show marked splenic involvement and although the spleen may be enlarged, the other signs of cirrhosis are not present. As a rule of thumb, the spleen is more severely involved than the liver with transfusional iron overload, whereas the reverse is the case in GH. Siderotic nodules in both liver and spleen may be regarded as an incidental finding in the cirrhotic patient, since their significance as potential sites of malignant change remains uncertain. For further discussion of the choice of sequences for detecting iron deposition and for using iron contrast agents, see chapters 2 and 3.

BUDD-CHIARI SYNDROME

This term is used rather loosely to cover thrombotic occlusions of the hepatic veins, hepatic venous obstruction caused by webs, stenoses or membranes in the veins themselves or in the adjacent part of the inferior vena cava, and also includes varieties of hepatic veno-occlusive disease which primarily involve the small peripheral branches of the hepatic venous system. In the Western hemisphere, the most common causes of Budd-Chiari syndrome are haematological disorders associated with a thrombotic tendency, including both congenital and acquired coagulopathies and myelodysplastic syndromes. In Oriental populations, the commonest cause is a membrane or web which may sited at the ostia of the hepatic veins, or within the cava itself. Local stenosis of the cava is also commonly associated. Direct invasion of hepatic veins by HCC provides a third major cause, particularly relevant in countries where HCC is common. In a significant proportion of cases, the cause of hepatic vein thrombosis is not clear but associations are described with numerous other conditions including Bechet's disease, chronic infections, extra-hepatic malignancies, chronic hepatitis, pregnancy, and intravenous drug abuse.

Acute presentation is typically with liver enlargement, ascites of sudden onset, and abdominal pain. However, most cases are diagnosed in sub-acute or chronic phases. Ascites is a constant feature, but liver size is variable and changes in lobar architecture are almost invariably seen. Enlargement of the caudate lobe (segment 1) is almost invariably present in acute cases, and is commonly seen in chronic cases. Marked atrophy may affect either left or right lobes, more commonly the right. In sub-acute and chronic cases, secondary portal hypertension is often found with imaging evidence of varices and splenomegaly. Patients are often jaundiced with abnormal liver function tests. Quite commonly, hepatic vein thrombosis involves only part of the liver and in the chronic phase this leads to atrophy of the affected segments and hypertrophy of the unaffected areas.

MRI Appearances

Imaging findings are widely variable, depending on the extent of liver involvement and the timescale of onset—whether acute, sub-acute or chronic. Most patients show enlargement of the embryological dorsal liver—ie the caudate lobe and the pericaval (central) portions of the right lobe segments. Diffuse congestion causes liver enlargement in the acute phase, while atrophy of the peripheral areas of the affected lobes or segments is more common in the chronic phase. Relative hypertrophy of the left lobe is seen in about half of chronic cases.

Ascites is almost invariably present, while features of secondary portal hypertension are fairly common, including splenomegaly, and varices. Enlargement of the azygous and hemi-azygous veins is a useful pointer to this complication.

The appearances on unenhanced images reflect the distribution of edema resulting from venous congestion within the liver, which is manifest as areas of relative hypointensity on T1w and hyperintensity on T2w images. The distribution and severity of the signal change varies with the extent and the timescale of the disease. In the acute phase, the abnormal signal is most marked around the periphery of the liver and may also be seen surrounding the hepatic vein branches producing a feathery pattern. This feature is best demonstrated in the portal phase of post-Gd T1w imaging, when normal enhancement around the portal tracts contrasts with the diminished enhancement around the hepatic vein radicals. In the more common sub-acute and chronic phases, the changes of local edema and perfusion abnormalities are usually more patchy, although the anatomic distribution may be correlated with segmental or lobar venous occlusions. In well-established chronic cases, the parenchymal liver signal may be normal on unenhanced images, with homogenous enhancement on post-Gd T1w imaging indicating uniform perfusion. Chronic cases often show collateral veins bridging between the portal inflow and systemic outflow routes which bypass the occluded hepatic veins. Most commonly these collaterals are seen over the liver surface, but bridging veins may also be seen within the liver parenchyma. In chronic cases, regenerative nodules are frequently found. These are areas of hyperplastic liver parenchyma which histologically resemble focal nodular hyperplasia. The nodules are most often of sub-cm size, but may be up to 3–4 cm diameter. They appear mildly hyperintense or isointense on T1w, and usually isointense on T2w imaging. On post-Gd T1w images the nodules are most commonly hypervascular in the arterial phase, but if malignancy is suspected, their benign nature can be confirmed by their normal uptake of SPIO contrast.

The hepatic veins may be shown to contain uniformly hypointense material which does not enhance on post-Gd T1w images, indicating thrombus, but quite frequently the veins cannot be distinguished from the surrounding liver parenchyma. Patent hepatic veins in the presence of other features of Budd-Chiari syndrome should prompt a search for a web either at the ostia of the veins or in the adjacent sub-diaphragmatic cava. The intra-hepatic segment of the cava is usually compressed side-to-side to leave only a narrow slit. If this part of the cava remains widely open, it is again suggestive of a web or stenosis more superiorly, typically just below the diaphragm.

In those cases of Budd-Chiari syndrome in which the etiology is uncertain, a search must be made for potential causes, particularly focal malignancy either within the liver or elsewhere in the upper abdomen. In patients with a thrombotic tendency, venous occlusions should be sought in the portal system, particularly as their presence may influence the possibility of surgical or endovascular interventional treatment.

CIRRHOSIS

Cirrhosis is a chronic disorder of the liver characterized by liver cell damage, regeneration, and fibrosis. The objectives of imaging in cirrhosis are firstly to seek morphologic evidence of the disease including changes in the size and shape of the liver, nodularity of the liver architecture, and the presence of portal hypertension manifested by ascites, splenomegaly, and varices. Secondly, although in most cases the cause of cirrhosis is determined from clinical and immunologic examination, specific MRI appearances are found in cirrhosis occurring with hemochromatosis or primary sclerosing cholangitis (PSC). A third objective is to detect the development of HCC, discussed in the next chapter.

Lobar Morphology in Cirrhosis

As cirrhosis progresses, the liver typically becomes smaller although occasionally normal liver size is maintained in late stage disease. In the majority of cases the right lobe undergoes more severe shrinkage than the left, so the left appears relatively large and sometimes there is genuine hypertrophy of the left lobe. This common discrepancy between left and right lobes may be the result of laminar flow in the portal vein causing toxins or infectious agents from the intestine preferentially to enter the right lobe, but this explanation fails to account for the relative predominance of the left lobe in patients with late stage sclerosing cholangitis or biliary cirrhosis, so other mechanisms are probably at work as well.

Occasionally, the left lobe may be particularly atrophied. Enlargement of the caudate lobe (segment 1) is a very common feature in patients with Budd-Chiari syndrome, probably because the venous drainage of this segment involves several small veins directly entering the intrahepatic inferior vena cava. However, hypertrophy of the caudate lobe also occurs in a substantial proportion of patients with advanced cirrhosis from other causes and may occur in patients with non-cirrhotic portal hypertension where patterns of portal flow are disturbed. Shrinkage of the liver in cirrhosis often produces a gap between the left and right lobes—the "expanded gallbladder fossa" sign—which is usually filled by the hepatic flexure of the colon.

The Nodular Architecture of the Cirrhotic Liver

Once cirrhosis is well-established, bands of fibrosis separate nodules of regenerating liver tissue which may vary from a few mm to several cm in size. Fibrotic change in the liver begins at a microscopic level and progresses by coalescence of areas of fibrosis to isolate nodules of macroscopic size. At the time of diagnosis, cirrhosis may be described as micro-nodular (the majority of nodules smaller than 3–5 mm size) or macro-nodular with individual nodules varying in size up to several cm diameter. On unenhanced MR images, fibrosis first appears as areas of hypointensity on T1w imaging, and at a more advanced stage becomes visible as a hyperintense network on T2w images. The fibrotic tissue enhances slowly with gadolinium so the recticular pattern is often less apparent on early post-Gd acquisitions than on unenhanced T1w images, but becomes clearer on delayed images when the parenchymal enhancement has faded and the fibrotic elements remain enhanced. The most effective demonstration of the liver architecture is seen after SPIO contrast, when the islands of liver tissue show very low signal separated by bright bands of fibrosis, an appearance reminiscent of CT of the lung with interstitial fibrosis. Whatever size they are, benign regenerative nodules show similar characteristics. They typically show the same signal intensity as normal liver on unenhanced T1w and T2w images, uniform enhancement in the portal venous phase following gadolinium, and uniform uptake of SPIO. Recent explant evidence has highlighted a minority of regenerative nodules which show hyperintensity on T1w imaging, although they remain isointense on T2w images and show portal phase enhancement after gadolinium.

PORTAL HYPERTENSION AND PORTAL VEIN THROMBOSIS

In the Western hemisphere, portal hypertension is most commonly the result of chronic liver disease, usually cirrhosis, occasionally secondary to Budd-Chiari syndrome or portal vein involvement by hepatic tumors. In a minority of cases, portal hypertension results from extra-hepatic causes, usually either as a complication of umbilical vein catheterization in infancy, or of gastro-intestinal sepsis in childhood or adult life. Left-sided varices typically result from inflammatory or neoplastic disease of the pancreas, and sporadic cases of portal thrombosis are seen in patients with thrombotic tendencies of any cause. In demonstrating the major features of portal hypertension—ascites, splenomegaly, and varices—MRI adds little to the information available from CT, while sonography is the first choice procedure for demonstrating the patency of the main vessels and the adequacy of flow within them. However, a demonstration of the anatomy and abnormalities of the portal venous system can be obtained without additional sequences or contrast injections, so this aspect can form part of the routine assessment of the liver by MRI.

MRI Appearances

Ascitic fluid shows uniformly high signal on T2w and low signal on T1w images. When the volume is large, pulsation or eddy currents within the fluid may mimic filling defects, particularly on GRE T2w images. Moderate or severe splenic enlargement is readily recognized, but mild degrees may be difficult to distinguish from the normal range. The spleen gradually diminishes in size with increasing age from early adult-hood onwards, and also varies in volume in proportion to the size of the patient. As a rough guide, the inferior pole of the spleen rarely projects anterior to the mid-axillary line in normal subjects.

Varices and porto-systemic shunts occur in numerous sites and only the most clinically significant will be discussed here. Varices in the wall of the lower oesophagus, around the gastric cardia and along the lesser curve of the stomach form the major source of gastrointestinal hemorrhage in patients with liver disease. These veins develop from collateral pathways between the short gastric veins communicating between the stomach and the spleen, and the gastric coronary (left gastric) vein which normally drains blood from the lesser curve of the stomach to join the portal vein just above the confluence of splenic and superior mesenteric veins. Superiorly, gastroesophageal varices drain into the azygous and hemi-azygous systems. The right anterior oblique coronal plane usually gives a good demonstration of esophageal varices in post-Gd T1w imaging. At the opposite end of the GI tract, collaterals may develop between peripheral branches of the inferior mesenteric vein around the rectum and distal colon, and perineal veins draining into the internal iliac veins. When manifest as haemorrhoids, these varices are not a problem for imaging, but when they occur in the sigmoid colon or elsewhere in the pelvis, they present an opportunity for misdiagnosis as a vascular tumor, and can incur a risk of post-operative bleeding in patients undergoing liver resection or transplantation. On coronal post-Gd T1w imaging, a clue to the presence of pelvic varices is often provided by the presence of large abnormal vessels with a non-anatomic orientation. A further common site of porto-systemic shunting develops when varices around the hilum of the spleen and the tail of the pancreas connect via retroperitoneal branches and drain into the left renal vein (spontaneous spleno-renal shunt). The main significance of this shunt is that if the flow through it is large, a "steal" phenomenon may develop leading to reduced portal venous inflow after transplantation, with the associated risk of portal vein thrombosis. If the shunt is recognized on pre-operative imaging, it can be closed surgically at the time of transplantation. In some such cases, post-Gd T1w images in the coronal plane will show large varices draining directly into the left renal vein. In other cases the communication can be indirectly detected by the presence of an abnormally distended left renal vein along with large varices in the left upper quadrant, even if the actual communication is not visualized. Another common site of porto-systemic shunting is the para-umbilical venous system. In patients with portal hypertension, these veins drain blood from the left portal vein near the left margin of segment 4 and track alongside the falciform ligament to communicate with veins in the abdominal wall in the region of the umbilicus. Less commonly, communication between the intrahepatic portal vein branches and systemic veins in the abdominal and chest wall develop by enlargement of the superior epigastric vein, the veins of Bulow, and the superior and inferior veins of Sappey.

With variceal porto-systemic shunts draining more and more of the portal venous blood as the severity of portal hypertension increases, flow through the main portal vein becomes less and less, and eventually the direction of flow may reverse when fibrosis causes sinusoidal pressure to exceed portal venous inflow pressure. Sluggish or reversed flow incurs a high risk of venous thrombosis, which should be demonstrated by imaging before therapeutic manoeuvres such as TIPSS placement or liver transplantation. The portal vein is a common site for non-occlusive thrombosis, which often appears as an eccentric filling defect reducing the lumen to a thin slit on one side of the vein. The thrombus may extend into intrahepatic portal branches, or into the termination of the superior mesenteric vein. Occasionally focal thrombi are seen within the intrahepatic portal branches, or localized to either splenic or superior mesenteric veins. With total occlusion of the portal vein, collateral flow typically develops in peri-portal veins giving the appearance described as cavernous transformation. The veins usually involved represent the peri-biliary plexus described by Couinaud and possibly the vasa vasorum of the portal vein itself. Occasionally varices may themselves become thrombosed.

In patients with advanced cirrhosis, bland thrombus in the portal vein or its divisions must be distinguished from tumor invasion. The main diagnostic features are that tumor thrombi tend to expand the veins which they invade, and show at least some degree of patchy enhancement on post-Gd T1w imaging. Bland thrombus does not enhance (except during recanalization), and only rarely expands the lumen of the affected veins. Bland thrombus is usually uniformly hypointense on T1w imaging, although if acute it may contain areas of relative hyperintensity. Whenever portal vein thrombosis is seen in a cirrhotic patient, a careful search should be made for an underlying HCC.

OTHER NON-CIRRHOTIC CONDITIONS CAUSING DISTURBED LIVER ARCHITECTURE

The liver is sometimes described as a chemical factory, because of its central role in metabolism and biosynthesis. As in other chemical factories, these processes produce toxic waste, which accounts for the relatively short lifespan of hepatocytes. Rapid regeneration of liver parenchyma is a normal response to liver cell injury of any type, so perhaps it is not surprising that several different abnormalities of liver architecture can be produced by a wide range of causes. All the conditions described below can produce local, regional or diffuse structural change in the liver, but are distinguishable from cirrhosis. In most cases the pathogenesis of these conditions is not well understood, but two of the processes which appear to be involved are desmoplastic fibrosis, and hyperplastic vascular regeneration at lobular or sinusoidal level. The exact cause of most of these conditions remains uncertain, but associations with chronic systemic illness, autoimmune disorders, infections, malignancies, and external toxins are all well established.

NODULAR REGENERATIVE HYPERPLASIA

This condition is characterized by the presence of regenerative nodules of liver parenchyma, but differs from cirrhosis in that there is little or no fibrosis. The hepatocytes are usually normal, although some dysplastic features have been described. When fibrosis does occur, it is usually located around the portal tracts, and obliteration of portal vein radicles can lead to portal hypertension. More commonly, the patients are asymptomatic and the condition is discovered incidentally. The nodules vary from a few mm to several cm in size and when small may be undetectable on imaging. NRH probably develops as a hyperplastic response to local blood flow changes within the liver, but the exact mechanism is uncertain. Cases have been described in association with exposure to toxic drugs or chemicals, systemic autoimmune disorders, myeloproliferative, and lymphoproliferative disorders, bowel cancer, and following transplantation of bone marrow and kidney.

MRI Appearances

Reported experience with imaging and in particular with MRI is limited to small numbers of cases. In some patients, particularly those with micronodular disease, the liver appears normal. Visible nodules have most often been hypo- or isoattenuating on CT. Signal intensity on unenhanced T1w and T2w imaging has been variously described as hypo-, iso- or hyperintense to adjacent liver. Enhancement of the nodules with gadolinium may be similar to that of normal liver, but some nodules show increased enhancement either diffusely or around the periphery of the lesion. Peripheral peliotic change has been reported histologically in conjunction with a hyper-enhancing rim. In our experience, the uptake of liver-specific contrast agents into the nodules is similar to that of normal liver.

Differential diagnosis from cirrhotic nodules is usually clear from the clinical context and the lack of fibrosis between the nodules on imaging, while the behavior of the nodules with liver-specific contrast agents allows them to be differentiated from malignant tumors.

PELIOSIS

This rare condition is manifest by the presence of dilated vascular spaces which may be multifocal or diffuse throughout the liver. Pathology shows areas of sinusoidal dilatation associated with enlarged feeding vessels and arteriovenous shunts. As with NRH, the pathogenesis is not clear. Causative factors include therapy with anabolic or contraceptive steroids, HIV-related bacterial infections, and other wasting diseases, particularly tuberculosis or malignancy.

MRI Appearances

In the few cases described so far, attention has been drawn to multiple foci which are hypointense on T1w and hyperintense on T2w imaging. Pronounced portal phase enhancement in these areas occurs with post-Gd T1w imaging and in some cases arterial phase hyperintensity has been shown. Peliosis may be associated with regenerative nodules, producing an appearance which could be suggestive of malignancy. However, uptake of liver-specific contrast agents into the nodular components will indicate their benign nature.

HEREDITARY HAEMORRHAGIC TELANGIECTASIA

Hereditary haemorrhagic telangiectasia (HHT) is a familial disorder with autosomal dominant transmission in which vascular malformations develop in multiple sites. The liver is involved in about 30% of cases. The vascular anomalies cause arteriovenous shunting which leads to the typical clinical presentation of high output cardiac failure. Pulmonary hypertension is not infrequent. When the liver is involved, portal hypertension may develop, probably as a result of arterio-portal shunting within the liver.

MRI Appearances

As with peliosis, the characteristic appearance is of multiple vascular malformations scattered through the liver. Increased hepatic arterial flow may be detected on Doppler sonography, CT or angiography. MRI shows numerous irregular foci of hypointensity on T1w and hyperintensity on T2w images, with prominence of the hepatic arteries and marked portal phase enhancement in the vascular lesions on post-Gd T1w images.

PSEUDO-CIRRHOSIS

In this rare condition an appearance which on imaging is indistinguishable from cirrhosis develops during or after chemotherapy for malignant disease. In the weeks or months following commencement of chemotherapy, the liver becomes nodular in contour with widespread fibrosis and areas of regeneration. Portal hypertension may develop and liver function tests may show the typical abnormalities of cirrhosis. This condition has been most often seen in patients with breast carcinoma, also with lymphoma. Histologically, the appearances are very similar to those of established cirrhosis, the main distinguishing feature being the absence of bridging fibrosis between the portal tracts. In most cases histology shows evidence of diffuse tumor infiltration, but the condition has also been described in patients undergoing chemotherapy in the absence of liver metastasis.

Anecdotal observations suggest a milder form of this condition occurs in some patients undergoing chemotherapy for metastatic liver disease from colorectal cancer, particularly when platinum-based drugs are being used. The livers often show a degree of fatty change, the liver parenchyma appears friable at surgery, and transient fibrosis has been observed during the chemotherapy.

A further manifestation of a fibrotic response to malignancy is seen in some patients with liver metastases in whom a desmoplastic reaction takes place around the tumor deposits. In combination with tumor shrinkage during chemotherapy, the fibrosis can result in the liver developing a heterogeneous appearance on imaging with patchy fibrosis but no visible residual tumor (see also chapter 12).

POST-NECROTIC SCARRING

In patients with very severe hepatitis, either infective or induced by alcohol or toxic drugs, acute hepatic necrosis may occur. If the patient survives, healing often results in extensive scarring producing bands of dense fibrosis separated by nodules of regenerating liver tissue, giving a similar macroscopic appearance to cirrhosis. The clinical presentation should give an indication of the diagnosis, but distinction between fulminant hepatitis and acute alcoholic hepatitis superimposed on cirrhosis may be impossible without histology.

ILLUSTRATIVE FIGURES

Fibrosis and edema—Figures 1–12
Iron deposition—Figures 13–21
Hepatic vein occlusion—Figures 22–29
Cirrhosis—lobar changes—Figures 30–38
Cirrhosis—nodular architecture—Figures 39–48
Portal hypertension—varices and shunts—Figures 49–58
Portal hypertension—venous occlusion—Figures 59–69
Mimics of cirrhosis—Figures 70–77

REFERENCES

1. Ito K, Mitchell DG, Siegelman ES. Cirrhosis: MR imaging features. Magn Reson Imaging Clin N Am 2002; 10:75–92.
2. Kanematsu M, Danet MI, Leonardou P, et al. Early hetereogeneous enhancement of the liver: magnetic resonance imaging findings and clinical significance. J Magn Reson Imaging 2004; 20:242–249.
3. Martin DR, Seibert D, Yang M, et al. Reversible heterogeneous arterial phase liver perfusion associated with transient acute hepatitis: findings on gadolinium-enhanced MRI. J Magn Reson Imaging 2004; 20:838–842.
4. Pomeranz S, Siegelman ES. MR imaging of iron depositional disease. Magn Reson Imaging Clin N Am 2002; 10:105–120.

5. Alustiza JM, Artetxe J, Castiella A, et al. MR quantification of hepatic iron concentration. Radiology 2004; 230:479–484.

6. Gandon Y, Olivie D, Guyader D, et al. Non-invasive assessment of hepatic iron stores by MRI. Lancet 2004; 363:357–362.

7. Noone TC, Semelka RC, Siegelman ES, et al. Budd-Chiari syndrome: spectrum of appearances of acute, subacute and chronic disease with magnetic resonance imaging. Magn Reson Imaging 2000; 11:44–50.

8. Cazals-Hatem D, Vilgrain V, Genin P, et al. Arterial and portal circulation and parenchymal changes in Budd-Chiari syndrome: a study of 17 explanted livers. Hepatology 2003; 37:510–519.

9. Casillas C, Marti-Bonmati L, Galant J. Pseudotumoral presentation of nodular regenerative hyperplasia of the liver: imaging in five patients including MR imaging. Eur Radiol 1997; 7:654–658.

10. Verswijvel G, Janssens F, Colla P, et al. Peliosis hepatis presenting as a multifocal hepatic pseudotumor: MR findings in two cases. Eur Radiol 2003; 4:L40–L44.

11. Gupta AA, Kim DC, Krinsky GA, et al. CT and MRT of cirrhosis and its mimics. AJR 2004; 183:1595–1601.

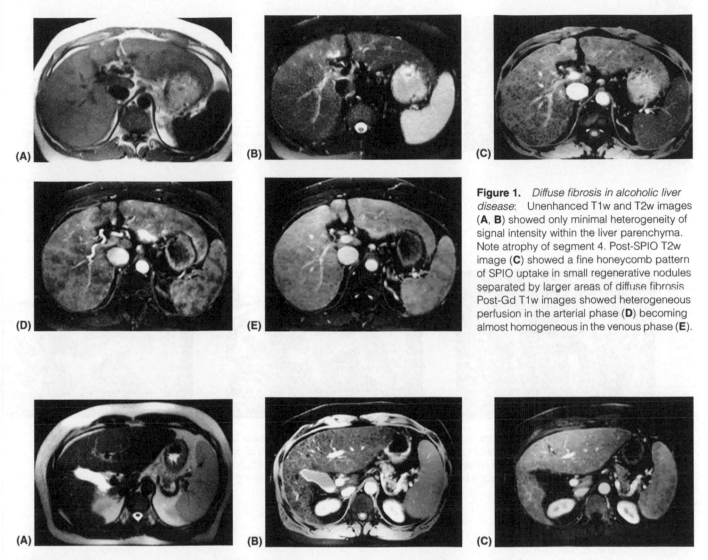

Figure 1. *Diffuse fibrosis in alcoholic liver disease:* Unenhanced T1w and T2w images (**A**, **B**) showed only minimal heterogeneity of signal intensity within the liver parenchyma. Note atrophy of segment 4. Post-SPIO T2w image (**C**) showed a fine honeycomb pattern of SPIO uptake in small regenerative nodules separated by larger areas of diffuse fibrosis. Post-Gd T1w images showed heterogeneous perfusion in the arterial phase (**D**) becoming almost homogeneous in the venous phase (**E**).

Figure 2. *Diffuse fibrosis from hepatitis C:* T2w image (**A**) showed splenomegaly and marked atrophy of the right lobe, but the liver signal was homogeneous. Post-SPIO T2w imaging (**B**) showed small foci of normal SPIO contrast uptake separated by large areas of diminished uptake. Post-Gd T1w portal phase image (**C**) showed homogenous enhancement, suggesting the patchy loss of function in the liver tissue was due to inflammatory change or fine fibrosis.

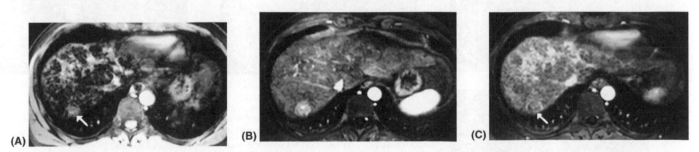

Figure 3. *Patchy fibrosis and HCC:* In a patient with established cirrhosis, post-SPIO T2w imaging (**A**) showed bands and streaks of non-functioning liver tissue, most marked in segments 8 and 4; note also the tumor nodule at the posterior aspect of segment 7 (arrow). Post-Gd arterial phase T1w imaging (**B**) showed a hypervascular nodule posteriorly, but only moderate heterogeneity of perfusion elsewhere. The delayed image (**C**) showed late enhancement of the fibrotic areas in segments 8 and 4, while the hepatocellular carcinoma in segment 7 (arrow) returned almost to isointensity.

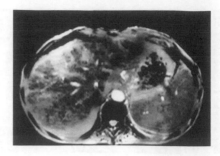

Figure 4.   *Patchy fibrosis*:   In this cirrhotic patient, post-SPIO T2w imaging showed multiple peripheral areas of loss of function indicating wedges of fibrosis radiating out from the porta.

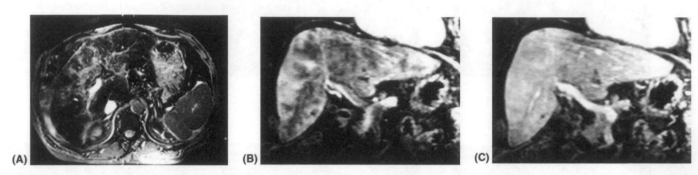

(A)   **(B)**   **(C)**

Figure 5.   *Patchy fibrosis*:   In a patient with alcoholic liver disease, post-SPIO T2w image (**A**) showed ill-defined bands of streaky fibrosis separating areas of relatively normal liver tissue. Coronal oblique post-Gd T1w images showed patchy peripheral enhancement in the arterial phase (**B**) with relative lack of enhancement of the perivenular parenchyma, but by the portal phase more homogeneous enhancement developed (**C**).

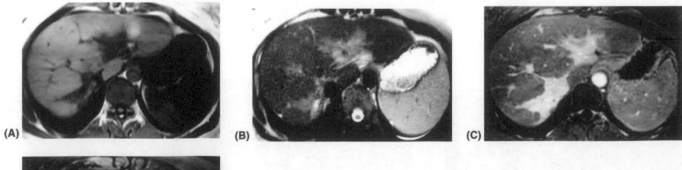

(A)   **(B)**   **(C)**

(D)

Figure 6.   *Perivascular fibrosis*:   Unenhanced T1w and T2w images (**A**, **B**) showed ill-defined areas of hypo- and hyperintensity respectively, surrounding the hepatic veins and IVC, and encompassing the main portal divisions near the liver hilum. Delayed post-Gd T1w images (**C**) showed persistent enhancement in these same areas, suggesting fibrotic change. Post-SPIO T2w imaging (**D**) showed the true extent of the fibrosis to be less marked than on (**C**). The difference in the extent of abnormality shown on (**C**) and (**D**) is explained by the persistent post-Gd enhancement of inflamed liver parenchyma, which nevertheless takes up SPIO almost normally, whereas fibrotic tissue—which also shows persistent post-Gd enhancement—takes up no SPIO.

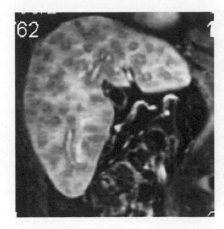

Figure 7. *Perivenular fibrosis*: Venous phase post-Gd T1w imaging showed a characteristic pattern of diminished enhancement surrounding small hepatic vein branches throughout the liver. The venules are clearly patent in this case, otherwise the appearances are very similar to those seen transiently in post-Gd images in Budd-Chiari syndrome. Biopsy confirmed perivenular fibrosis.

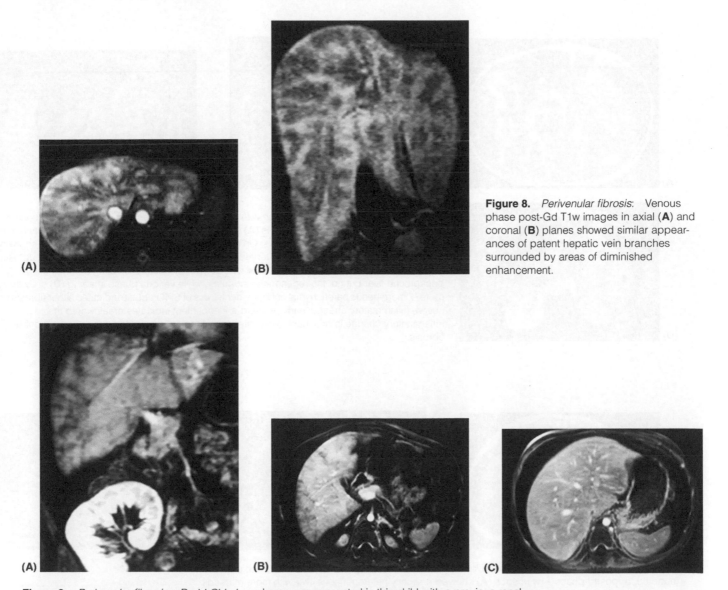

Figure 8. *Perivenular fibrosis*: Venous phase post-Gd T1w images in axial (**A**) and coronal (**B**) planes showed similar appearances of patent hepatic vein branches surrounded by areas of diminished enhancement.

Figure 9. *Perivenular fibrosis*: Budd-Chiari syndrome was suspected in this child with a previous renal transplant; coronal (**A**) and axial (**B**) post-Gd T1w venous phase images showed patent hepatic vein branches, but persistent heterogeneity of peripheral perfusion, which became homogeneous by 10 minutes after injection (**C**). Biopsy confirmed perivenular fibrosis with patent hepatic venules.

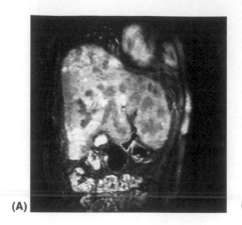

(A)

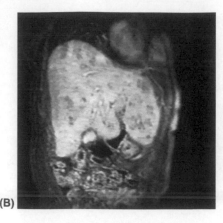

(B)

Figure 10. *Perivenular fibrosis*: In a cirrhotic patient post-Gd T1w coronal images showed heterogeneous enhancement in the early venous phase (**A**) with non-enhancing areas surrounding hepatic vein branches, and although the venules are shown to be patent in the later venous image (**B**), there is still a cuff of perivascular non-enhancing tissue around them.

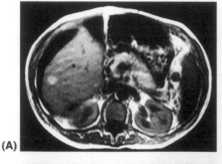

(A)

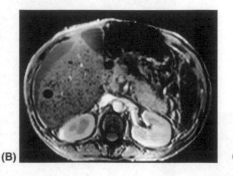

(B)

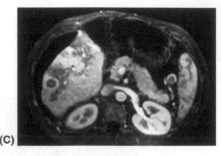

(C)

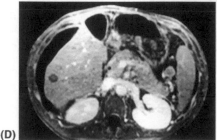

(D)

Figure 11. *Fibrosis and inflammation with regenerative nodules*: In a patient with alcoholic liver disease, unenhanced T1w images (**A**) showed mild heterogeneity of signal intensity of the liver with several hyperintense nodules. On post-SPIO T2w imaging (**B**) the nodules all showed normal uptake of contrast, while the intervening liver tissue showed severely diminished uptake. Post-Gd T1w arterial phase imaging (**C**) showed hypervascularity affecting much of the background liver but not the regenerative nodules, while venous phase imaging (**D**) showed a more homogeneous parenchymal enhancement. Loss of SPIO uptake indicates either fibrosis or severe inflammatory change; early post-Gd enhancement indicates areas where the inflammatory change is dominant, while later enhancement suggests a major component of fibrosis.

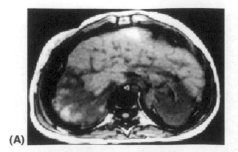

(A)

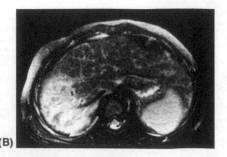

(B)

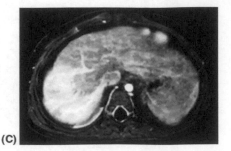

(C)

Figure 12. *Fibrosis and inflammation in lobular hepatitis*: In a 3-year-old child with acute onset of jaundice, opposed-phase T1w images (**A**) showed a slightly heterogeneous liver with more marked hypointensity in the right lobe. T2w imaging showed marked but heterogeneous hyperintensity affecting the right lobe with a little streaky hyperintensity elsewhere in the liver. Post-Gd T1w venous phase images (**C**) showed hypervascularity in the affected area of the right lobe and in the streaky fibrotic areas in the left lobe. Biopsy confirmed lobular hepatitis with a fibrotic component as well as a major inflammatory element.

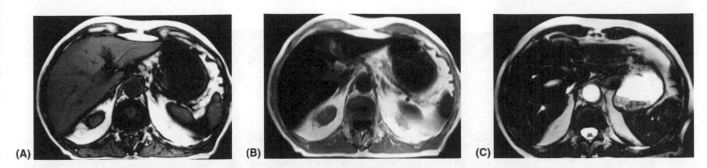

Figure 13. *Genetic hemochromatosis*: Opposed-phase T1w imaging (**A**) showed liver signal intensity to be approximately equal to that of kidney and muscle. On the in-phase T1w images (**B**), the liver parenchyma was markedly hypointense to kidney and muscle, indicating diffuse iron deposition. Liver signal intensity was also less than usual on the true FISP image (**C**). The loss of signal caused by iron deposition increases with TE—the echo times of (**A**), (**B**) and (**C**) were 2.4, 4.7 and 3.5 m sec respectively.

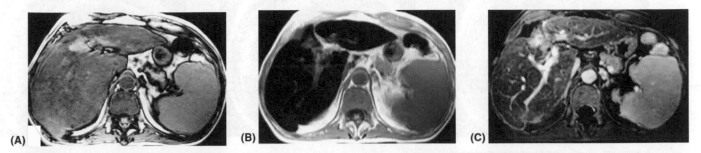

Figure 14. *Diffuse iron overload*: Opposed-phase T1w image (**A**) showed mild hypointensity of the liver parenchyma compared to spleen. In-phase T1w imaging (**B**) showed dramatic signal loss throughout the liver. Post-Gd T1w images (**C**) showed relatively normal enhancement. Note the mild left lobe atrophy with particular shrinkage of segment 4, which also contains an area of fibrosis with marked venous phase enhancement after gadolinium, and no iron deposition.

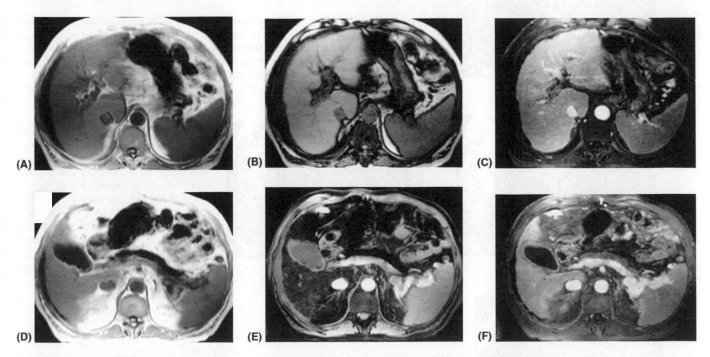

Figure 15. *Genetic hemochromatosis with pancreatic involvement*: In-phase, opposed-phase and post-Gd T1w images (**A**, **B**, **C**) showed cirrhotic changes with nodular liver contour and a little ascites. The liver parenchyma showed only a mild signal loss on the in-phase image, so the degree of iron deposition would be in keeping with cirrhosis from non-GH causes. However, the T1w in-phase images through the pancreas (**D**) showed extreme hypointensity of the pancreatic parenchyma which was confirmed on unenhanced GRE T2W images (**E**), also with sub-normal pancreatic enhancement on post-Gd T1w imaging (**F**).

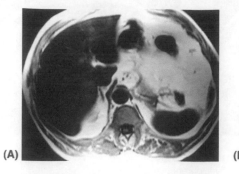

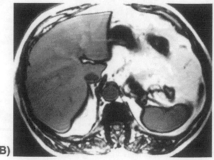

Figure 16. *Genetic hemochromatosis*: No signs of cirrhosis were found in this patient with a moderate degree of hypointensity on the in-phase (**A**) compared with the opposed-phase (**B**) T1w images; on other slices an advanced hepatocellular carcinoma was shown.

(A)   (B)

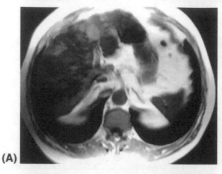

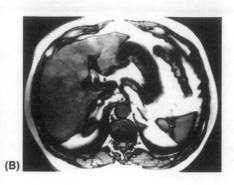

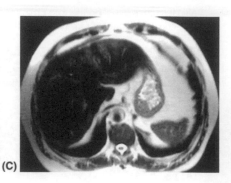

(A)   (B)   (C)

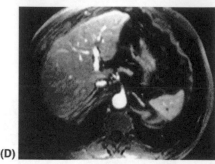

(D)

Figure 17. *Combined iron and fat deposits*: In a patient with alcoholic liver disease, in-phase T1w imaging (**A**) showed patchy areas of hypo- and hyperintensity compared with the opposed-phase image (**B**). HASTE images (**C**) also showed a mild heterogeneity of liver parenchyma suggesting patchy edema or inflammatory change. Post-Gd T1w imaging (**D**) showed persistent but minimal heterogeneity of the parenchyma.

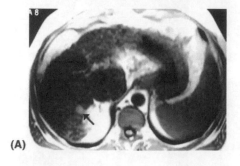

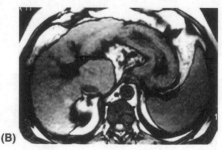

(A)   (B)

Figure 18. *Mild iron deposition in cirrhosis*: In a patient with morphologic changes of cirrhosis (atrophic liver with hypertrophied caudate lobe, nodular contour, heterogeneous architecture and splenomegaly), diffuse iron deposition was indicated by the generalised hypointensity of liver tissue on T1w in-phase images (**A**) compared with opposed-phase images (**B**). Note also the nodule on the medial aspect of segment 7, suspicious for HCC (arrow).

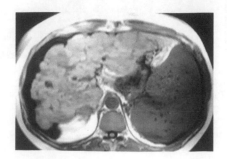

Figure 19. *Gamna-Gandy bodies*: In this patient with advanced cirrhosis, in-phase T1w imaging showed numerous sub-cm nodules of marked hypointensity within the spleen. They probably represent foci of previous hemorrhage and hemosiderin deposition.

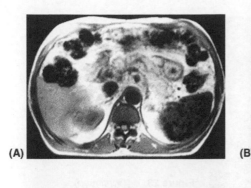

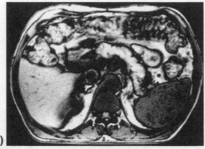

Figure 20. *Gamna-Gandy bodies*: T1w in-phase (**A**) and opposed-phase (**B**) images both show numerous nodules of marked hypointensity scattered through the spleen in this patient with chronic hepatitis C and cirrhosis.

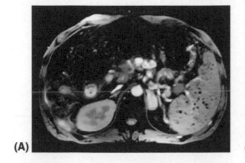

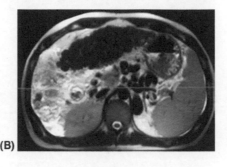

Figure 21. *Gamna-Gandy bodies*: In this patient with siderotic nodules in both liver and spleen, unenhanced T2w GRE images (**A**) showed markedly hypointense foci; on the FSE T2w image at the same level (**B**), the iron deposits were barely visible.

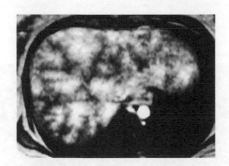

Figure 22. *Acute Budd-Chiari syndrome*: Because the venous occlusion in this young female patient was acute, the liver morphology was normal. This post-Gd T1w image in the portal phase showed the typical feathery pattern of peri-portal enhancement with lack of enhancement around the hepatic vein radicals and no enhancement within the hepatic veins themselves.

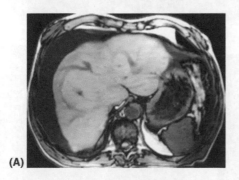

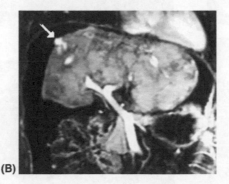

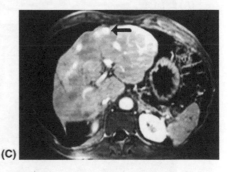

Figure 23. *Chronic Budd-Chiari syndrome*: In this patient with chronic occlusion of the right and middle hepatic veins, unenhanced T1w images (**A**) showed relative shrinkage of the right lobe with distortion of the course of the main vessels suggesting hypertrophy of the central part of the liver, and also marked ascites. Coronal and axial T1w post-Gd images in the portal phase (**B**, **C**) showed heterogeneous perfusion throughout the liver, with prominent collateral vessels over the diaphragmatic surface of the right lobe [arrow in (**B**)] and adjacent to the falciform ligament [arrow in (**C**)]. A further post-Gd venous phase coronal image through the periphery of the right lobe (**D**) again showed a superficial collateral vein. Portal phase MIP image (**E**) confirmed collateral flow from the patent portal system into prominent superficial veins, and also showed the patent left hepatic vein (arrowheads), but no filling of the right or middle hepatic veins. (*Continued*)

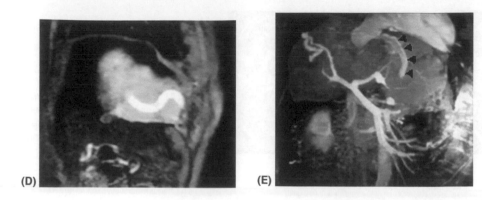

(D) (E) **Figure 23.** (*Continued*)

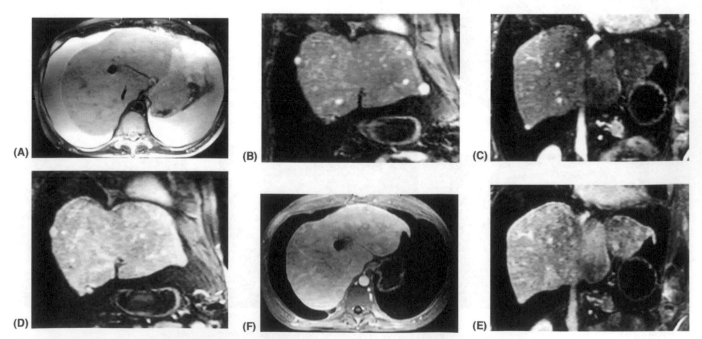

(A) (B) (C)

(D) (F) (E)

Figure 24. *Chronic Budd-Chiari syndrome*: T2w imaging (**A**) showed a small, but diffusely hyperintense liver with substantial ascites. The circular area of signal drop-out was caused by the presence of a TIPSS. Coronal oblique arterial phase post-Gd T1w images (**B**, **C**) showed numerous hypervascular nodules mostly close to the liver surface. Venous phase images (**D**, **E**) showed persistent moderate enhancement in the nodules with heterogeneous enhancement in the remaining liver parenchyma. Axial delayed (10 minutes) image (**F**) showed persisting heterogeneity of parenchymal enhancement with some of the nodules then appearing less enhanced than the adjacent liver. In the context of cirrhosis, these nodules would be suspicious for hepatocellular carcinoma, but in Budd-Chiari syndrome they are a recognized feature of liver regeneration.

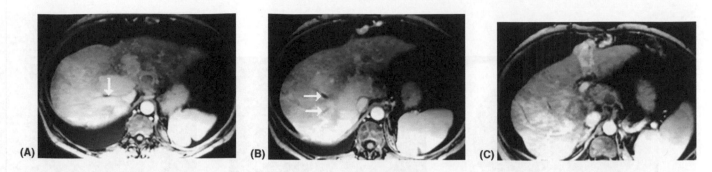

Figure 25. *Chronic Budd-Chiari syndrome:* Venous phase post-Gd T1w images at three different levels (**A**, **B**, **C**) showed persisting heterogeneous enhancement of the liver parenchyma with the most marked enhancement in the region of liver adjacent to the inferior vena cava (the embryological "dorsal liver"). The un-opacified right hepatic vein can be seen traversing this area [arrows in (**A**, **B**)]. Prominent collateral flow through vessels in and around the falciform ligament is shown in (**B**) and (**C**).

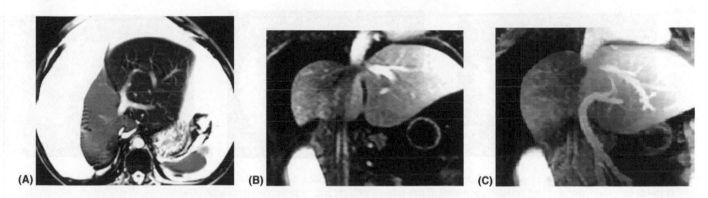

Figure 26. *Partial Budd-Chiari syndrome:* Axial T2w image (**A**) showed normal architecture in the left lobe but a severely atrophied right lobe with no visible internal architecture or vessels. Note the gross ascites but no splenic enlargement. Coronal post-Gd T1w image in the venous phase (**B**) confirmed patency of the left hepatic vein but diminished enhancement in the atrophic right lobe with an occluded right hepatic vein. MIP image from the same series (**C**) also confirmed occlusion of the right main portal vein branch.

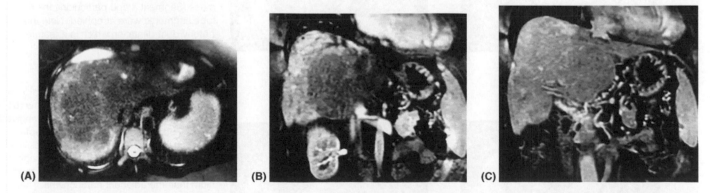

Figure 27. *Chronic Budd-Chiari syndrome with portal vein occlusion:* In this patient with a thrombogenic disorder causing occlusion of the hepatic veins, peripheral edema was shown as an ill-defined area of hyperintensity around the liver margin on T2w images (**A**). Early post-Gd T1w images in the coronal plane (**B**) showed relative hyper-perfusion of the peripheral liver parenchyma which persisted to a lesser degree in the venous phase (**C**) which also demonstrated cavernous transformation of the portal vein.

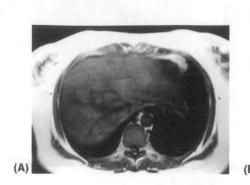
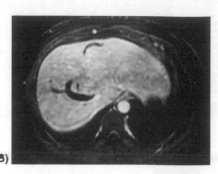
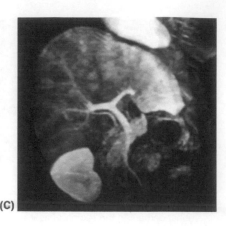

(A) (B) (C)

Figure 28. *Partial Budd-Chiari syndrome:* Unenhanced T1w image (**A**) showed relative atrophy of the right lobe with prominent vascular channels. Post-Gd T1w imaging (**B**) showed rather heterogeneous perfusion with well-defined areas of complete occlusion by thrombosis in some—but not all—of the hepatic veins. Early venous phase MIP image (**C**) showed the typical feathery pattern of peri-portal enhancement with reduced enhancement around the hepatic vein radicals.

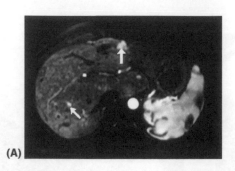
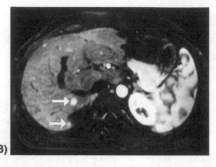
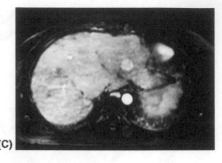

(A) (B) (C)

Figure 29. *Hypervascular nodules in Budd-Chiari syndrome:* Arterial phase post-Gd T1w images (**A, B**) showed several hypervascular nodules (arrowed) in this patient with chronic hepatic vein occlusion. The venous phase images (**C**) showed persistent heterogeneity of perfusion with the nodules fading to isointensity.

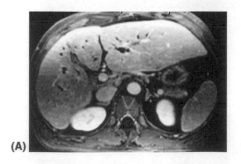
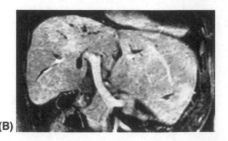

(A) (B)

Figure 30. *Right lobe atrophy:* Axial (**A**) and coronal (**B**) portal phase post-Gd T1w images in a patient with cirrhosis associated with primary sclerosing cholangitis (PSC); segments 2 and 3 were considerably hypertrophied, forming about half of the total liver mass. Segment 4 and particularly the right lobe segments were atrophied. Note the patchy duct dilatation which is a feature of PSC.

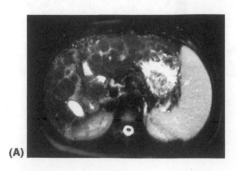
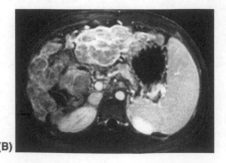

(A) (B)

Figure 31. *Right lobe atrophy:* Axial T2w (**A**) and post-Gd equilibrium phase T1w (**B**) images in a patient with cystic fibrosis showed macro-nodular change with fibrous septa between the large regenerative nodules which had relatively higher signal on T2w imaging and more marked enhancement with gadolinium than the adjacent parenchyma. There was gross atrophy of the right lobe such that the gallbladder lay immediately adjacent to the right kidney. The spleen was substantially enlarged and small varices were visible in (**B**) anterior to the left lobe of liver, and in the pancreatic bed.

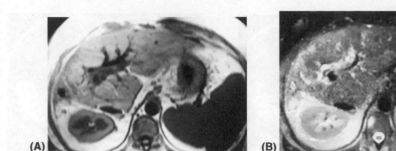

Figure 32. *Severe atrophy of right lobe:* Unenhanced T1w and T2w images (**A**, **B**) showed a slightly heterogeneous liver parenchyma with moderate splenic enlargement and almost total atrophy of the right lobe of the liver. The patient had previously undergone thrombotic occlusion of the right portal vein branch. Post-Gd T1w image (**C**) showed a non-occluding thrombus within the left portal branch (arrow).

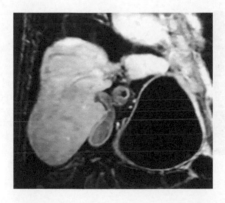

Figure 33. *Left lobe atrophy:* In a patient with end stage alcoholic cirrhosis, coronal post-Gd T1w imaging showed a tiny left lobe, hypertrophied right lobe, and surrounding ascites. The unusual feature of left lobe shrinkage in this patient was probably the result of occlusion of the left main portal vein branch.

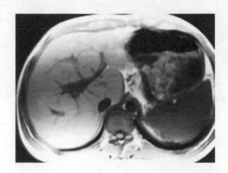

Figure 34. *Enlarged caudate lobe:* Unenhanced T1w image showed an enlarged caudate lobe in a patient aged 18 with non-cirrhotic portal hypertension. Biopsy showed normal histology.

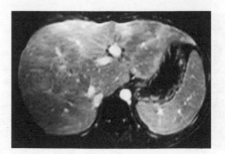

Figure 35. *Enlarged caudate lobe:* Axial post-Gd T1w image showed an enlarged caudate lobe and mildly enlarged spleen in a patient with Budd-Chiari syndrome caused by hepatic vein webs.

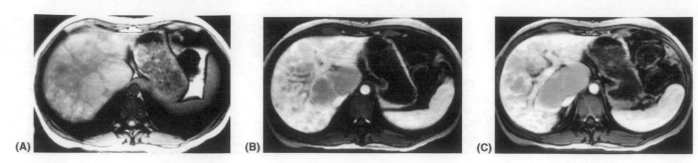

Figure 36. *Enlarged caudate lobe*: In a 22-year-old patient with auto-immune hepatitis associated with celiac disease, unenhanced T1w imaging (**A**) showed nodules of different sizes separated by intervening bands of inflammatory and fibrotic tissue which were hypointense to the liver parenchyma. Post-Gd T1w images (**B**, **C**) showed very patchy enhancement predominantly in the areas which had low signal pre-contrast. Explant histology revealed acute on chronic hepatitis and the large caudate lobe which has a tumor-like appearance on these images was made up of coalescent regenerative nodules.

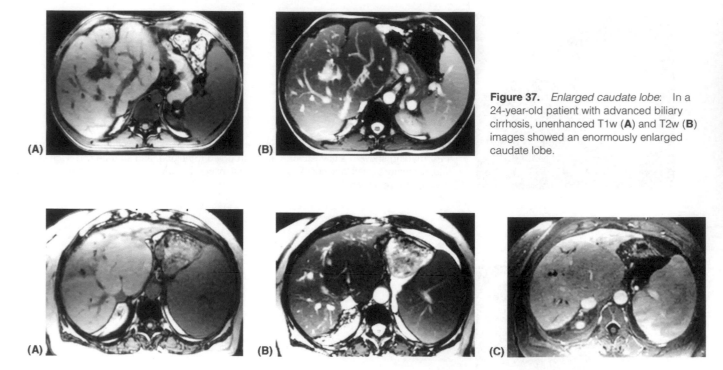

Figure 37. *Enlarged caudate lobe*: In a 24-year-old patient with advanced biliary cirrhosis, unenhanced T1w (**A**) and T2w (**B**) images showed an enormously enlarged caudate lobe.

Figure 38. *Enlarged caudate lobe*: In a patient with advanced cirrhosis and severe portal hypertension, unenhanced T1w (**A**) and True FISP (**B**) images showed a grossly enlarged caudate lobe mimicking a tumor, although normal vessels were visible within it. Post-Gd T1w imaging (**C**) showed distension of the intrahepatic bile ducts resulting from the ducts being stretched over the large caudate, which showed uniform enhancement.

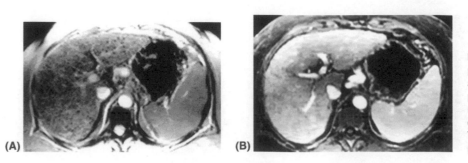

Figure 39. *Fine nodular architecture*: In a patient with alcoholic cirrhosis, micro-nodular architecture was best appreciated on the post-SPIO T2w images (**A**), showing a fine reticular pattern of fibrosis surrounding islands of liver parenchyma which have lower signal. The nodular structure was less clear on the post-Gd T1w image (**B**).

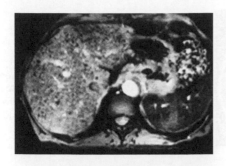

Figure 40. *Fine nodular architecture*: Post-SPIO T2w image in a patient with micro-nodular cirrhosis showed the typical fine reticular pattern of fibrosis surrounding small regenerative nodules.

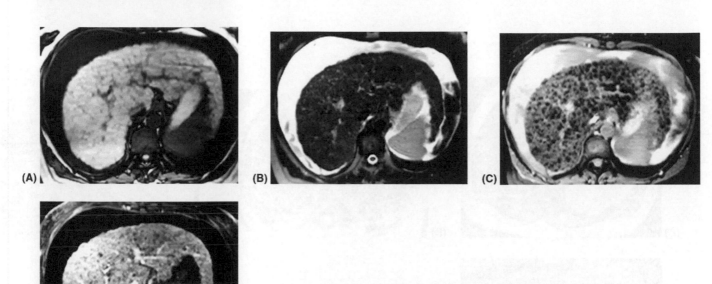

Figure 41. *Fine nodular architecture*: In a patient with late stage cirrhosis and ascites, unenhanced T1w imaging (**A**) showed a reticular pattern with the regenerative nodules appearing hyperintense to the intervening bands of fibrosis. The fibrosis was not visible on the unenhanced T2w image (**B**), but was clear on the post-SPIO T2w image (**C**) and showed more enhancement than adjacent liver on the post-Gd equilibrium phase T1w image (**D**).

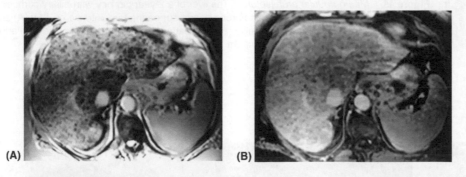

Figure 42. *Fine nodular architecture*: Advanced cirrhosis with fine nodular architecture was shown on both the post-SPIO T2w image (**A**) and the post-Gd T1w image (**B**). Note the central area of reduced signal surrounding the vena cava in (**A**)—this corresponds to the embryological dorsal liver, which may have a separate venous drainage from the rest of the liver, and is sometimes referred to as "segment 9".

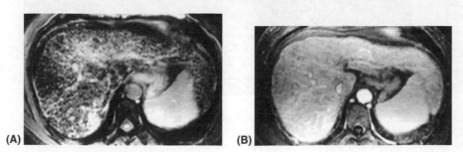

Figure 43. *Fine nodular architecture*: Micro-nodular cirrhosis with a reticular pattern of fibrosis and regenerative nodules of a few millimeters size, was best seen on the post-SPIO T2w image (**A**), but was also visible on the post-Gd T1w image (**B**).

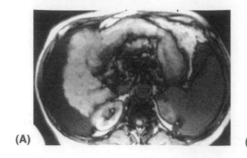
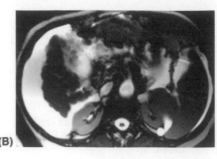

Figure 44. *Macro-nodular architecture:* In a patient with end-stage cirrhosis, a severely shrunken liver was shown on axial T1w (**A**) and true FISP (**B**) images; note the nodular liver contour, substantial volume of ascites and the expanded gallbladder fossa shown in (**B**).

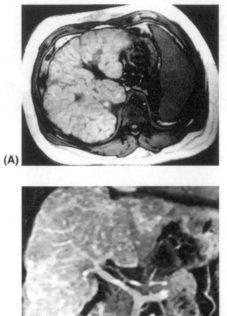
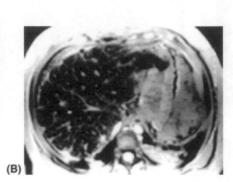
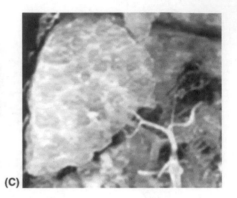

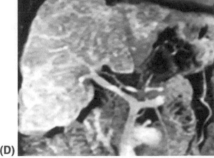

Figure 45. *Macro-nodular architecture:* The liver of a 2-year-old boy with biliary cirrhosis showed a coarse reticular pattern, with fibrotic bands appearing hypointense on T1w (**A**) and hyperintense on T2w (**B**) images; a similar reticular pattern of enhancement was seen in arterial (**C**) and venous (**D**) phase coronal post-Gd T1w images.

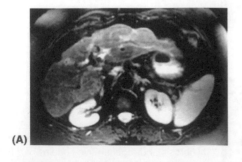
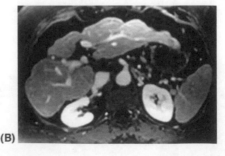
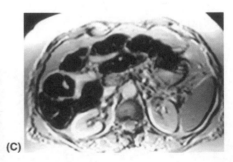

Figure 46. *Macro-nodular architecture in non-cirrhotic liver:* In a patient with alcoholic liver disease, axial T2w (**A**), post-Gd T1w (**B**) and post-SPIO T2w (**C**) images all showed a coarsely nodular liver but with very little fibrosis; the patient's liver function remained stable for more than 7 years of subsequent follow up.

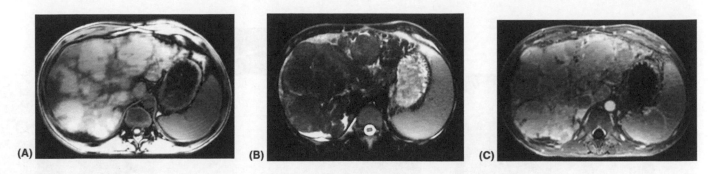

Figure 47. *Macro-nodular architecture:* In a 13-year-old patient with cystic fibrosis, the liver showed a coarse pattern of patchy fibrosis which appeared hypointense on T1w (**A**) and slightly hyperintense on T2w (**B**) images; post-Gd T1w imaging (**C**) showed patchy enhancement of the fibrotic areas together with irregular dilatation of intrahepatic bile duct branches. Explant histology showed the biliary cirrhosis typically associated with cystic fibrosis.

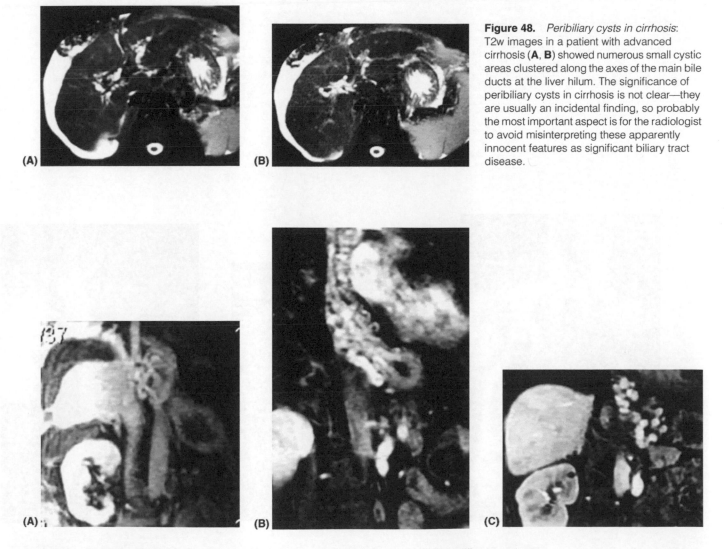

Figure 48. *Peribiliary cysts in cirrhosis:* T2w images in a patient with advanced cirrhosis (**A, B**) showed numerous small cystic areas clustered along the axes of the main bile ducts at the liver hilum. The significance of peribiliary cysts in cirrhosis is not clear—they are usually an incidental finding, so probably the most important aspect is for the radiologist to avoid misinterpreting these apparently innocent features as significant biliary tract disease.

Figure 49. *Esophageal varices:* Post-Gd T1w right anterior oblique coronal images in six different patients (**A–F**) showing varying patterns of varices around the lower esophagus and gastric cardia. (*Continued*)

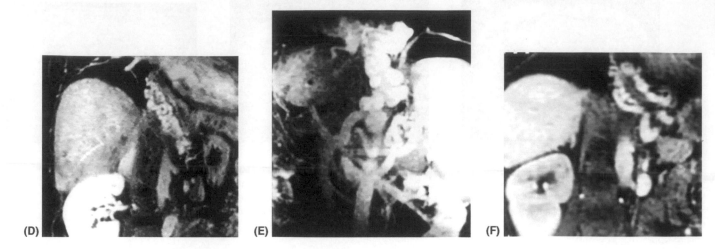

Figure 49.   (*Continued*)

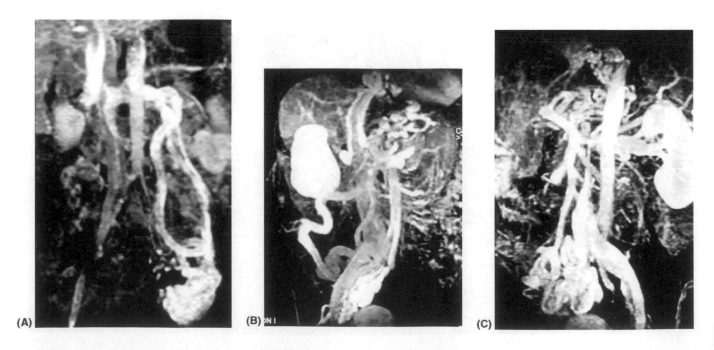

Figure 50.   *Pelvic varices*:   Post-Gd T1w coronal MIP images showing three examples of large varices in the pelvis draining to the renal (**A**), lumbar (**B**), and iliac (**C**) veins.

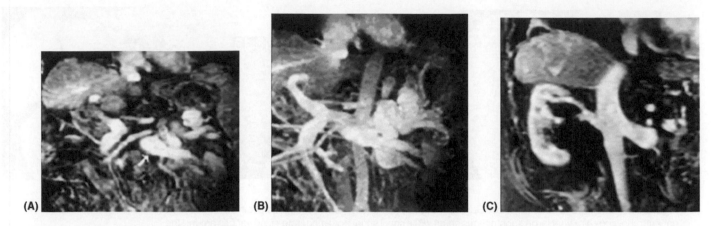

Figure 51. *Spleno-renal shunt.* Coronal post-Gd T1w venous phase image (**A**) showed a distended segment of the left renal vein (arrow) with large varices adjacent to it. The coronal MIP image (**B**) showed the dilated renal vein together with numerous adjacent varices draining from the left upper quadrant. Sometimes the first clue to the presence of a spontaneous spleno-renal shunt is the presence of a dilated left renal vein, as shown in this more posterior image (**C**) from the same acquisition as (**A**).

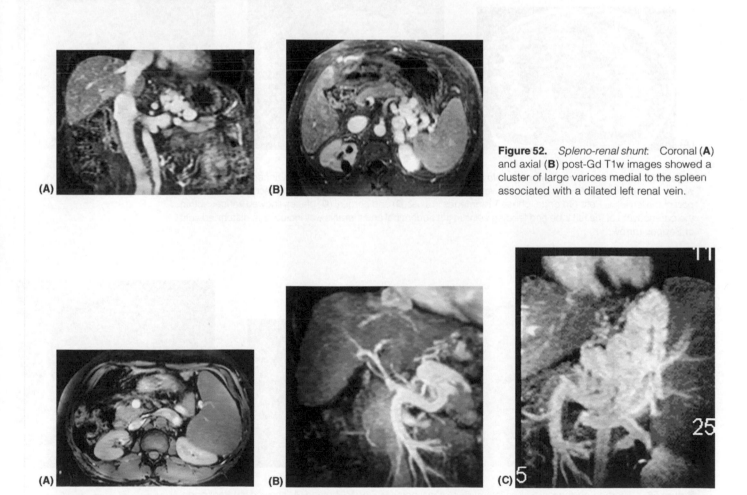

Figure 52. *Spleno-renal shunt.* Coronal (**A**) and axial (**B**) post-Gd T1w images showed a cluster of large varices medial to the spleen associated with a dilated left renal vein.

Figure 53. *Spleno-renal shunt.* Axial post-Gd T1w image (**A**) showed a large left renal vein, splenomegaly and a patent superior mesenteric vein, but no adjacent varices. Right anterior oblique MIP image (**B**) showed the portal vein to be patent but very narrow, with much larger splenic and mesenteric veins. The left anterior oblique coronal MIP image (**C**) confirmed huge varices around the hilum of the spleen and communication with the left renal vein.

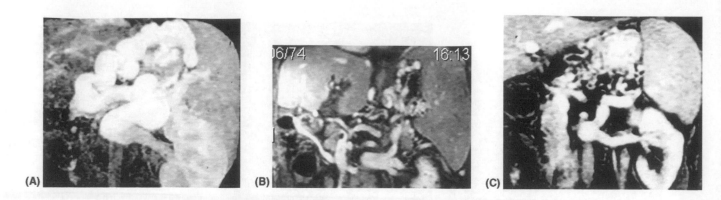

Figure 54. *Spleno-renal shunts*:   Post-Gd T1w images in left anterior coronal oblique position in three patients showing (**A**) a very large spontaneous shunt, (**B**) a small shunt from moderate-sized varices around the splenic hilum and tail of pancreas, (**C**) a medium-sized spleno-renal shunt.

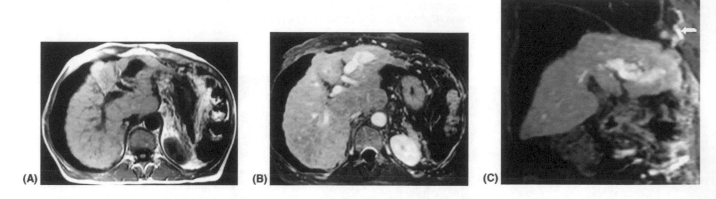

Figure 55. *Aberrant venous drainage into the left portal vein*:   In this patient with advanced cirrhosis and previous splenectomy, T1w image (**A**) showed a small nodular liver with markedly dilated vessels in the anterior part of the left lobe. Post-Gd portal phase T1w images in axial (**B**) and coronal (**C**) planes showed varices within the parenchyma of the left lobe and feeding veins in the abdominal and thoracic wall including a distended vein of Sappey (arrow).

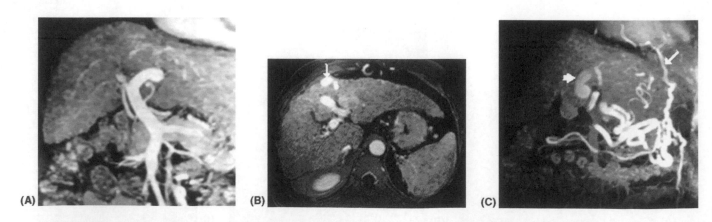

Figure 56. *Thoraco-abdominal wall collaterals*:   Coronal post-Gd T1w MIP image (**A**) showed a patent portal system with distension of the left portal branch within a small nodular liver. Axial venous phase image (**B**) showed the distended left portal vein to be associated with superficial collaterals adjacent to the falciform ligament with a prominent para-umbilical vein (arrow). A more anterior coronal MIP image (**C**) showed numerous collaterals including an enlarged vein of Sappey (arrow) draining blood from the dilated left portal vein branch (arrowhead).

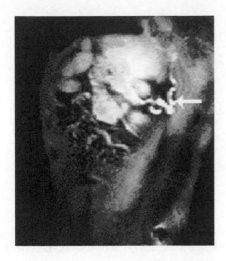

Figure 57. *Dilated vein of Sappey:* Right anterior oblique coronal post-Gd T1w image showing a distended vein of Sappey (arrow) acting as a collateral channel in a patient with severe atrophy and fibrosis.

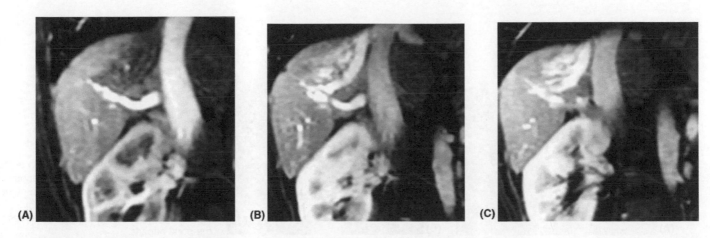

(A)   (B)   (C)

Figure 58. *Intrahepatic shunting:* In a patient with established cirrhosis, coronal post-Gd T1w imaging in the early portal phase (**A**) showed marked enhancement in the right portal vein but no hepatic venous enhancement. Later venous phase images (**B**, **C**) showed filling of disproportionately enlarged right hepatic vein branches between the porta hepatis and IVC, indicating direct portal venous-hepatic venous shunting.

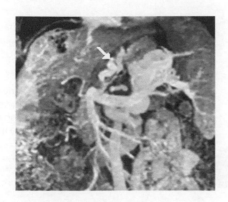

Figure 59. *Complete occlusion of the main portal vein:* Coronal post-Gd MIP image showed normal splenic and superior mesenteric veins with collaterals running along the lesser curve of stomach (arrow), but no filling of the portal vein or its branches in the liver.

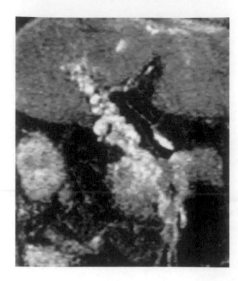

Figure 60.   *Cavernous transformation of the portal vein:*   Coronal post-Gd MIP image showed the portal vein to be replaced by varicose collaterals producing the typical appearance of "cavernous transformation."

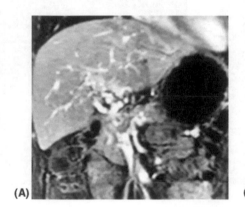

(A)

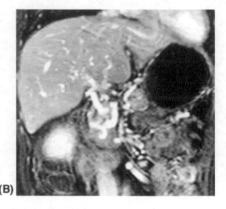

(B)

Figure 61.   *Cavernous transformation of the portal vein:*   Coronal post-Gd T1w venous phase images (**A**, **B**) showed no filling of the main portal vein which was replaced by numerous medium-sized collaterals across the porta hepatis.

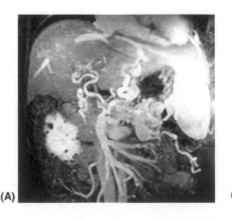

(A)

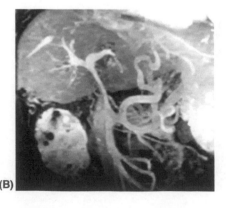

(B)

Figure 62.   *Non-occlusive portal vein thrombosis:*   Post-Gd MIP images in early (**A**) and late (**B**) venous phase showed numerous collaterals both near the liver hilum, along the lesser curve of stomach and adjacent to the spleen. Although the main portal vein remained patent, its lumen was diffusely narrowed by thrombus adherent to the vein wall.

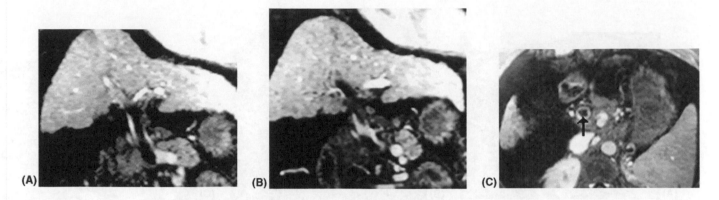

Figure 63. *Non-occlusive thrombosis of the main portal vein:* Coronal post-Gd T1w images in the venous phase (**A**, **B**) showed on adjacent slices a single thrombus filling the whole of the main portal vein and extending a short way into the intrahepatic divisions. Axial post-Gd T1w imaging at the level of the pancreatic head also showed non-occlusive thrombus lying centrally within the vein (arrow).

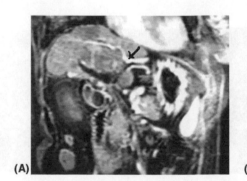

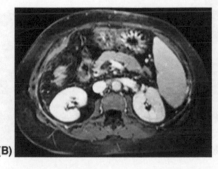

Figure 64. *Complete thrombosis of main portal vein and its intrahepatic branches:* Coronal (**A**) and axial (**B**) post-Gd T1w images showed the main portal vein to be completely occluded by thrombus from its junction with the splenic vein (**B**). The thrombus extended well into the right portal vein branch (**A**)—note superficial varices over the liver surface (arrow) taking collateral flow.

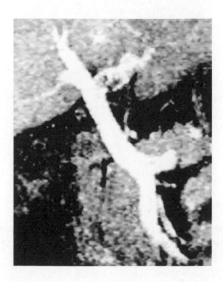

Figure 65. *Non-occluding thrombus limited to left portal vein branch:* Coronal venous phase post-Gd T1w image showed an ill-defined filling defect occupying but not occluding the main stem of the left portal vein branch.

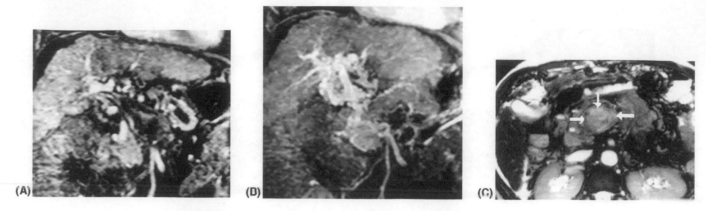

Figure 66. *Bland thrombus expanding the portal vein:* In a cirrhotic patient with no evidence of malignancy, coronal post-Gd T1w imaging showed extensive occlusion of the portal, splenic and termination of superior mesenteric veins (**A**) with dense collateral flow around the porta hepatis (**B**). Axial True FISP imaging at the level of the pancreatic head (**C**) showed the portal vein to be considerably expanded by heterogeneous thrombus (arrows) suggesting an acute event.

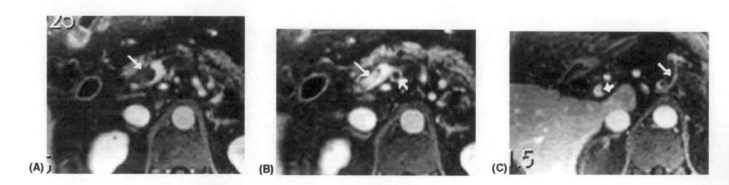

Figure 67. *Thrombosis of portal vein and coronary vein:* In a patient with established cirrhosis and varices, axial post-Gd T1w images at the level of the pancreatic head showed a large but non-occluding thrombus in the main portal vein [arrow in (**A**)]. Slightly cranial to this level (**B**), eccentric thrombus was still visible in the portal vein (large arrow), but the portal end of the gastric coronary vein also contained non-occlusive thrombus (small arrow). At a more cranial level still (**C**), further thrombus was shown within the coronary vein (large arrow), while the main portal vein showed a small area of thrombus adjacent to the medial wall (small arrow).

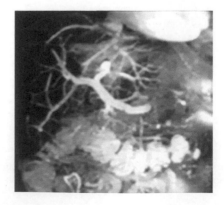

Figure 68. *Superior mesenteric vein thrombosis:* Coronal post-Gd MIP image showed a patent portal vein, and intrahepatic divisions, a patent termination of the splenic vein (the distal part of the splenic vein was outside the acquisition slab), but no filling of the superior mesenteric vein.

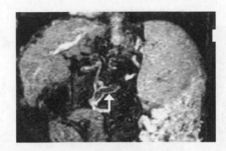

Figure 69. *Splenic vein thrombosis*:   In a cirrhotic patient, left anterior oblique coronal post-Gd T1w image showed non-occlusive thrombus within a segment of the main splenic vein (arrow). Also note large varices surrounding the inferior pole of the spleen.

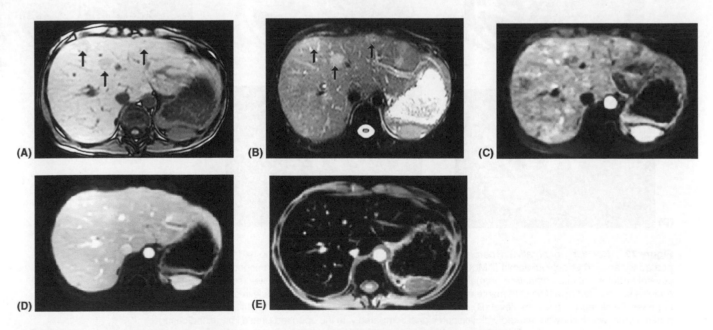

Figure 70. *Nodular regenerative hyperplasia*:   In a 36-year-old renal transplant patient with unexplained elevation of serum alkaline phosphatase, sonography and CT were normal but MR showed multiple nodules (arrows) which were mildly hypointense on T1w (**A**) and hyperintense on T2w (**B**) images. The nodules remained hypointense on arterial phase post-Gd T1w images (**C**), but showed faintly increased enhancement in the portal phase (**D**). The nodules became almost invisible on post-SPIO T2w images (**E**) confirming their benign hepatocellular nature. The appearances were unchanged on follow-up MRI 3 months and 10 months later.

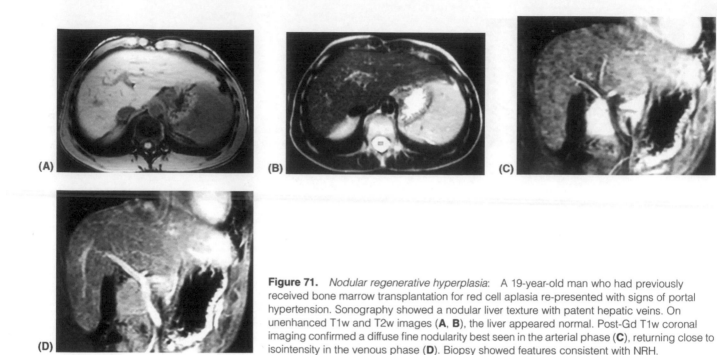

Figure 71. *Nodular regenerative hyperplasia:* A 19-year-old man who had previously received bone marrow transplantation for red cell aplasia re-presented with signs of portal hypertension. Sonography showed a nodular liver texture with patent hepatic veins. On unenhanced T1w and T2w images (**A**, **B**), the liver appeared normal. Post-Gd T1w coronal imaging confirmed a diffuse fine nodularity best seen in the arterial phase (**C**), returning close to isointensity in the venous phase (**D**). Biopsy showed features consistent with NRH.

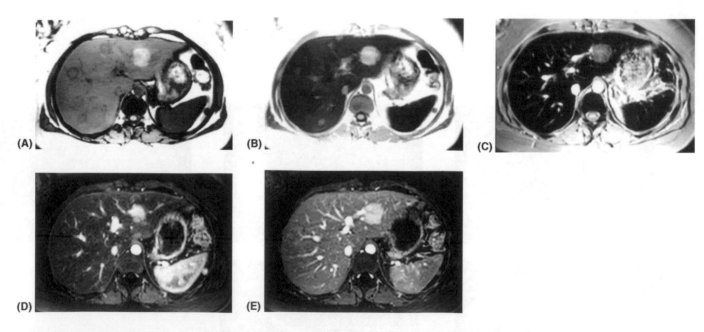

Figure 72. *Nodular regenerative hyperplasia and FNH:* In a 23-year-old woman who had been previously treated for acute myeloid leukaemia (AML) by bone marrow transplantation, screening sonography showed several nodules within an otherwise normal liver. Opposed-phase T1w images (**A**) showed several isointense nodules surrounded by a halo of hypointensity, together with a single hyperintense nodule in segment 2/3. The in-phase T1w image at the same level (**B**) showed all the nodules to be hyperintense relative to the liver parenchyma, which showed markedly diminished signal compared with the opposed-phase image, indicating diffuse iron deposition. Similar signal loss was shown in the normal-sized spleen, but not in the pancreas. Unenhanced T2w GRE images (**C**) showed diffuse signal loss in the parenchyma of the liver and spleen consequent upon iron deposition, the left lobe nodule remaining hyperintense while the other nodules were invisible. Post-Gd T1w imaging in arterial (**D**) and venous (**E**) phases showed marked enhancement of the left lobe nodule with a small central scar, typical of FNH. The nodules elsewhere in the liver remained isointense at all phases of enhancement. Hemosiderosis is a recognized complication of treated AML. NRH is said to occur in about 20% of patients after marrow transplantation. The lesions remained stable during follow up.

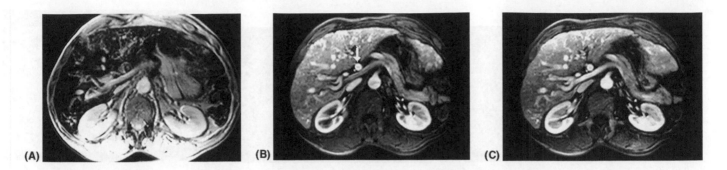

Figure 73. *Hereditary hemorrhagic telangiectasia (HHT):* In a patient with abnormal liver architecture shown on sonography, post-SPIO T2w imaging (**A**), and unenhanced images (not illustrated) were suggestive of patchy fibrosis, with ill-defined linear areas of abnormal signal intensity scattered through liver parenchyma. Post-Gd T1w images in arterial (**B**) and venous (**C**) phases showed the areas of abnormal signal to be related to dilated vascular channels producing scattered hypervascular nodules throughout the periphery. Note the immensely dilated hepatic artery [arrow in (**B**)]. HHT is associated with multiple arterio-venous or venous-venous shunts within the liver. Biopsy confirmed the features of HHT.

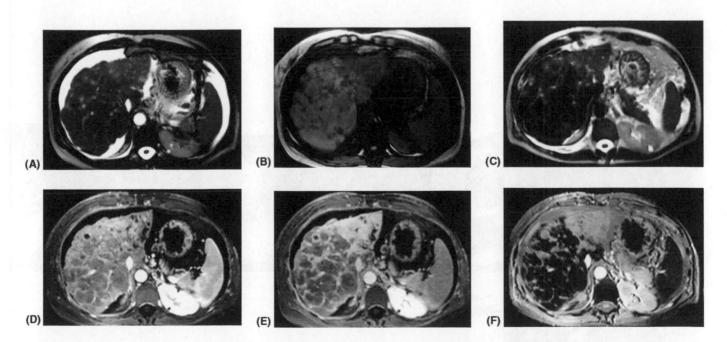

Figure 74. *Pseudo-cirrhosis in breast cancer.* In a middle-aged patient who was receiving chemotherapy for breast carcinoma, true FISP (**A**), T1w (**B**) and T2W (**C**) images all showed a shrunken liver with a nodular contour and ascites, with patchy hypointensity on T1w and hyperintensity on T2w imaging. Early and delayed post-Gd T1w imaging (**D**, **E**), and post-SPIO T2w imaging (**F**) confirmed the nodular architecture with linear fibrosis affecting the right lobe and more dense confluent fibrosis in the left lobe. The appearance was indistinguishable from that of advanced cirrhosis, but laparoscopic biopsy confirmed adenocarcinoma of breast origin.

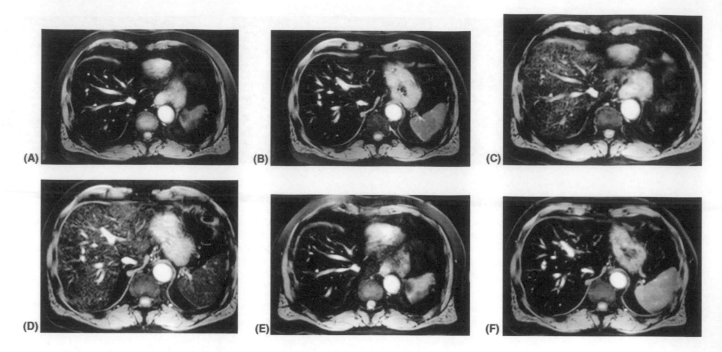

Figure 75. *Transient liver fibrosis associated with chemotherapy:* A patient with colorectal cancer underwent SPIO-enhanced MRI before, during and after the cessation of chemotherapy. Post-SPIO T2w images before treatment (**A**, **B**) showed homogeneously normal parenchymal signal intensity. Post-SPIO T2w images obtained during chemotherapy (**C**, **D**) showed a fine honeycomb pattern of relative hyperintensity similar to that seen with lobular fibrosis in patients with early cirrhosis. Images obtained after the cessation of chemotherapy (**E**, **F**) showed that the liver architecture had returned to normal.

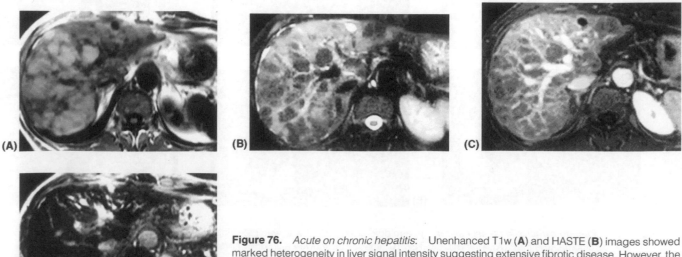

Figure 76. *Acute on chronic hepatitis:* Unenhanced T1w (**A**) and HASTE (**B**) images showed marked heterogeneity in liver signal intensity suggesting extensive fibrotic disease. However, the heterogeneity was largely lost on post-Gd T1w venous phase imaging (**C**), and on post-SPIO T2w images (**D**) the areas which were abnormal on the unenhanced images showed normal uptake of contrast, suggesting the initial abnormalities were caused by edema rather than fibrosis. Biopsy confirmed acute on chronic hepatitis.

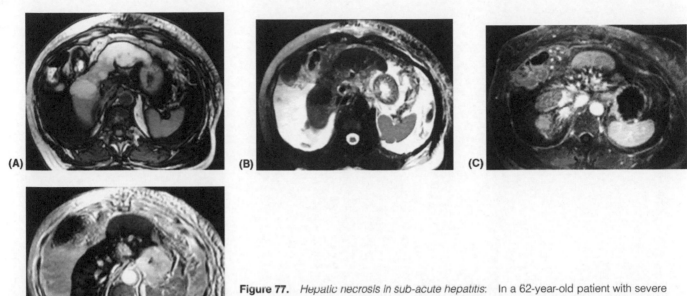

Figure 77. *Hepatic necrosis in sub-acute hepatitis:* In a 62-year-old patient with severe seronegative hepatitis, T1w (**A**), HASTE (**B**), post-Gd T1w (**C**), and post-SPIO T2w (**D**) images all showed marked shrinkage of the liver with a coarse nodular architecture and gross ascites. Note the absence of splenomegaly, and only a few small mesenteric varices in (**C**). Biopsy confirmed panacinar necrosis.

CHAPTER 9

Detecting Hepatocellular Carcinoma in the Cirrhotic Liver

I n some patients with cirrhosis hepatocellular carcinoma (HCC) develops by a stepwise process of de-differentiation from benign regenerative nodules to malignant HCC. The nomenclature of nodules in the cirrhotic liver has been confusing, but the older terms of "adenomatous hyperplasia," "macroregenerative nodule," and "adenomatous hyperplasia with atypia" have been superseded by the single category of dyplastic or borderline nodule. A major objective of imaging is to detect the presence of malignant change in the cirrhotic liver, and to determine what interventional treatments are feasible: assessing the resectability of tumors or their suitability for percutaneous ablation or chemoembolization, and exploring the vascular anatomy of the liver as a prelude to liver transplantation.

DYSPLASTIC NODULES

Pathology

The pathologic diagnosis of dysplasia in a nodule is a judgement based on multiple criteria some of which are qualitative, others quantitative. The cellular features include large cell change, small cell change, nuclear atypia, fat inclusions, clear-cell change and the presence of copper-associated protein. The architectural features include larger nodule size, thicker cellular plates, loss of reticulin, reduced number of portal tracts, and increased number of unpaired arteries. These nodules are borderline lesions which may have only subtle differences from regenerative nodules so the diagnosis is often difficult even with the whole nodule available, and even more difficult with only biopsy material. When examining an entire explanted liver, it is impractical for the pathologist to carry out microscopic examination of every nodule, and sampling is based on selection of those nodules which appear suspicious or abnormal to the naked eye. Because of this approach, it is likely that the detection of dysplastic nodules in the cirrhotic liver currently under-estimates their true incidence.

MRI Appearances

On unenhanced T1w images, dysplastic nodules are typically hyperintense to normal liver, and are usually larger than surrounding regenerative nodules. The explanation for the hyperintensity is not yet clear. Possible factors include copper deposition and the accumulation of excess glycogen or fat, although frank fatty change within a dysplastic nodule is only rarely detectable on chemical shift imaging. On unenhanced T2w imaging, dysplastic nodules may be iso- or hypointense. They typically show portal phase enhancement with gadolinium, and normal uptake of SPIO, so the main differences from regenerative nodules are that dyplastic nodules are larger and hyperintense on unenhanced T1w images. However, correlation with explant pathology has shown recently that some nodules with hyperintensity on T1w imaging have been found to have no histologic features of dysplasia; in summary both regenerative and dysplastic nodules may be either iso- or hyperintense on T1w images. In about 5% of cases, pathologically proven dysplastic nodules have shown arterial hyperintensity with gadolinium, a feature usually associated with frank malignancy.

DYSPLASIA AND HCC

Both dysplastic nodules and HCC may be either solitary or multiple. Not uncommonly, HCC and dysplastic nodules co-exist in the same liver. Occasionally, a focus of HCC is seen developing within a dysplastic nodule, giving rise to the "nodule-in-nodule" sign which is characteristic of malignancy.

WHY LOOK FOR HCC IN CIRRHOSIS?

By the time they present with symptoms, most HCCs are well-advanced and untreated patients then have a median survival of only a few months. Systemic chemotherapy has so far proved largely unsuccessful. Transplantation is of little or no benefit when the tumor has invaded major hepatic vessels or in the presence of lymph node or distant metastases. However, when HCCs are detected at an early stage, patients may potentially be cured by resection or transplantation, while radiofrequency ablation, cryotherapy, percutaneous alcohol injection, or chemo-embolization are feasible options for palliation or obliteration of smaller lesions.

WHO IS AT HIGH RISK OF HCC IN CIRRHOSIS?

All types of cirrhosis predispose to HCC, but the patients particularly at risk are those who have chronic infection with hepatitis B or C, alcoholic liver disease, haemochromatosis, and male patients with primary biliary cirrhosis (PBC). Combination of these factors multiplies the risk level. The risk is less for females with PBC and for other forms of chronic auto-immune hepatitis, while patients with cirrhosis associated with primary sclerosing cholangitis are at risk of developing cholangiocarcinoma rather than HCC. With most causes of cirrhosis, the development of HCC is much more likely in the later stages of the disease (Child's grade B or C), but in patients with chronic hepatitis B infection, HCC may develop in advance of cirrhotic change. Further risk factors for HCC include age over 50, male gender, and macronodular change.

While percutaneous biopsy is still sometimes used for the histologic diagnosis of HCC, many patients with advanced liver disease have bleeding disorders or ascites, both of which increase the immediate risk of complications. The danger of tumor implantation in the needle track also weighs against the use of percutaneous biopsy which is rarely necessary with appropriate imaging.

HEPATOCELLULAR CARCINOMA

Like other malignant tumors, HCCs start out small. Multiple HCCs may develop simultaneously or sequentially, and intrahepatic metastasis of HCC is a common mode of spread, with tumor seeding along the portal tracts. Lymph node spread is typically to the porta hepatis, peripancreatic and celiac axis nodes, and also to the nodes in the right cardiophrenic angle just above the diaphragm.

HCC may be solitary or multiple. When multiple, the lesions are often of different sizes and may show different features on both unenhanced and post-Gd images. Nodules of HCC may coalesce to produce areas of massive tumor involvement and occasionally the appearances of diffuse liver replacement by tumor.

Local in-drawing of the liver capsule is seen only rarely with untreated HCC. It is more commonly associated with peripheral cholangiocarcinoma, epithelioid hemangioendothe-lioma, and also rarely with metastatic disease, but in the cirrhotic liver it is usually due to confluent fibrosis.

MRI Appearances

Unenhanced Imaging
On unenhanced T1w images, HCCs may show any type of signal. Most commonly, small lesions are hyper- or isointense, while the more advanced larger lesions are typically hypointense on T1w imaging. On T2w images, advanced HCC is usually hyperintense while smaller or well-differentiated lesions are more likely to be isointense. A focus of hyperintensity within an isointense nodule on T2w imaging (nodule-in-nodule sign) is strongly suggestive of HCC developing in a dysplastic lesion.

Post-Gd T1w Imaging

On post-Gd T1w images, the typical HCC appears hyperintense in the arterial phase and shows fairly rapid washout, becoming iso- or hypointense in the portal venous phase. A small minority of HCCs are iso- or even hypointense in the arterial phase of enhancement. Correlation with histology indicates that, as a general rule, the lesions which show the greatest arterialization are those which are least well-differentiated, i.e., the intensity of arterial phase enhancement correlates with the degree of malignancy. Exceptions to this may be seen with tumors containing a large proportion of fibrous tissue, which can also be relatively avascular with little or only delayed enhancement. Also in general, the greater the arterial enhancement, the faster the washout, so from being hyperintense in the arterial phase, high-grade HCCs become hypointense in the portal phase. Persistent hypointensity at all phases after gadolinium should not be taken to exclude malignancy—occasional HCCs (5% or so) are quite avascular.

Heterogeneity

When small (1–2 cm or less), HCCs usually show homogeneous signal intensity on both enhanced and unenhanced images. Larger lesions are commonly heterogeneous with patchy enhancement at different phases after contrast. On unenhanced images, heterogeneous tumors may show areas of fat deposition, demonstrated by the change in signal between in-phase and opposed-phase T1w images. Focal hemorrhage within an HCC will often produce areas of high signal on T1w imaging and either low or high signal—or occasionally both—on T2w images. Patchy central necrosis is relatively common with large HCCs producing areas of bright signal on unenhanced T2w images, low signal on T1w images and little or no early enhancement on post-Gd T1w images.

Capsule

A "capsule" enclosing the lesion is a common feature of HCCs which is not seen with either dysplastic or regenerative nodules. When well-developed, the capsule appears as a hypointense rim on both unenhanced T1w and T2w images, but in most cases the capsule is seen only on post-Gd T1w images where it appears as a brightly enhancing rim most marked in the venous or delayed phase. Although histologically these capsules usually incorporate some fibrous tissue, at least in part the rim of enhancement includes a layer of liver parenchyma adjacent to the tumor in which the blood supply has been modified by local arterio-portal shunting. This sometimes produces a "corona" of early enhancement around the lesion, in addition to the more clearly defined fibrous capsule.

Vascular Invasion

Vascular invasion is a characteristic microscopic feature of HCC, and is fairly frequently seen on a larger scale at imaging. Tumor extension into the portal vein results in a "cork in a bottle" appearance with a central plug of tumor projecting along the lumen of the vein. Similar changes may occur with invasion of the hepatic veins, and in such cases extension into the IVC or even into the right atrium may be shown. It is usually possible to distinguish between bland thrombus developing on the surface of an invading tumor, and a large plug of tumor within the lumen, since tumor thrombus characteristically shows patchy enhancement after gadolinium while bland thrombus shows no enhancement. Expansion of the lumen of the portal vein, hepatic vein or IVC is quite common with tumor thrombus, while venous occlusion by bland thrombus usually leads to diminution in the lumen rather than expansion, although occasionally, expanding bland thrombus may be found.

Hepatocyte-Specific Contrast Agents

HCCs often appear bile-stained when section at pathology, because although they contain no portal tracts and have no excretory biliary outlet, they may retain enough hepatocyte function to accumulate bile. Advanced HCCs take up little or no hepatocyte contrast agents, but well- or moderately well-differentiated tumors accumulate varying amounts, the uptake depending on the degree of differentiation of the tumor. Because the contrast is not excreted, the conspicuity of these lesions can increase for up to 24 hours after injection. Although such delayed images can be helpful in detecting small HCCs, their uptake of intracellular contrast means that they are difficult to distinguish from regenerative and dysplastic nodules.

SPIO Contrast

Because SPIO particles are taken up by reticuloendothelial cells, the contrast effect of SPIO is seen in normal liver parenchyma and in focal lesions which contain functioning Kupffer cells. These include regenerative nodules, focal nodular hyperplasia, some hepatocellular adenomas, and some well-differentiated HCCs. The degree of uptake of SPIO into HCCs is very variable. Typically the larger lesions show no uptake, and many small HCCs are also sufficiently de-differentiated to show no perceptible uptake of SPIO. Even so, careful measurement of the signal intensity using the same T2w sequence before and after SPIO administration will often show a small signal change in HCCs. It is exceptional for even a well-differentiated HCC to lose more than about 30% of its signal intensity between pre- and post-SPIO T2w acquisitions. Even in these cases, because the liver signal shows a greater decrease than the tumor the lesions become more conspicuous after SPIO. Regenerative and dysplastic nodules show a degree of SPIO uptake which is close to that of normal liver, so any cirrhotic nodule which fails to take up SPIO may be regarded as malignant.

Accuracy of MRI in Detecting HCC

Comparing dual contrast MRI with pathologic detection of HCCs after liver transplantation shows that almost all tumors larger than 1 cm size can be detected. Detection rates for sub-cm HCCs remain disappointingly low. One of the major difficulties arises when we try to identify, at pathologic examination of the explanted liver, individual small nodules which have been previously demonstrated on imaging in a diffusely nodular end-stage liver.

NON-HEPATOCELLULAR FOCAL LESIONS IN THE CIRRHOTIC LIVER

Benign cysts, hemangiomas, biliary adenomas and micro-hamartomas all occur occasionally in the cirrhotic liver. It is the authors' impression that cysts and hemangiomas—which are relatively common incidental findings in patients undergoing cross-sectional imaging for surveillance in malignant disease—are less commonly seen in late stage cirrhosis than in the general patient population, perhaps because the fibrotic process obliterates these benign malformations. Metastases (except from intrahepatic primary tumors), focal nodular hyperplasia, and adenoma are all rare in patients with well-advanced cirrhosis. In a patient with advanced cirrhosis and a known primary extrahepatic malignancy, multiple liver nodules with malignant features are more likely to be HCC—even if atypical—than metastatic disease.

AN APPROACH TO THE DIFFERENTIAL DIAGNOSIS OF CIRRHOTIC NODULES

As discussed earlier, the stepwise de-differentiation of regenerative nodules through dysplasia to frank malignancy leads to a continuous spectrum of appearances both histo-logically and on imaging. Some nodules are clearly in one category or the other, but in some cases the features overlap. At histology, individual features of de-differentiation may be present in varying combinations and may be expressed to different degrees.

When the pathologist examines a diffusely nodular end-stage liver, the selection of sampling sites for microscopic examination is based on the naked-eye appearances. The nodules which are specifically sampled are those which look different from the surrounding nodules, or are larger. In imaging, we take a similar approach, seeking characteristics which distinguish dysplastic and malignant lesions from benign regenerative nodules. With MRI, these features include the signal intensities on unenhanced T1w and T2w images, the presence of iron or fat deposits or hemorrhage, the degree of arterial and portal vascularity as shown by enhancement with gadolinium, and the degree of cellular function as shown by uptake of tissue-specific contrast agents.

Size

Small nodules (sub-cm) may be benign, dysplastic or malignant. With increasing size, the probability of malignancy rises. Regenerative nodules are rarely larger than 1–2 cm size, dysplastic nodules only occasionally reach 4–5 cms and any lesion larger than this will almost certainly be malignant (or contain foci of malignancy).

Appearance on Unenhanced T1w Images

Nodules which show uniform hyperintensity on T1w imaging are most often dysplastic or malignant, although occasional regenerative nodules show this feature. Areas of focal hyperintensity within an otherwise iso- or hypointense nodule may be due to local hemorrhage or fat deposition and are suggestive of malignancy. Focal fat is rarely recognized on imaging of dysplastic or regenerative nodules, and hemorrhage in benign nodules has been described only in patients with end stage disease and acute hypoperfusion of the liver. Nodules which are hypointense on T1w images are likely to be HCC, although differentiation must be made from liver cysts and hemangiomas, which show the same characteristics on T2w and post-Gd T1w imaging in cirrhosis as they do in the non-cirrhotic liver. Focal hypointensity in cirrhotic nodules is often caused by localized iron deposition which is a non-specific feature in differentiating benign from malignant nodules.

Appearance on T2w Images

Cysts and hemangiomas produce very bright and well-defined areas of hyperintensity on T2w images, but those cirrhotic nodules which are hyperintense on T2w imaging should be regarded as HCC, since this feature is not seen with regenerative or dysplastic nodules. Nodules which are isointense may be benign, dysplastic or malignant; those which are hypointense on T2w images are more likely to be dysplastic than malignant but could be either.

Chemical Shift Imaging

Although diffuse fatty infiltration is fairly common in patients with early cirrhosis, end-stage livers rarely contain sufficient fat to cause a major signal change between in-phase and opposed-phase T1w images. In these unusual cases, the presence of fat within nodules is non-specific and does not help to distinguish benign from malignant. However, in most cases fat deposition localized to individual nodules is a strong indicator of malignancy, although only a minority of HCCs contain enough fat to be recognized on imaging.

Enhancement with Gadolinium

Clear-cut nodules larger than 1 cm which show arterial-phase enhancement with gadolinium should be regarded as most likely to be HCCs. Areas of arterial enhancement which are not clear-cut nodules, particularly close to the liver surface, may be produced by focal vascular anomalies or superficial areas of non-portal venous inflow into the liver. Arterial hypervascularity in nodules of sub-cm size is still suggestive of malignancy but a degree of uncertainty remains about some of these small nodules, discussed further below. Arterial hyperintensity has been described with dysplastic nodules but is relatively rare.

Hyperintensity in the portal or delayed phases of enhancement should also be regarded as an indication of malignancy in a nodule, although this type of enhancement is much less common in HCC than the typical arterial blush. Finally, the absence of arterial or venous phase enhancement in a nodule should not be taken to exclude malignancy—occasional HCCs are quite avascular. In summary, any nodule which shows distinctly different enhancement characteristics from the rest of the liver should be regarded with utmost suspicion of being malignant, giving due consideration to the recognition of hemangiomas and other vascular malformations, and the small hypervascular lesions discussed below.

Appearances Following Tissue-Specific Contrast Agents

The uptake of tissue-specific contrast agents depends on the integrity of Kupffer cell function (for SPIO) and hepatocyte cell function (for the T1 agents). Although the histology of hepatocellular tumors shows a variable population of hepatocytes and Kupffer cells, their functional capacity is very variable. Few studies have investigated the phenomenon of functional dissociation between hepatocytes and Kupffer cells in liver disease, but MRI experience suggests that with progressive de-differentiation, hepatocyte function is preserved for longer than is Kupffer cell function, so some lesions which show no uptake of SPIO can still concentrate hepatocyte-specific T1 agents. This concept is supported by historic data from radionuclide imaging, where some hepatocellular tumors which showed no uptake of technetium-labelled colloid still had functional capacity to take up some technetium-labelled imino-diacetic acid derivatives targeted at hepatocytes. Because SPIO is a more sensitive discriminator between benign and malignant nodules than are the liver-specific T1 agents, the use of SPIO is preferred for the characterization of cirrhotic nodules, particularly when combined with gadolinium chelates in a dual-contrast approach.

SPIO

The uptake of SPIO in the cirrhotic liver, as measured by percentage signal intensity loss (PSIL) when pre- and post-contrast images are compared, is a little less than in the normal (non-cirrhotic) liver, but this does not usually influence the detectability of tumors. The relatively reduced uptake in cirrhosis is explained by a combination of factors including replacement of liver parenchyma by fibrosis, arterio-portal shunting within the cirrhotic liver, and a global reduction in liver perfusion with shift of the injected contrast to spleen and bone marrow. Histologic studies have shown that the number of Kupffer cells found in dysplastic nodules is similar to that of regenerative nodules, while with HCC, a reduction in Kupffer cells parallels the other features of de-differentiation. Nodules which take up no SPIO may be regarded as malignant, and those which take up the same amount as adjacent liver may be regarded as benign. Nodules which take up less SPIO than the adjacent liver—and it may be necessary to measure PSIL on pre- and post-SPIO images using the same GRE T2w sequence in order to show a small amount of uptake—are likely to be well-differentiated HCCs or high grade dysplastic nodules. A useful rule of thumb is that nodules which show increased lesion-to-liver contrast after SPIO should be regarded as HCCs until otherwise determined.

On post-SPIO T2w images, small HCCs need to be distinguished from vessels, cysts and hemangiomas which also show high signal. This can be clarified by comparison with the unenhanced images and if necessary with post-Gd images. Probably the most difficult differentials for HCC on post-SPIO T2w images are the dense areas of focal fibrosis which are sometimes coalescent in late stage cirrhosis. Again, careful comparison with unenhanced and post-Gd T1w images (especially delayed images) will usually clarify the distinction, but in occasional cases with focally-defined massive or nodular fibrosis, the distinction may be impossible.

Hepatocyte Agents

Mangafodipir and the hepatocyte-specific gadolinium chelates are accumulated to a normal degree in regenerative and dysplastic nodules. Their uptake in HCCs is related to the degree of differentiation, so that well-differentiated tumors may show marked enhancement with these agents which persists longer than in the adjacent liver, owing to the lack of a biliary excretion pathway from the tumor. Reduction or lack of uptake of T1 hepatocyte agents into a nodule is a good indicator of malignancy.

"UNIDENTIFIED BRIGHT OBJECTS"

Just as in MRI studies of the central nervous system, unidentified bright objects (UBOs) can be problematic in the diagnosis of liver tumors. Liver UBOs in cirrhosis are small hypervascular areas seen on post-Gd T1w images. They fall into two categories—anomalies of vascular perfusion with a local arterial blush, and small hyper-arterialised parenchymal nodules.

Anomalies of Vascular Perfusion

Focal vascular anomalies of the liver occur in all groups of patients, but are more often seen in cirrhotics, possibly because of the more rapid regeneration and turnover of liver parenchyma, combined with raised portal venous pressure. Non-portal venous inflow to the liver arrives by several routes including the parabiliary venous plexus surrounding the main extrahepatic bile ducts, the cholecystic veins draining the gallbladder, the inferior and superior veins of Sappey, and occasionally from anomalous right gastric or pancreatico-duodenal veins, most often seen after surgical procedures on the distal stomach. The effect of these vessels is manifest as an increased but transient arterial blush in the area of liver supplied by these veins, which becomes indistinguishable from the adjacent parenchyma in the portal venous phase of enhancement. Typically these areas are seen adjacent to the gallbladder fossa, on the anterior surface of segment 4 adjacent to the falciform ligament, on the posterior aspect of segment 4 adjacent to the porta hepatis, and over the bare area of the liver adjacent to the right hemidiaphragm. The characteristic feature of these lesions is that they show a triangular or irregular shape and they are always located alongside one of the surfaces of the liver. The term THID (transient hepatic intensity difference) can be used to describe these vascular changes, but is also applied in cases where similar focal areas of peripheral hyperintensity in the arterial phase occur at sites unassociated with anomalous venous inflow. These "lesions" are probably caused by the occlusion of a local portal vein radical with compensatory increase in arterial flow. Because a similar change can be produced by tumors occluding small portal vein radicles, a careful search must be made for mass lesions at the apex of THIDs which are usually cone- or wedge-shaped (see also chapter. 4). Similar perfusion anomalies may arise following needle biopsy of the liver, probably related to local portal vein branch thrombosis or arterio-portal shunting at the biopsy site (see also chap. 4). Arteriovenous malformations within the liver may also produce a hypervascular blush in the arterial phase of enhancement. These lesions are usually clear-cut and show low signal on unenhanced T1w imaging, with marked post-Gd enhancement which remains sequentially similar to that of the hepatic veins.

Benign Hypervascular Nodules

Although most nodules—including those of sub-cm size—which show arterial hypervascularity in the cirrhotic liver will be HCCs, recent surveillance studies have shown that a minority of small hypervascular nodules remain stable between consecutive imaging examinations, or even disappear completely. Consecutive imaging studies or histology after transplantation confirm that some of these nodules are malignant, but others which show benign behavior have largely similar imaging features. Most of these benign nodules are isointense on unenhanced T1w and T2w images, and they show normal uptake of SPIO, so the only abnormal feature is their arterial hypervascularity. Even after transplantation, in some cases these nodules show no distinctive features on naked eye examination of the explanted liver, so the pathologist may be unable to locate the nodule for histologic examination. The most effective discriminator is probably the lack of uptake of SPIO in malignant nodules. The pathologic and imaging diagnosis of small hypervascular nodules in cirrhosis remains challenging, and is discussed further in Chapter 14.

ILLUSTRATIVE FIGURES

Dysplastic nodule—Figures 1–5
Co-existent HCC and dysplastic nodule—Figures 6–10
Well-differentiated HCC—Figures 11–12
Solitary HCC—Figures 13–22
Hemangioma in cirrhosis—Figure 23
Multiple HCC—Figures 24–28
HCC with vascular invasion—Figures 29–33
HCC with capsule—Figures 34–38
HCC causing indrawn liver surface—Figure 39
HCC with nodal metastasis—Figure 40
HCC with fat—Figures 41–43
HCC in hemochromatosis—Figure 44–50
Benign hypervascular nodules—Figures 51–54

REFERENCES

1. Ward J, Robinson PJ. How to detect hepatocellular carcinoma in cirrhosis. Eur Radiol 2002; 12:2258–2272.
2. Matsui O, Kadoya M, Kameyama T, et al. Benign and malignant nodules in cirrhotic livers: distinction on blood supply. Radiology 1991; 178:493–497.
3. Earls JP, Theise ND, Weinreb JC, et al. Dysplastic nodules and hepatocellular carcinoma: thin-section MR imaging of explanted cirrhotic livers with pathologic correlation. Radiology 1996; 201:207–214.
4. Peterson MS, Baron RL, Murakami T. Hepatic malignancies: usefulness of acquisition of multiple arterial and portal venous phase images at dynamic gadolinium-enhanced MR imaging. Radiology 1996; 201:337–345.
5. Murakami T, Baron RL, Peterson MS, et al. Hepatocellular carcinoma: MR imaging with Mangafodipir Trisodium (Mn-DPDP). Radiology 1996; 200:69–77.
6. Rofsky NM, Weinreb JC, Bernardino ME, et al. Hepatocellular tumors: characterization with Mn-DPDP-enhanced MR imaging. Radiology 1993; 188:53–59.
7. Yamamoto H, Yamashita Y, Yoshimatsu S, et al. Hepatocellular carcinoma in cirrhotic livers: detection with unenhanced and iron oxide-enhanced MR imaging. Radiology 1995; 195:106–112.
8. Bhartia B, Ward J, Guthrie JA, et al. Hepatocellular carcinoma in cirrhotic livers: double-contrast thin-section MR imaging with pathologic correlation of explanted tissue. AJR 2003; 180:577–584.
9. Krinsky GA, Lee VS, Theise ND, et al. Hepatocellular carcinoma and dysplastic nodules in patients with cirrhosis: prospective diagnosis with MR imaging and explantation correlation. Radiology 2001; 219:445–454.
10. Ward J, Guthrie JA, Scott DJ, et al. Hepatocellular carcinoma in the cirrhotic liver: double-contrast MR imaging for diagnosis. Radiology 2000; 216:154–162.
11. Jeong YY, Mitchell DG, Kamashima T. Small (<20mm) enhancing hepatic nodules seen on arterial phase MR imaging of the cirrhotic liver: clinical implications. AJR 2002; 178:1327–1334.
12. Ito K, Fujita T, Shimizu A, et al. Multiarterial phase dynamic MRI of small early enhancing hepatic lesions in cirrhosis or chronic hepatitis: differentiating between hypervascular hepatocellular carcinomas and pseudolesions. AJR 2004; 183:699–705.
13. Kamura T, Kimura M, Sakai K, et al. Small hypervascular hepatocellular carcinoma versus hypervascular pseudolesions: differential diagnosis on MRI. Abdom Imaging 2002; 27:315–324.

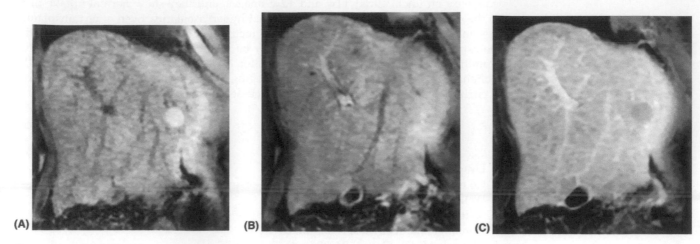

Figure 1. *Dysplastic nodule*: In a patient with primary biliary cirrhosis, coronal oblique T1w images before (**A**), in arterial phase (**B**), and in delayed phase (**C**) after Gd showed a diffuse finely nodular architecture. The 2 cm nodule in the left lobe was hyperintense on unenhanced T1w imaging (**A**), isointense during the arterial phase (**B**) and relatively hypointense on delayed post-Gd T1w images (**C**). The fibrotic tissue which comprises much of this enlarged liver enhanced more than the parenchyma on the later images.

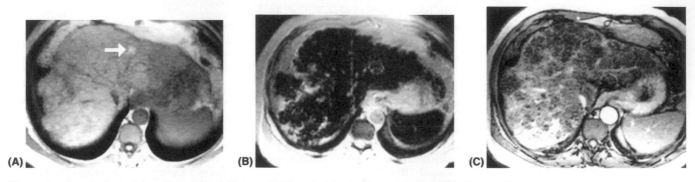

Figure 2. *Dysplastic nodule*: In a patient with hepatitis C and cirrhosis, the unenhanced T1w image (**A**) showed a single hyperintense nodule (arrow) in the left lobe; the post-SPIO T2w image (**B**) showed patchy fibrosis most marked in the right lobe, but the left lobe nodule took up SPIO normally. Post-Gd T1w imaging (**C**) showed no increased vascularity in the suspicious nodule.

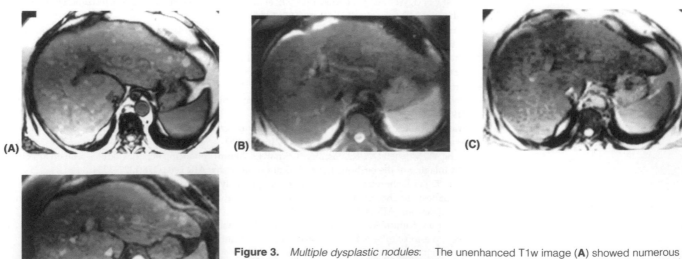

Figure 3. *Multiple dysplastic nodules*: The unenhanced T1w image (**A**) showed numerous small hyperintense nodules which appeared isointense on T2w images (**B**) and showed normal uptake of SPIO (**C**); in the arterial phase T1w images post-Gd (**D**), the nodules again appeared mildly hyperintense but comparison with the unenhanced image showed the degree of enhancement of the nodules was less than that of the surrounding liver.

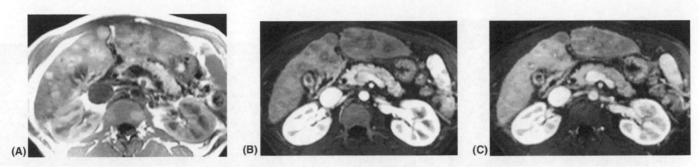

Figure 4. *Multiple dysplastic nodules:*   An unenhanced T1w image (**A**) showed numerous hyperintense nodules; post-Gd T1w images in arterial phase (**B**) and venous phase (**C**) showed no increased vascularity in these lesions.

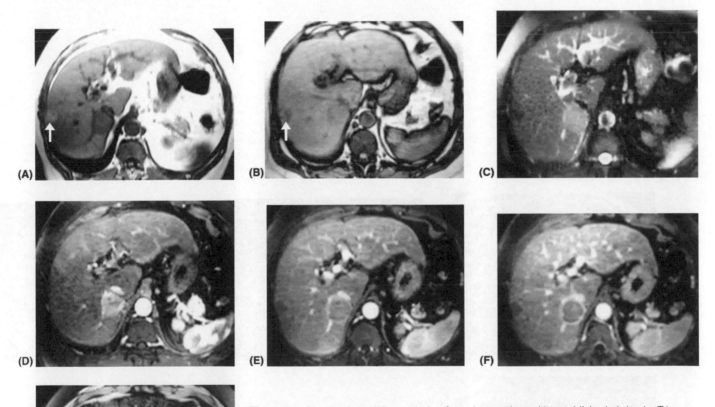

Figure 5. *Dysplastic nodule containing fat:*   In a patient with established cirrhosis, T1w images showed a 3 cm slightly hypointense lesion in the medial aspect of the right lobe posterior to the IVC, and also a 1.5 cm lesion laterally which was hyperintense on in-phase (**A**) and hypointense on opposed-phase (**B**) T1w images (arrow in **A**, **B**). The larger lesion was hyperintense on T2w imaging, the smaller lesion isointense (**C**). On post-Gd T1w images, the larger lesion showed arterial hypervascularity (**D**), faded to isointensity in the venous phase (**E**) with an enhancing caspsule on delayed images (**F**), and it did not take up SPIO contrast as shown by post-SPIO T2w images (**G**). The smaller lesion remained almost isointense with liver on all sequences after both Gd and SPIO. Explant histology confirmed the larger lesion to be HCC and the smaller lesion to be a dysplastic nodule with the unusual feature of fatty infiltration.

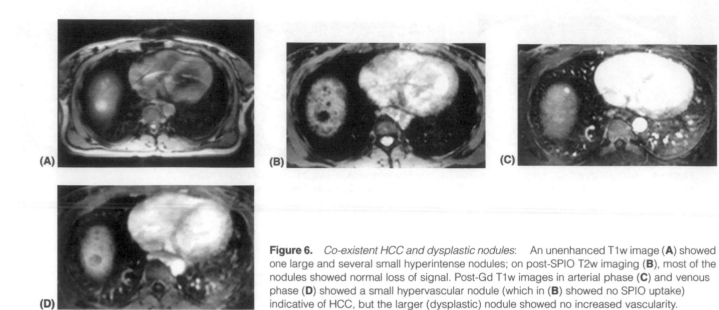

Figure 6. *Co-existent HCC and dysplastic nodules*:   An unenhanced T1w image (**A**) showed one large and several small hyperintense nodules; on post-SPIO T2w imaging (**B**), most of the nodules showed normal loss of signal. Post-Gd T1w images in arterial phase (**C**) and venous phase (**D**) showed a small hypervascular nodule (which in (**B**) showed no SPIO uptake) indicative of HCC, but the larger (dysplastic) nodule showed no increased vascularity.

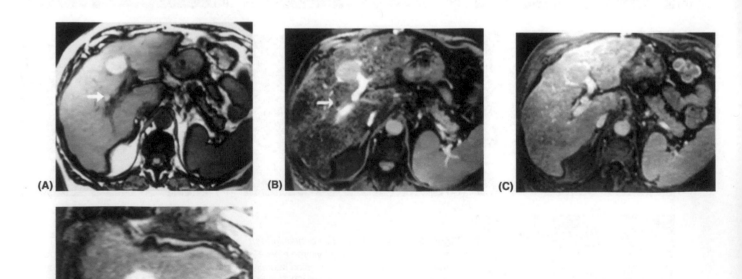

Figure 7. *Co-existent HCC and dysplastic nodule*:   An unenhanced T1w image (**A**) showed a 3 cm hyperintense nodule in segment 4 and a 1 cm nodule adjacent to the porta hepatis (arrow); on post-SPIO T2w imaging (**B**), the larger nodule showed diminished uptake of SPIO suggesting malignancy, the smaller nodule showed normal uptake, indicating dysplasia (arrow). Both nodules were isointense on the venous phase post-Gd T1w images (**C**), but the coronal images obtained in the arterial phase (**D**) showed the larger nodule to be hypervascular.

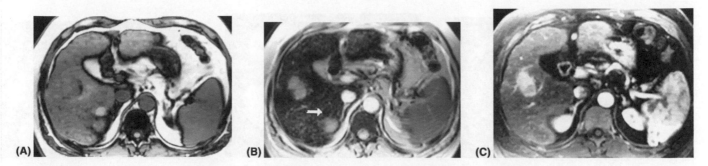

Figure 8. *Co-existent HCC and dysplastic nodule:* An unenhanced T1w image (**A**) showed a hyperintense nodule in segment 6, also an ill-defined larger abnormality fairly centrally in segments 5 and 6. The post-SPIO T2w images (**B**) showed normal uptake in the segment 6 dysplastic nodule (arrow), while the larger abnormality in segments 5 and 6 showed little or no SPIO uptake. Arterial phase post-Gd T1w images (**C**) confirmed the larger lesion was a hypervascular HCC, while there was no increase in vascularity in the segment 5/6 dysplastic nodule.

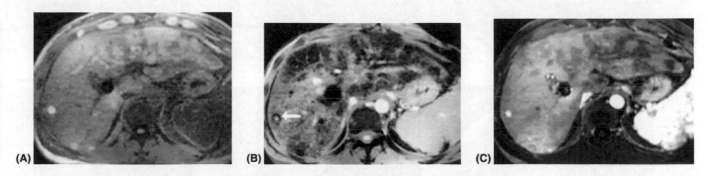

Figure 9. *Nodule-in-nodule:* An unenhanced T1w image (**A**) showed several hyperintense nodules of 1 cm or less. Post-SPIO T2w images (**B**) showed normal iron uptake in all of these nodules, but with a small high signal focus in the center of the largest nodule (arrow). Arterial phase post-Gd T1w images (**C**) showed a hypervascular lesion which appears smaller than the nodule in (**A**) and (**B**). Histology confirmed a focus of HCC within a dysplastic nodule.

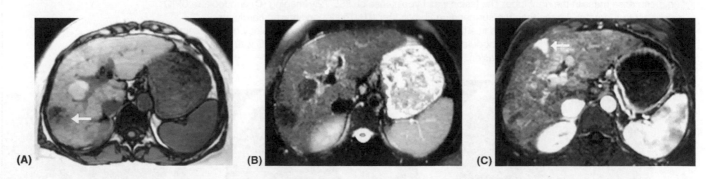

Figure 10. *Nodule-in-nodule:* Multiple nodules in a patient with advanced cirrhosis showed different characteristics; on the unenhanced T1w image (**A**) the nodule adjacent to the right portal division was hyperintense, while the more peripheral nodule in segment 6/7 (arrow) showed patchy hypointensity. The corresponding T2w image (**B**) showed both nodules to be uniformly hypointense. The arterial phase post-Gd T1w image (**C**) showed a small central focus of early enhancement in the more central nodule, while the peripheral nodule showed patchy arterialization. Note also the wedge-shaped THID (arrowed) in segment 4. The post-SPIO T2w image (**D**) again showed the nodule-in-nodule appearance of the central lesion, typical of a focus of HCC developing in a dysplastic nodule. Further areas of reduced iron uptake were present in the more peripheral nodule and also just anterior to the left portal vein branch (arrow), suggesting further malignancy here. Arterial phase images at other levels (**E**, **F**) showed additional hypervascular tumors confirmed as multiple HCC. (*Continued*)

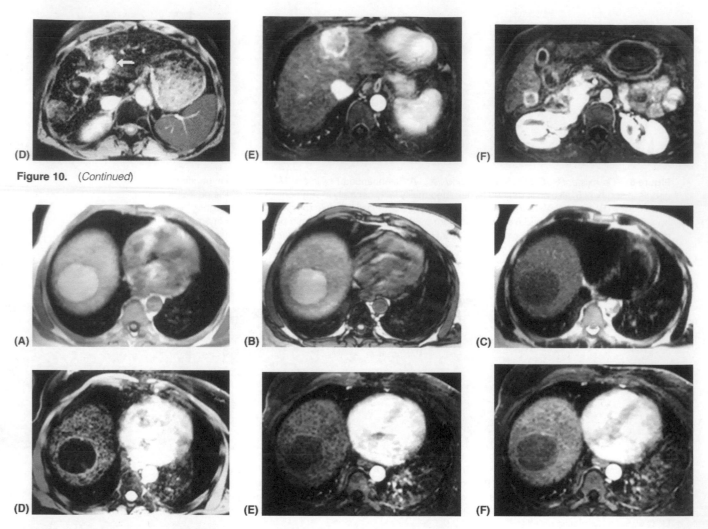

Figure 10. (*Continued*)

Figure 11. *Homogeneously hyperplastic, well-differentiated HCC of benign type*: In a patient with hepatitis B-related cirrhosis, both in-phase and opposed-phase T1w images (**A**, **B**) showed a 5 cm hyperintense mass in the right lobe. The lesion was hypointense on FSE T2w imaging (**C**) and took up SPIO contrast to a greater degree than the surrounding fibrotic liver (**D**). The lesion showed hardly any enhancement on post-Gd T1w images in either arterial (**E**) or venous (**F**) phases. Histology of the resected specimen showed a large dysplastic nodule containing areas of well-differentiated HCC with uniform hyperplasia and no microvascular invasion.

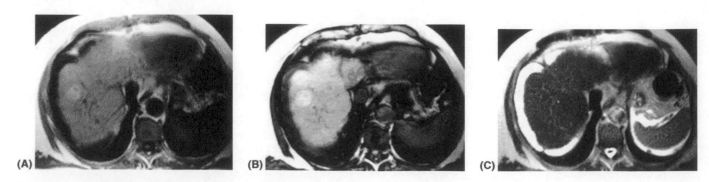

Figure 12. *Well-differentiated HCC*: In a late stage cirrhotic liver, a hyperintense 3 cm nodule was shown on both in-phase and opposed-phase T1w images (**A**, **B**). The lesion was isointense on FSE T2w images (**C**) and showed heterogeneous uptake of SPIO contrast (**D**). Post-Gd T1w images showed the lesion to be hypervascular in the arterial phase (**E**) and isointense on the venous phase (**F**). Histology showed a well-differentiated HCC with no microvascular invasion. (*Continued*)

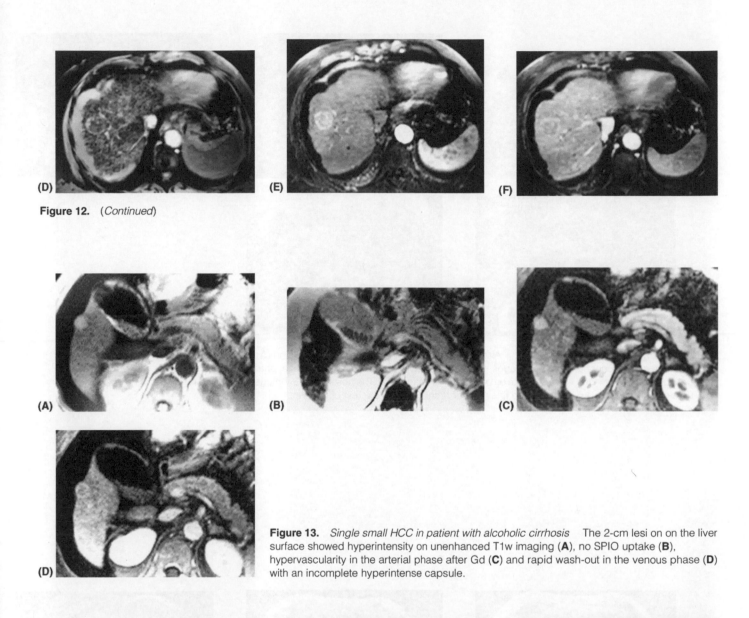

Figure 12. (*Continued*)

Figure 13. *Single small HCC in patient with alcoholic cirrhosis* The 2-cm lesi on on the liver surface showed hyperintensity on unenhanced T1w imaging (**A**), no SPIO uptake (**B**), hypervascularity in the arterial phase after Gd (**C**) and rapid wash-out in the venous phase (**D**) with an incomplete hyperintense capsule.

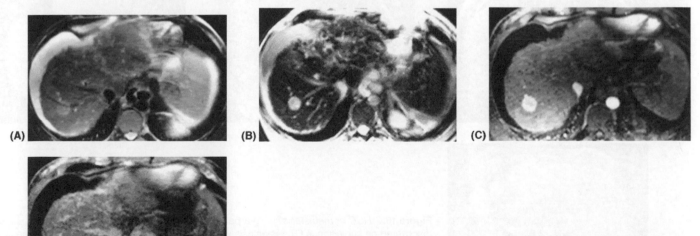

Figure 14. *Solitary HCC in a patient with cirrhosis from chronic hepatitis B:* The lesion of 2.5 cm was barely visible on the unenhanced T2w image (**A**), but was well seen after SPIO (**B**); it showed hypervascularity in the post-Gd arterial phase T1w images (**C**), but became isointense in the venous phase (**D**).

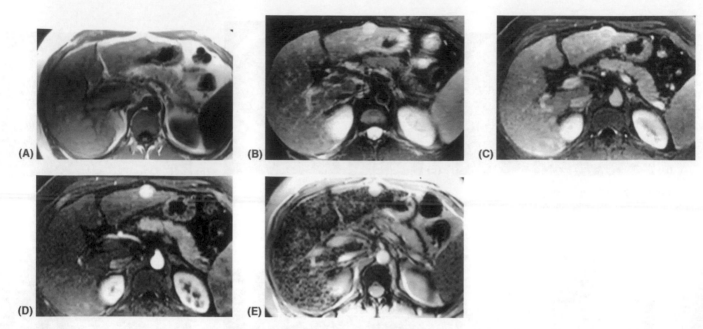

Figure 15. *Small HCC in segment 3*: Although isointense on unenhanced T1w imaging (**A**), the lesion was hyperintense on unenhanced T2w images (**B**); it showed hypervascularity in the arterial phase (**C**) and became isointense in the venous phase on post-Gd T1w images (**D**). The post-SPIO T2w image (**E**) showed no uptake in the lesion, but illustrates the fine nodular architecture of the rest of the liver.

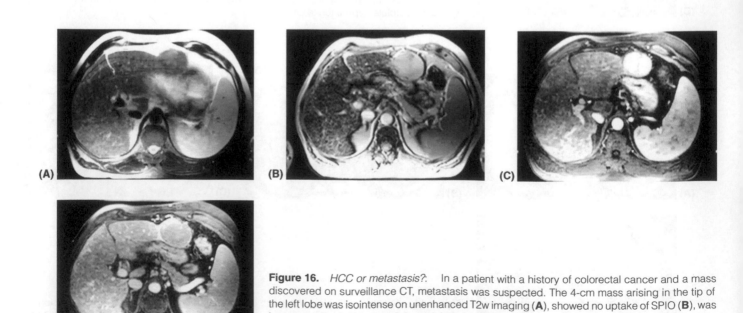

Figure 16. *HCC or metastasis?*: In a patient with a history of colorectal cancer and a mass discovered on surveillance CT, metastasis was suspected. The 4-cm mass arising in the tip of the left lobe was isointense on unenhanced T2w imaging (**A**), showed no uptake of SPIO (**B**), was hypervascular in the post-Gd arterial phase imaging (**C**) and became isointense with an enhancing capsule in the venous phase (**D**)—all typical features of HCC, confirmed on histology. Note the fine nodular architecture of the liver and the enlarged spleen, indicative of cirrhosis.

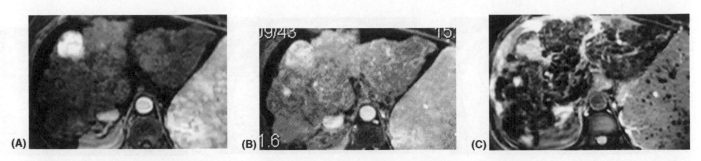

Figure 17. *HCC in cirrhosis from Budd-Chiari syndrome*: In a grossly nodular liver, an arterial phase post-Gd T1w image (**A**) showed a hypervascular mass in segment 4 with incomplete wash-out in the venous phase (**B**). The heterogeneity of enhancement indicates HCC rather than the regenerative hyperplastic nodules which occur in chronic Budd-Chiari, and this was confirmed by the absence of SPIO uptake in the mass (**C**).

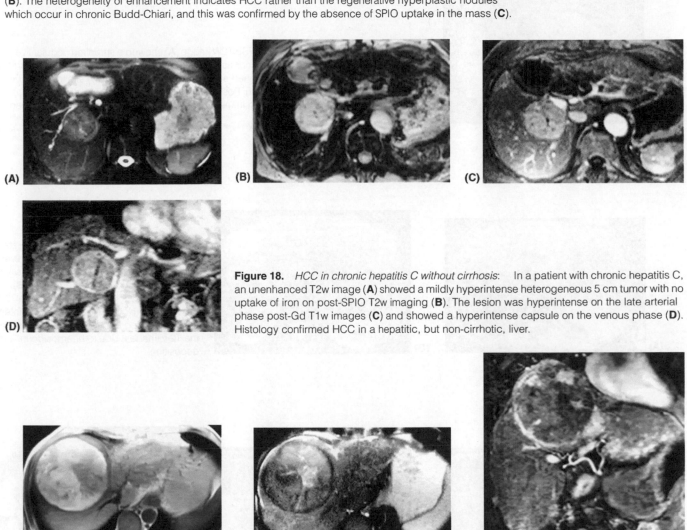

Figure 18. *HCC in chronic hepatitis C without cirrhosis*: In a patient with chronic hepatitis C, an unenhanced T2w image (**A**) showed a mildly hyperintense heterogeneous 5 cm tumor with no uptake of iron on post-SPIO T2w imaging (**B**). The lesion was hyperintense on the late arterial phase post-Gd T1w images (**C**) and showed a hyperintense capsule on the venous phase (**D**). Histology confirmed HCC in a hepatitic, but non-cirrhotic, liver.

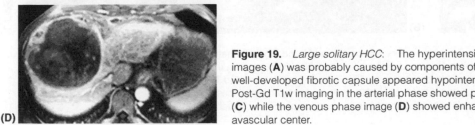

Figure 19. *Large solitary HCC*: The hyperintensity of the lesion shown on unenhanced T1w images (**A**) was probably caused by components of both hemorrhage and fat in the lesion; the well-developed fibrotic capsule appeared hypointense on the unenhanced T2w images (**B**). Post-Gd T1w imaging in the arterial phase showed patchy peripheral and central enhancement (**C**) while the venous phase image (**D**) showed enhancement of the capsule with a relatively avascular center.

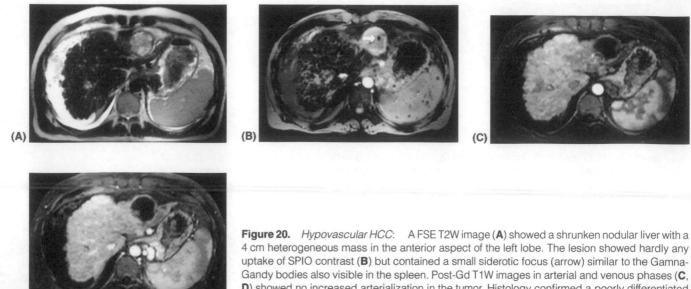

Figure 20. *Hypovascular HCC*:   A FSE T2W image (**A**) showed a shrunken nodular liver with a 4 cm heterogeneous mass in the anterior aspect of the left lobe. The lesion showed hardly any uptake of SPIO contrast (**B**) but contained a small siderotic focus (arrow) similar to the Gamna-Gandy bodies also visible in the spleen. Post-Gd T1W images in arterial and venous phases (**C**, **D**) showed no increased arterialization in the tumor. Histology confirmed a poorly differentiated HCC with extensive necrosis.

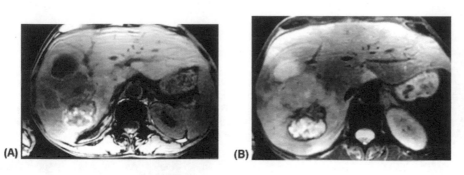

Figure 21. *Hemorrhage in HCC*:   Extensive tumor within the right lobe of the liver enclosed a central area of hyperintensity on both unenhanced T1w (**A**) and T2w (**B**) images, indicating recent intra-tumoral hemorrhage. Note the markedly hypointense rim surrounding the hyperintense center on the T2w images, due to haemosiderin deposition.

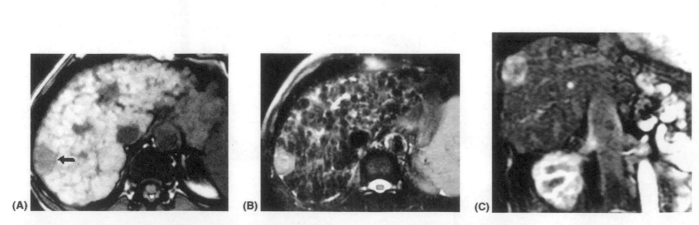

Figure 22. *HCC developing during surveillance*:   Unenhanced T1w (**A**) and T2w (**B**) images in a patient with cryptogenic cirrhosis showed a well-defined nodular architecture with a 3 cm mass in the right lobe (arrow) which was hypointense on T1w and hyperintense on T2w images. Coronal post-Gd T1w images showed the lesion to be hypervascular in the arterial phase (**C**) and isointense in the venous phase (**D**). Figure 22 (**E**) is from the arterial phase of the MRI study obtained one year previously, which showed no evidence of malignancy. (*Continued*)

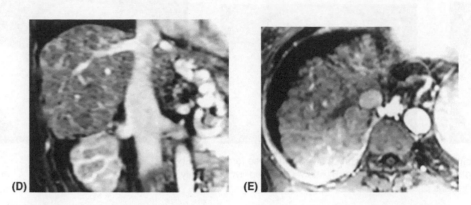

Figure 22. (*Continued*)

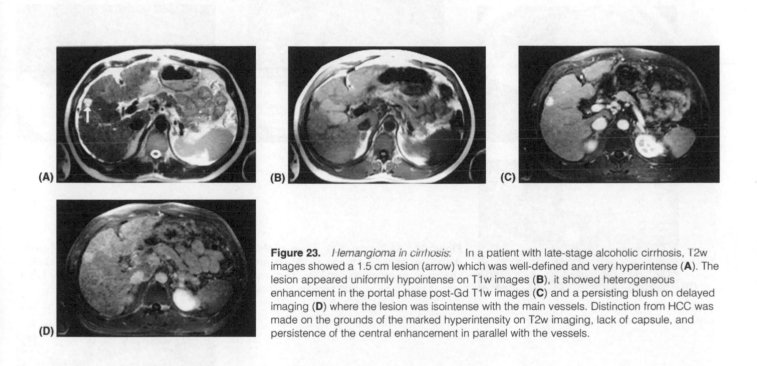

Figure 23. *Hemangioma in cirrhosis:*   In a patient with late-stage alcoholic cirrhosis, T2w images showed a 1.5 cm lesion (arrow) which was well-defined and very hyperintense (**A**). The lesion appeared uniformly hypointense on T1w images (**B**), it showed heterogeneous enhancement in the portal phase post-Gd T1w images (**C**) and a persisting blush on delayed imaging (**D**) where the lesion was isointense with the main vessels. Distinction from HCC was made on the grounds of the marked hyperintensity on T2w imaging, lack of capsule, and persistence of the central enhancement in parallel with the vessels.

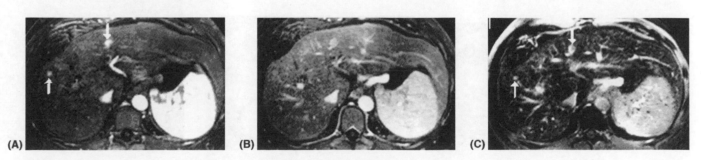

Figure 24. *Multiple HCC:*   In a patient with well-compensated cirrhosis, progressively rising alpha-fetoprotein levels and normal sonography, two hypervascular nodules of sub-cm size (arrows) were particularly conspicuous on arterial phase post-Gd T1W imaging (**A**) acquired 15 minutes after prior injection of SPIO, due to a synergistic increase in contrast between the high signal intensity of enhancing lesions and the low signal intensity of background liver after SPIO. The lesions remained faintly visible on the venous phase image (**B**). The post-SPIO image T2w (**C**) showed no SPIO uptake in these nodules (arrows), confirming their malignant character. Similar HCC nodules were present elsewhere in the liver.

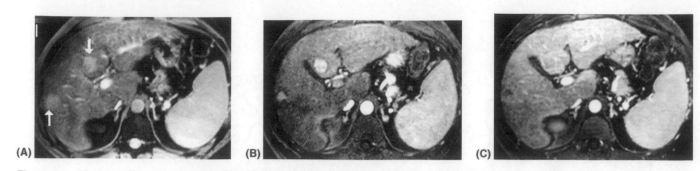

Figure 25. *Multiple HCC:*   Two nodules of 2-3 cm size appeared slightly hyperintense (arrows) on the unenhanced T2w image (**A**). The arterial phase post-Gd T1w image (**B**) showed marked hyperintensity in the lesions with rapid wash-out shown on the venous phase image (**C**).

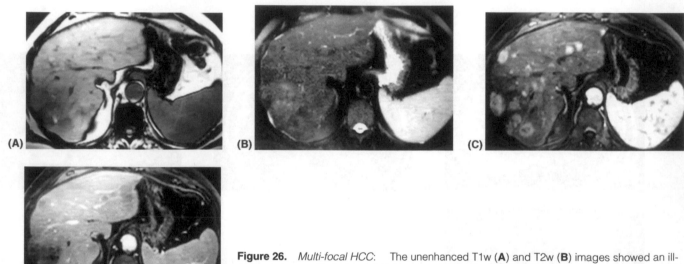

Figure 26. *Multi-focal HCC:*   The unenhanced T1w (**A**) and T2w (**B**) images showed an ill-defined abnormality in the right lobe. The arterial phase (**C**) and venous phase (**D**) post-Gd T1w images confirmed a multi-nodular hypervascular tumor in the lateral aspect of segment 7, but also showed several small nodules of similar character in the left lobe.

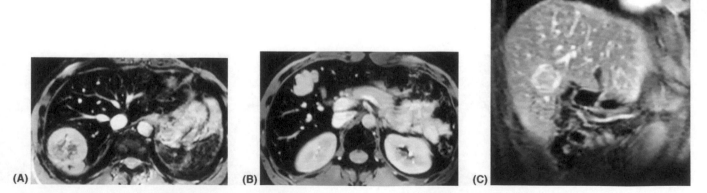

Figure 27. *Multiple HCC in hepatitis B, non-cirrhotic liver.*   Post-SPIO T2w images (**A, B**) showed two lobulated tumors centerd in segments 7 and 4. Note the underlying architecture of the liver was normal, the spleen size was also normal and there was no ascites. The venous phase post-Gd T1w images in RAO coronal view (**C, D**) showed the typical hypervascular capsule of HCC. Following resection of these tumors, liver histology confirmed chronic hepatitis B, but no cirrhosis. Patients with chronic hepatitis B infection are at considerable risk of HCC in the pre-cirrhotic stage, while those with hepatitis C or alcoholic liver disease rarely develop HCC until cirrhosis is established. (*Continued*)

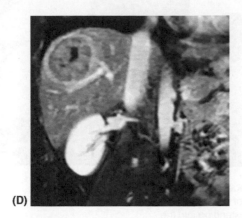

(D)

Figure 27. (*Continued*)

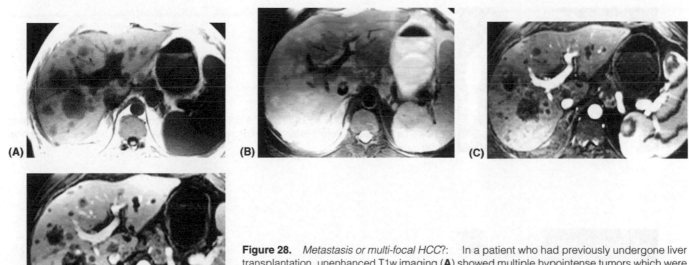

(A) (B) (C)

(D)

Figure 28. *Metastasis or multi-focal HCC?*:   In a patient who had previously undergone liver transplantation, unenhanced T1w imaging (**A**) showed multiple hypointense tumors which were mildly hyperintense on the unenhanced T2w image (**B**). The arterial phase (**C**) and venous phase (**D**) post-Gd T1w images showed numerous hypointense tumors, some of which showed a continuous rim of enhancement in the arterial phase to give an appearance identical with that of metastatic disease. Histology showed poorly differentiated HCC.

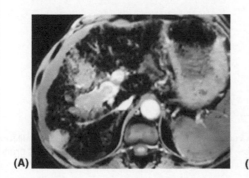

(A)

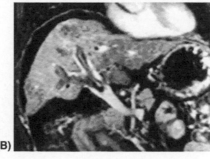

(B)

Figure 29. *HCC invading portal vein*:   The post-SPIO T2w image (**A**) showed multi-focal tumor with extension along the right main portal vein branch. The venous phase post-Gd T1w coronal image (**B**) showed extensive tumor within a nodular liver and non-occlusive filling defects within the right portal vein branches extending down the main portal vein. Patchy enhancement was shown within the filling defect, indicating that this was tumor rather than bland thrombus.

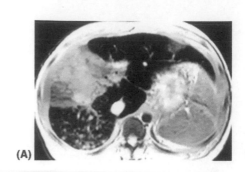

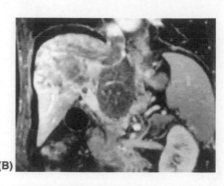

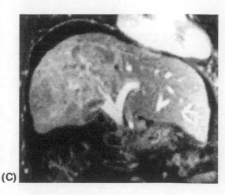

(A)   (B)   (C)

Figure 30. *HCC extending into portal vein, hepatic vein, and IVC:*   A post-SPIO T2w image (**A**) showed a large area of tumor centered on segment 4, but encompassing both left and right branches of the main portal vein. The coronal post-Gd T1w images (**B**, **C**) showed a large heterogeneous tumor mass extending into the main portal vein, and via the right hepatic vein into the IVC.

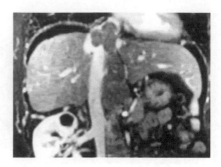

Figure 31. *HCC extending into IVC:*   A coronal oblique venous phase post-Gd T1w image showed a large filling defect extending from the left hepatic vein into the IVC from an ill-defined left lobe tumor.

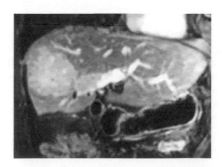

Figure 32. *HCC extending into portal vein:*   A venous phase post-Gd T1w image showed continuity between the right lobe tumor and the large filling defect in the right main portal vein branch.

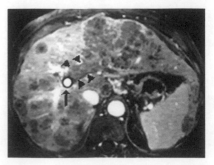

Figure 33. *HCC invading portal vein:*   A venous phase post-Gd T1w image showed multifocal HCC with replacement of much of the left lobe; tumor was growing along the left main portal branch (arrowheads) to reach a TIPSS (arrow) which remained patent.

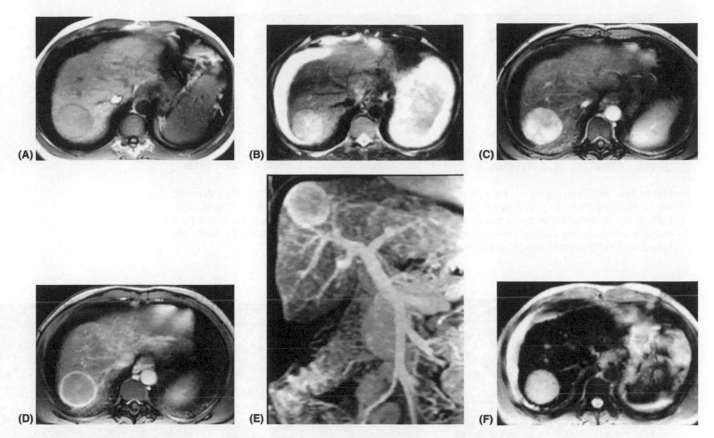

Figure 34. *HCC with capsule*: Unenhanced T1w and T2w images (**A**, **B**) showed a well-defined rounded mass in the right lobe with underlying nodular liver architecture and ascites, resulting from hepatitis C. The capsule surrounding the tumor appeared hypointense on both T1w and T2w images, suggesting fibrous tissue. The post-Gd arterial phase T1w image (**C**) showed intense enhancement in both tumor and capsule, while the venous phase image (**D**) showed rapid wash-out from the tumor but persistent hyperintensity in the capsule, also illustrated in the venous phase MIP image (**E**). The post-SPIO T2w image (**F**) showed the tumor to be apparently smaller than on the arterial phase image, confirming that the rim of tissue surrounding the tumor which forms the "capsule" was part of the adjacent liver rather than part of the tumor.

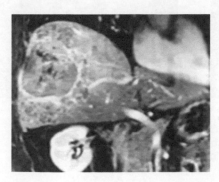

Figure 35. *HCC with capsule*: An RAO coronal venous phase post-Gd T1w image showed a rim of peripheral enhancement surrounding the right lobe tumor.

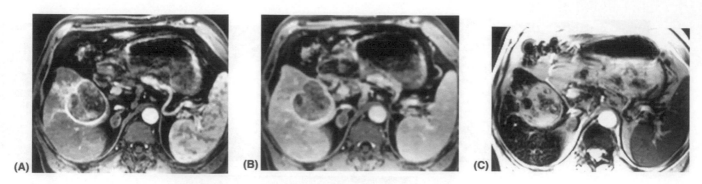

Figure 36. *HCC with capsule*:   An arterial phase post-Gd T1w image (**A**) showed a brightly enhancing rim surrounding the tumor in segment 5. In the venous phase (**B**) the enhancement faded a little, but the capsule still remained hyperintense to surrounding liver. The post-SPIO T2w image (**C**) confirmed that the rim of tissue which showed the bright enhancement was in the liver adjacent to the tumor, not in the tumor itself. Note also a right adrenal metastasis showing similar signal to the HCC.

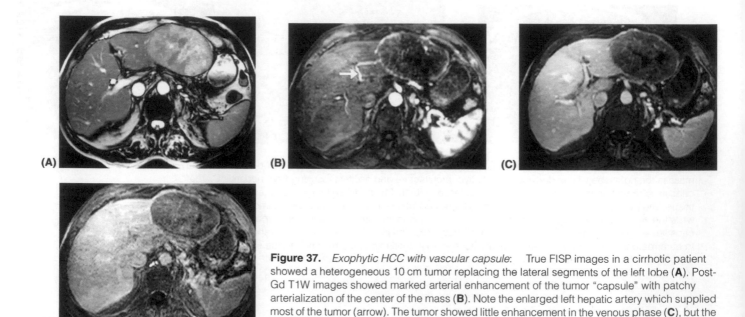

Figure 37. *Exophytic HCC with vascular capsule*:   True FISP images in a cirrhotic patient showed a heterogeneous 10 cm tumor replacing the lateral segments of the left lobe (**A**). Post-Gd T1W images showed marked arterial enhancement of the tumor "capsule" with patchy arterialization of the center of the mass (**B**). Note the enlarged left hepatic artery which supplied most of the tumor (arrow). The tumor showed little enhancement in the venous phase (**C**), but the capsule again became hyperintense on the delayed images (**D**).

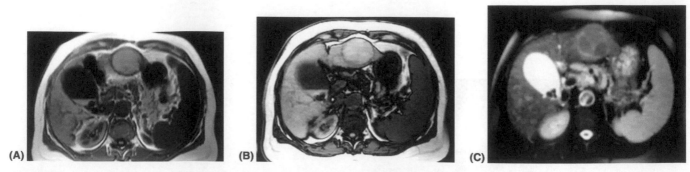

Figure 38. *HCC with fibrotic capsule*:   Both in-phase and opposed-phase T1W images (**A**, **B**) showed a hyperintense 5 cm mass arising in segment 3. The low signal intensity capsule was particularly clear on the in-phase image. The lesion was largely isointense on HASTE imaging (**C**), but took up no SPIO contrast (**D**). Delayed post-Gd T1W images in coronal and axial planes (**E**, **F**) showed hyperintensity of the fibrous capsule around the tumor. (*Continued*)

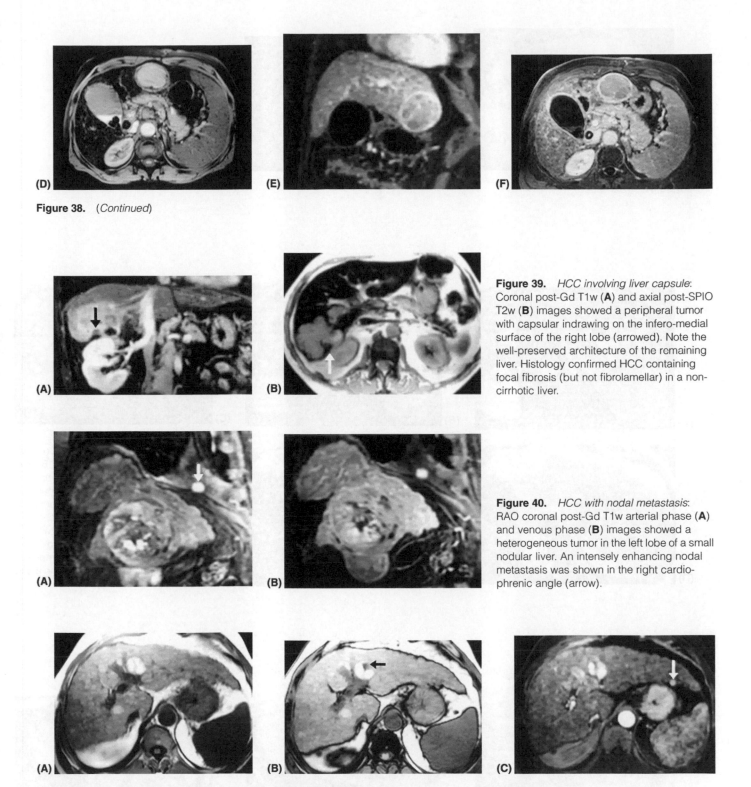

Figure 38. (*Continued*)

Figure 39. *HCC involving liver capsule*: Coronal post-Gd T1w (**A**) and axial post-SPIO T2w (**B**) images showed a peripheral tumor with capsular indrawing on the infero-medial surface of the right lobe (arrowed). Note the well-preserved architecture of the remaining liver. Histology confirmed HCC containing focal fibrosis (but not fibrolamellar) in a non-cirrhotic liver.

Figure 40. *HCC with nodal metastasis*: RAO coronal post-Gd T1w arterial phase (**A**) and venous phase (**B**) images showed a heterogeneous tumor in the left lobe of a small nodular liver. An intensely enhancing nodal metastasis was shown in the right cardio-phrenic angle (arrow).

Figure 41. *HCC with fat*: An in-phase unenhanced T1w image (**A**) showed several hyperintense nodules, the largest of 3 cm in segment 3. The opposed-phase T1w image (**B**) showed similar hyperintensity in the smaller nodules, but a sector of the segment 3 mass showed signal dropout indicative of fatty change (arrow). The post-Gd T1w arterial phase (**C**) and venous phase (**D**) images showed typical enhancement characteristics of HCC in the segment 3 nodule, while the other nodules in segment 6 showed normal vascularity. The post-SPIO T2w image (**E**) showed normal uptake in the segment 6 nodules but reduced uptake in the larger segment 3 lesion. Explant histology confirmed HCC in segment 3 with dysplastic nodules in segments 3 and 6. Note the sub-cm arterialised nodule on the posterior surface of segment 3 (arrow) which was only visible in the arterial phase - its histology showed dysplasia but no HCC. (*Continued*)

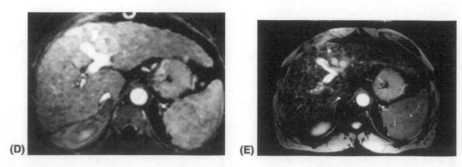

Figure 41. (*Continued*)

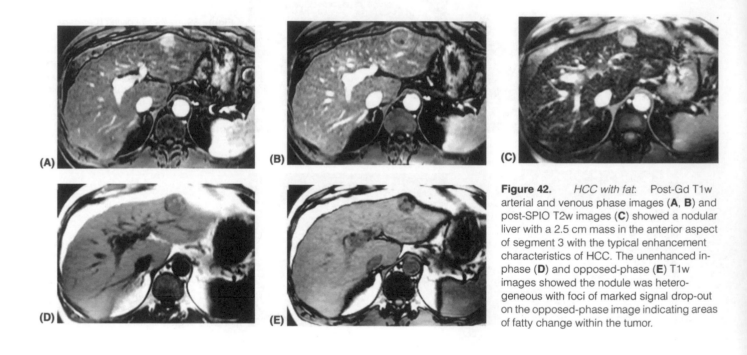

Figure 42. *HCC with fat*: Post-Gd T1w arterial and venous phase images (**A**, **B**) and post-SPIO T2w images (**C**) showed a nodular liver with a 2.5 cm mass in the anterior aspect of segment 3 with the typical enhancement characteristics of HCC. The unenhanced in-phase (**D**) and opposed-phase (**E**) T1w images showed the nodule was heterogeneous with foci of marked signal drop-out on the opposed-phase image indicating areas of fatty change within the tumor.

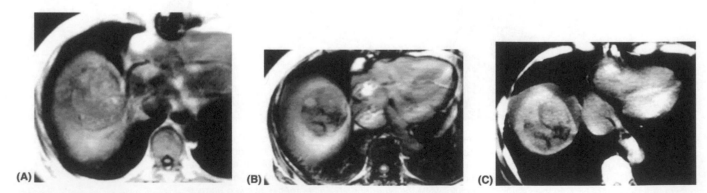

Figure 43. *HCC with fat*: Unenhanced in-phase (**A**) and opposed-phase (**B**) T1w images showed a heterogeneous tumor near the diaphragmatic surface of the right lobe containing extensive areas of low signal on the opposed-phase image. CT in the same patient (**C**) showed similar low attenuation areas indicating seams of fat within the tumor.

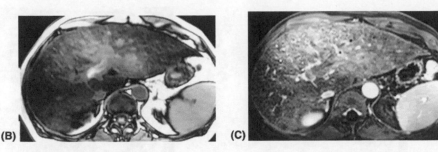

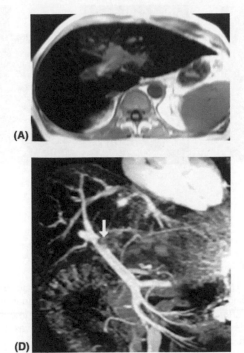

Figure 44. *HCC in hemochromatosis:* Unenhanced in-phase (**A**) and opposed-phase (**B**) T1w images showed a multi-focal tumor centered around the left portal vein branch. The background liver showed reduced signal intensity on the opposed phase image, but on the in-phase image—because of the longer TE—the liver signal was much lower owing to iron deposition. The post-Gd venous phase T1w image (**C**) showed an ill-defined central tumor with an enhancing component extending into and filling the lumen of the left portal vein. The coronal MIP image in the portal venous phase (**D**) showed tumor in the left portal branch intruding into the main portal vein lumen (arrow).

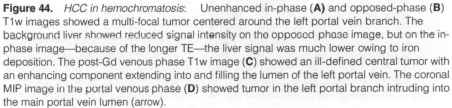

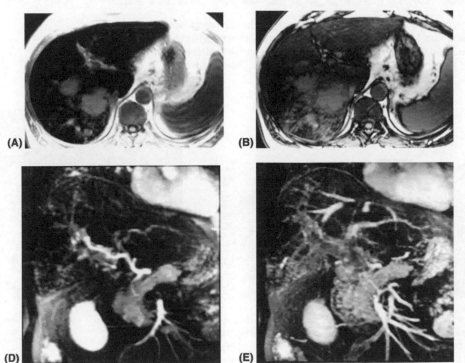

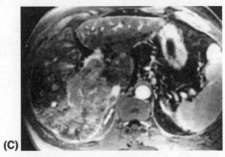

Figure 45. *HCC in hemochromatosis:* Unenhanced in-phase (**A**) and opposed-phase (**B**) T1w images showed multi-focal tumor occupying the right lobe, with diffuse signal loss in the background liver, more marked on the in-phase image. The post-Gd venous phase T1w image (**C**) showed multi-focal tumor with growth along the right portal vein. RAO coronal MIP images from the arterial phase (**D**) and venous phase (**E**) showed tumor entirely filling the main portal vein and its right branches. Note patchy enhancement within the intravascular portion of the tumor, confirming this was not bland thrombus.

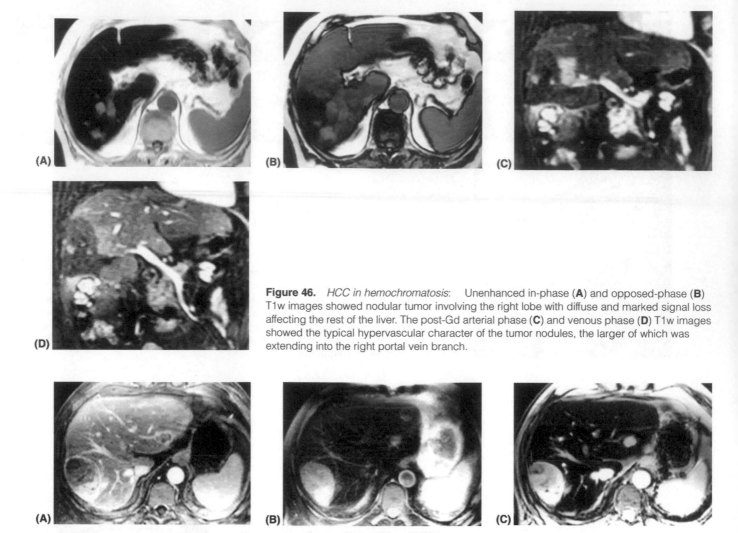

Figure 46. *HCC in hemochromatosis:* Unenhanced in-phase (**A**) and opposed-phase (**B**) T1w images showed nodular tumor involving the right lobe with diffuse and marked signal loss affecting the rest of the liver. The post-Gd arterial phase (**C**) and venous phase (**D**) T1w images showed the typical hypervascular character of the tumor nodules, the larger of which was extending into the right portal vein branch.

Figure 47. *HCC in hemochromatosis:* A post-Gd venous phase T1w image (**A**) showed heterogeneous tumors with rim enhancement in both left and right lobes. The same two lesions were shown on unenhanced FSE T2w (**B**) and GRE T2w (**C**) images; because the GRE sequence is much more sensitive to susceptibility effects than the FSE acquisition, the signal loss from the background liver and contrast between liver and lesions is much greater on the GRE image.

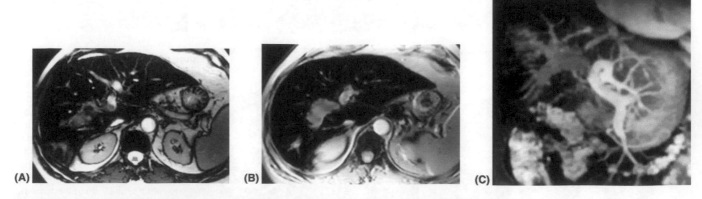

Figure 48. *HCC in hemochromatosis:* In a patient with diffuse signal loss from iron deposition, true FISP (**A**) and gradient-echo T2w (**B**) images showed tumor extending from the periphery of the right lobe into the right portal vein. The post-Gd RAO coronal venous phase T1w MIP image (**C**) showed patency of the main portal vein and the left branch with obliteration of the lumen of the right portal vein and its main divisions by tumor.

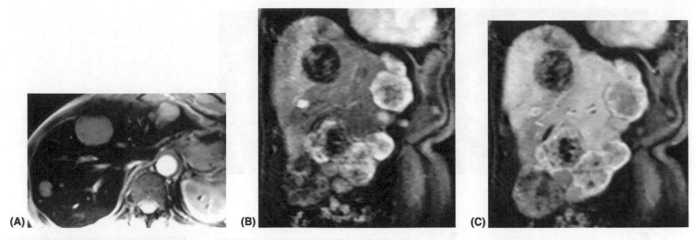

Figure 49. *HCC in hemochromatosis*:   A GRE T2w image (**A**) showed multiple tumor nodules with diffuse loss of signal from the background liver. The RAO coronal arterial phase (**B**) and venous phase (**C**) post-Gd T1w images showed multiple tumors with varying degrees of vascularity.

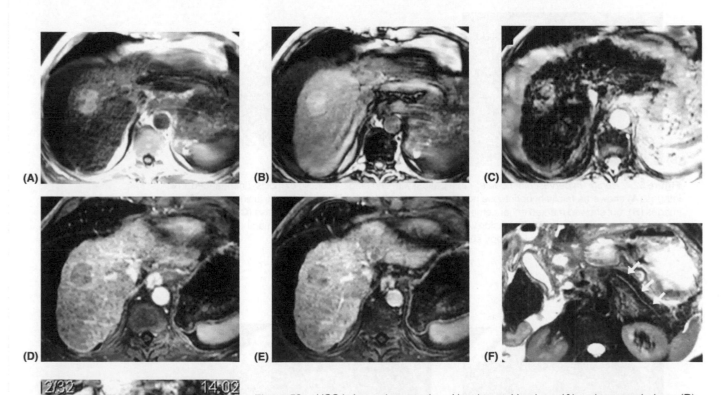

Figure 50. *HCC in hemochromatosis*:   Unenhanced in-phase (**A**) and opposed-phase (**B**) T1w images, and GRE T2w (**C**) images showed a small liver with finely nodular architecture and abnormally low signal on both T2w and in-phase T1w images, indicating iron deposition. A 3 cm tumor nodule showed heterogeneous hyperintensity on all sequences. The post-Gd arterial phase (**D**) and venous phase (**E**) T1w images showed the lesion was not hypervascular. The GRE T2w image through the pancreas (**F**) showed evidence of diffuse iron deposition with loss of signal in the pancreatic parenchyma (arrows); a post-Gd T1w image at the same level (**G**) showed normal enhancement of the gland.

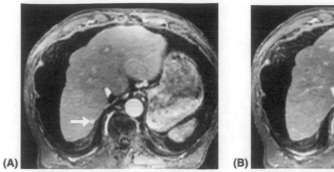
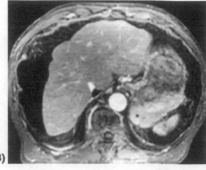

Figure 51. *Benign hypervascular nodule*: In a patient with late stage cirrhosis, post-Gd T1w images showed a 7 mm nodule which was brightly hyperintense (arrow) in the arterial phase (**A**) with incomplete washout by the portal phase (**B**). Explant histology showed no evidence of malignancy.

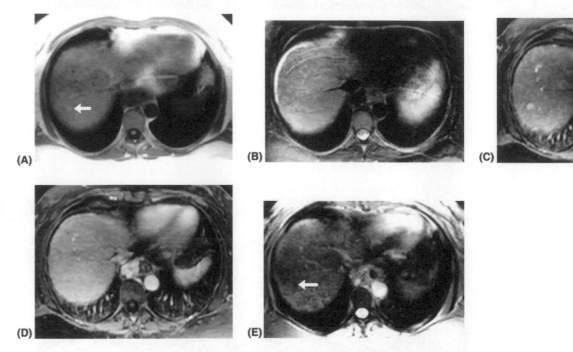

Figure 52. *Benign hypervascular nodule*: In a patient with end stage alcoholic cirrhosis, unenhanced T1w images (**A**) showed a faintly hyperintense nodule in segment 7 (arrow). The nodule was isointense on T2w images (**B**), but showed marked enhancement on post-Gd T1w images in the arterial phase (**C**) with complete washout by the portal phase (**D**). The lesion was hypointense (arrow) on post-SPIO T2w imaging (**E**), indicating normal uptake of SPIO. Explant histology showed no evidence of malignancy.

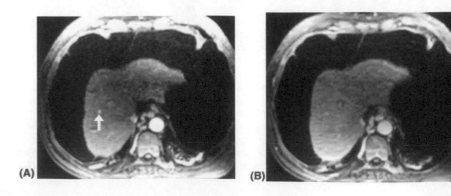

Figure 53. *Benign hypervascular nodule*: In a patient with end stage alcoholic cirrhosis, a 6 mm hypervascular nodule (arrow) was shown in segment 8 in the arterial phase (**A**) of post-Gd T1w imaging, with incomplete wash-out in the portal phase (**B**). Explant histology showed no malignancy.

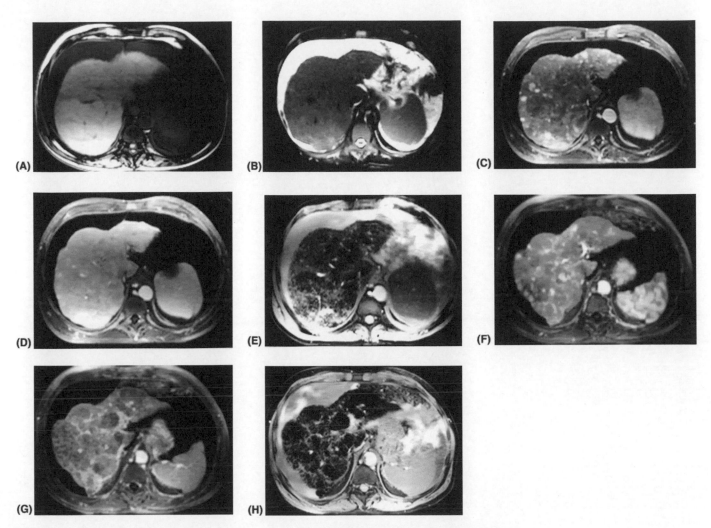

Figure 54. *Multiple hypervascular nodules with benign course:* In a patient with alcoholic liver disease, MRI showed a small nodular liver with fairly uniform signal on unenhanced T1w and T2w images (**A**, **B**). Post-Gd T1w imaging showed numerous hypervascular nodules in the arterial phase (**C**), fading close to isointensity on the portal phase (**D**). On post-SPIO T2w images (**E**), it was difficult to be sure whether or not the nodules had take up contrast because of the presence of widespread patchy fibrosis. Multiple HCC was suspected, but the patient remained fairly well and at repeat examination 2½ years later, multiple hypervascular nodules were again present in the arterial phase post-Gd T1w imaging (**F**), rapidly fading to isointensity on the portal phase (**G**). Post-SPIO T2w imaging (**H**) this time showed less fibrosis, and no non-functioning nodules were visible.

CHAPTER 10

Early Detection of Liver Metastases by MRI

THE ROLE AND VALUE OF IMAGING

Metastatic spread of tumors to the liver is common, with a high incidence from primary sites in the colon, oesophagus, pancreas, stomach, and lungs, and moderately frequent incidence from other primaries, including breast, melanoma, ovary, and kidney. 10–20% of patients with colorectal cancer have synchronous liver metastases at the time of their primary resection and about 50% of patients will develop metastases at some stage of the disease. Surgical resection or ablation of the liver lesions provides the only means of long term survival in these patients, but treatment success is dependant on the detection of all sites of intra-hepatic disease and the exclusion of disease outside the liver. Incomplete resection of intra-hepatic disease has no clinical benefit and does not prolong survival. Patients with fewer, small metachronous metastases have been found to have the most favourable prognosis, but recent data indicate that patients with more extensive disease may still benefit from resection. Consequently, surgery is becoming more aggressive, and the proportion of patients being referred for surgical consideration is rising. Moreover, since patients are being referred with earlier disease, often with multiple small lesions, the task of imaging is becoming more demanding. The role of preoperative imaging is to identify patients who will most benefit from hepatic resection by correctly locating all the metastases. Lesion characterization is as important as lesion detection in determining the management of these patients since a high proportion of small liver lesions, even in patients with a primary malignancy elsewhere, are benign. While failure to detect benign lesions doesn't alter patient management, the incorrect interpretation of benign lesions as malignant may lead to an inappropriate surgical approach, or may wrongly preclude surgery as an option.

MICROSCOPIC METASTASES

All liver metastases start out as tumors of microscopic size. They arrive as cellular emboli via the bloodstream and lodge in the pre-sinusoidal arterioles, in the terminal portal venules, in the sinusoids themselves and in the adjacent spaces of Disse. Metastases of 50–100 μm diameter are often reported in histological studies and although the time period between the seeding of a metastasis and the time it becomes visible on imaging varies, surveillance studies estimate that the mean age of synchronous metastases at the time of surgery for the primary tumor is about 2–3 years.

THE TRUE ACCURACY OF IMAGING

There is no expectation that current imaging techniques will resolve metastases of millimeter size, yet detection rates of 85–90% are consistently reported for CT and MR. Much of the literature on liver imaging is limited by inadequate methods for verification of findings, which make it inevitable that reported sensitivities are overestimated and that the true incidence of disease is underestimated. Recent follow-up studies confirm that a substantial proportion of small metastases are undetected by imaging, IOUS, and surgery and even when histological examination of the resected liver is used as the gold standard, the verification of millimeter and sub-millimeter lesions is questionable since the specimens are traditionally sliced at 1 cm intervals.

In two recent multi-observer studies which evaluated current MR and CT techniques for detecting colorectal metastases, approximately 15% of patients were found to have 'new' metastases on follow up CT performed 4–6 months after hepatic resection. These lesions were very likely to have been present at the time of surgery, and missed both by pre-operative imaging and by surgical inspection with IOUS. Most metastases larger than 1 cm are identifiable with current CT and MR techniques but detection of smaller lesions is still relatively poor. In the two studies referred to above—both of which performed a meticulous correlation with surgery and histology of the resected specimen sectioned at 3 mm intervals—24% (19/80) and 18% (5/27) of sub-cm lesions were not detected by any imaging technique. Moreover, these results compare favourably with earlier studies which have specifically measured the detection rate for surgically confirmed small lesions. Nevertheless, although the detection of small lesions remains disappointing, detection rates continue to improve and development in this field is rapid. There is now good evidence that MR imaging enhanced with liver specific contrast agents is one of the most sensitive methods for detecting liver metastases but reported sensitivities are still likely to be artificially elevated.

OPTIMIZING MR TECHNIQUE FOR DETECTING SMALL METASTASES

Unenhanced Images

The best results so far have been achieved using a field strength of 1.5T with a phased array multi-coil and optimized imaging parameters. Breathhold sequences should be used whenever possible because they are the most effective means of eliminating motion artifact. Unenhanced images are an essential component of liver MRI. Unenhanced T2w images are important in characterizing lesions, particularly distinguishing solid and non-solid tumors, while in-phase and opposed-phase T1w GRE images provide a definitive diagnosis of focal or diffuse fatty infiltration. This is particularly relevant in patients being considered for hepatic resection since severe fatty change—which is not uncommon with chemotherapy—may compromise hepatic function postoperatively. Further, the interpretation of both sonography and CT may be hampered by fat deposition. Tumors in a fatty liver may be inconspicuous on CT and sonography, and areas of focal fat or focal fatty sparing may mimic metastases. Conversely, fatty change is not a diagnostic problem for MR; in- and opposed-phase T1w imaging is regarded as the most accurate technique for differentiating metastases and focal fatty change. Liver-to-tumor contrast is often low on breathhold FSE T2w sequences due to magnetization transfer and reduced susceptibility effects, and our experience is that with current sequences metastases are often more conspicuous on T1w than on FSE T2w images. However, breathhold STIR is probably the most sensitive unenhanced sequence for depicting metastatic disease. Its combination of T1 and T2 weighting provide high contrast leading to a further increase in the conspicuity of small lesions (see also chapter 2).

Dynamic Gd-Enhancement

Dynamic Gd-enhanced imaging (DGEI) using conventional 2D sequences has been shown to be superior to unenhanced imaging and helical CT for detecting metastatic disease. The conspicuity of lesions depends on the differences in perfusion between normal liver and tumor, so multi-phasic imaging is essential. While some (hypervascular) metastases are best seen at the arterial phase when there is only minimal enhancement of background liver, most (hypovascular) lesions are best demonstrated at the portal phase when liver enhancement is maximum. The arterial phase is the most crucial acquisition and should be optimized with test bolusing. Even hypovascular metastases have a characteristic enhancing rim which may only be seen at the arterial phase. Not only does this rim enhancement allow metastases to be distinguished from benign lesions, but also it often improves the conspicuity of small lesions which become less distinct and apparently become smaller on later acquisitions.

DGEI with fat suppression is the technique of choice for demonstrating small metastases on the liver surface. Fat suppression is critically important because it accentuates Gd enhancement and suppresses the competing high signal of intra-abdominal fat adjacent to the liver surface. Surface deposits are often best seen on delayed images acquired 5–10 minutes after injection when they become hyperintense due to slow accumulation of contrast within the tumor.

In patients with metastatic disease probably the main role of DGEI however, is to differentiate benign from malignant lesions. DGEI is the most reliable method for determining the nature of a lesion and is recommended for all surgical candidates with equivocal lesions in a location which is likely to influence the surgical approach. By observing the perfusion and extraction characteristics of tissues at the different phases of enhancement, the typical appearance of cysts, hemangiomas, FNH, and metastases can be recognized and a specific diagnosis achieved in almost all cases.

Tissue-Specific Contrast Agents

Liver-specific contrast agents were developed to produce greater and more prolonged lesion-to-liver contrast than is achievable with the ECF agents. On DGEI a minority of lesions remain occult because they have perfusion characteristics similar to normal liver. Also, many small metastases are invisible by the equilibrium phase when contrast is evenly distributed between intravascular and extracellular spaces. All of the currently available liver-specific agents produce high tissue contrast and significantly improve the detection of focal liver lesions compared with unenhanced MR, with enhanced MR using ECF agents with 2D GRE sequences, and with contrast-enhanced CT. Two types of agents are available—those which target the hepatocytes and produce positive enhancement on T1w images (gadobenate, gadoxetic acid, mangafodipir) and the superparamagnetic iron oxide (SPIO) agents (ferumoxides, ferucarbotran) which target the Kupffer cells and cause a marked signal loss on T2w GRE. Gadobenate and gadoxetic acid have a biphasic function. Both behave like ECF Gd agents in the first few minutes after injection and exhibit hepatocyte selectivity on delayed phase images. Both phases are recommended for maximum sensitivity but the detection of small metastases is significantly better on delayed images than in the early vascular phases. Compared with unenhanced images lesion detection is also considerably improved with mangafodipir. With this agent, peak liver enhancement occurs approximately 15 minutes after slow intravenous infusion or injection, but imaging at 24 hours has been shown to improve the detection of small metastases due to delayed washout around their periphery.

At the time of writing no comparative studies have evaluated the accuracy of these agents using high-resolution 3D T1w GRE imaging but it would be reasonable to expect improvements in the detection of sub-cm lesions with the better spatial resolution provided by this sequence.

Probably the most sensitive method for detecting hepatic metastases is MRI enhanced with SPIO. Although few studies have compared the different liver specific agents against each other, SPIO-enhanced MRI has demonstrated varying degrees of superiority, particularly for small lesions. Moreover SPIO-enhanced MR has been shown to have a sensitivity similar to CTAP and to be at least as accurate with fewer false-positive calls. However, the effective use of SPIO enhancement depends on the appropriate choice of sequence parameters. We have compared the accuracy of optimized T2w breathhold SPIO-enhanced FSE and various GRE sequences with unenhanced images, for the detection of surgically confirmed metastases. While the best GRE sequence produced accuracies of 93% and 82% for all lesions and for lesions <1 cm respectively, breathhold FSE produced accuracies of only 82% and 64% and offered no improvement over unenhanced sequences (details of the optimized T2W GRE sequence are given in chapter 3). The same SPIO-enhanced GRE technique with fat suppression is also of value in depicting lesions on the surface of the liver and extra-hepatic deposits in adjacent structures (peritoneum, lymph nodes, adrenals), which become highly conspicuous against the suppressed signal of intra-abdominal fat and the reduced signal of liver after SPIO. The choice of SPIO agent is also influential. Ferucarbotran is administered as a bolus and provides the opportunity to obtain dynamic T1w images in the first few minutes after injection. At this time the iron oxide particles are distributed throughout the intra-vascular space and being less concentrated they produce positive enhancement on T1w images. Although liver-to-lesion contrast is much greater on T2w GRE delayed images, this early T1 enhancement on high resolution 3D FS T1w images is particularly valuable for depicting sub-cm tumors. In most patients the T1 effect is distinctly less than that of ECF Gd agents but this can be beneficial in the setting of metastatic disease. Liver and vessels often show a similar signal intensity during the first-pass phase with SPIO which produces a virtual 'blank canvas' against which small metastases are very conspicuous. Lesions are also readily distinguished from adjacent vessels which otherwise may obscure very small tumors on T2w images. After ferucarbotran we now routinely obtain dynamic high resolution 3D FS T1w images followed by delayed T2w GRE imaging in all surgical patients with metastatic disease. We believe that this combination increases diagnostic confidence and is more sensitive for small lesion detection than delayed T2w images alone, although currently there is little published data to support this view.

Relative Performance of Dynamic Gd-Enhanced Imaging and Post-Superparamagnetic Iron Oxide Imaging

Of major interest is the relative capability of DGEI using high-resolution 3D FS T1W GRE sequences and SPIO-enhanced MRI using optimized T2W GRE sequences. Compared with 2D methods, 3D sequences improve the detection of small lesions because they allow the liver to be imaged with thinner sections, no inter-slice gap, higher signal-to-noise ratio and improved spatial resolution. While most focal liver lesions can be characterized with DGEI on the basis of their perfusion patterns, on post-SPIO T2w images cysts, hemangiomas, and metastases may all be hyperintense and can be indistinguishable. Since lesion detection and characterization are both important in determining the correct management of surgical patients, DGEI would be the technique of choice if lesion detection was equal to that achieved with SPIO. Using histopathology and surgery with IOUS as the reference standard for detecting metastases, we recently compared dynamic contrast-enhanced thin slice helical CT, high resolution 3D T1w DGEI and SPIO-enhanced T2w MR using our optimized gradient echo sequence. Both MR techniques were significantly more accurate than CT, but the detection of lesions 1 cm or smaller was better with SPIO than with DGEI. Further, in this analysis only the delayed T2w GRE images were included when SPIO was used, and as discussed above we now believe that the addition of dynamic 3D T1w imaging further improves the detection of sub-cm lesions on post-SPIO images. All the benign lesions in the study were correctly characterized on both MR techniques by combined review of post-contrast images with unenhanced T1w and T2w images. We found the pre-contrast HASTE sequence to be effective in demonstrating the high fluid content associated with cysts and hemangiomas, allowing the correct diagnosis in all cases. CT produced the highest number of false positive calls and nearly half of these were due to small benign lesions being wrongly interpreted as metastases. False positive findings with both MR techniques were very few.

RECOMMENDATIONS

On the basis of these results, our current practise in patients who are surgical candidates is to perform unenhanced in- and opposed-phase T1w GRE and HASTE sequences followed by dynamic SPIO-enhanced 3D FS T1w GRE imaging and delayed T2w GRE sequences. If a lesion in a location which may alter the surgical approach has benign characteristics on HASTE images, we perform DGEI immediately after SPIO-enhanced imaging for further characterization. With tumors which are closely related to major vessels, DGEI in the coronal oblique plane can be added to define the surgical anatomy more clearly. In non-surgical patients or patients with rising tumor markers, unenhanced imaging followed by DGEI is preferred.

ILLUSTRATIVE FIGURES

Natural history of surgically treated metastases—Figures 1, 2
Fatty change and diagnosis of metastases—Figures 3, 4
Choice of unenhanced sequences—Figures 5, 6
Technical aspects of the use of ECF gadolinium agents—Figures 7–10
Technical aspects of the use of tissue-specific T1 agents—Figures 11–13
Technical aspects of the use of SPIO—Figures 14–22
Value of the combined use of ECF gadolinium with SPIO—Figures 23, 24

REFERENCES

1. Cameron GR. The liver as a site and source of cancer. BMJ 1954; 4858:347–353.
2. Campani D, Caligo MO, Esposito I, Bevilacqua G. Epidemiology & pathology of liver metastases. In: Bartolozzi C, Lencioni R, eds. Liver Malignancies Diagnostic and Interventional Radiology. Berlin: Springer-Verlag, 1999.
3. Pistolesi GF, Caudana R, Marana G. Magnetic resonance imaging of liver metastases. In: Bartolozzi C, Lencioni R, eds. Liver Malignancies Diagnostic and Interventional Radiology. Berlin: Springer-Verlag, 1999.
4. Huppertz A, Balzer T, Blakeborough A, et al. Improved detection of focal liver lesions at MR imaging: multicenter comparison of gadoxetic acid-enhanced MR images with intraoperative findings. Radiology 2004; 230:266–275.
5. Imam K, Bluemke DA. MR imaging in the evaluation of hepatic metastases. Magn Reson Imaging Clin N Am 2000; 8:741–756.
6. Kim MJ, Kim JH, Lim JS, et al. Detection and characterization of focal hepatic lesions mangafodipir versus. superparamagnetic iron oxide-enhanced magnetic resonance imaging. J Mag Reson Imag 2004; 20:612–621.
7. Kim YK, Lee JM, Kim CS, et al. Detection of liver metastases: gadobenate dimeglumine-enhanced three-dimensional dynamic phases and one-hour delayed phase MR imaging versus superparamagnetic iron oxide-enhanced MR imaging. Eur Radiol 2005; 15:220–228.
8. Lencioni R, Della Pina C, Bruix J, et al. Clinical management of hepatic malignancies: ferucarbotran-enhanced magnetic resonance imaging versus contrast-enhanced spiral computed tomography. Dig Dis Sci 2005; 50:533–537.
9. Reimer P, Jähnke N, Fiebich M, et al. Hepatic lesion detection and characterization: value of nonenahnced MR imaging, superparamagnetic iron oxide-enhanced MR imaging and spiral CT-ROC analysis. Radiology 2000; 217:152–158.
10. Robinson PJA. The liver. In: Husband JE, Reznek RH, eds. Imaging in Oncology. 2nd ed. London: Taylor & Francis, 2004.
11. Semelka RC, Braga L, Armao D, et al. Diseases of the hepatic parenchyma. In: Semelka RC, ed. Abdominal-Pelvic MR. New York: Wiley-Liss, 2002.
12. Sica GT, Ji H, Ros PR. CT and MR imaging of hepatic metastases. Am J Roentgenol 2000; 174:691–698.
13. Vidiri A, Carpanese L, Annibale MD, et al. Evaluation of hepatic metastases from colorectal carcinoma with MR-superparamagnetic iron oxide. J Exp Clin Cancer Res 2004; 23:53–60.
14. Ward J, Guthrie JA, Wilson D, et al. Colorectal hepatic metastases, detection with SPIO-enhanced breathhold imaging: comparison of optimized sequences at 1.5T. Radiology 2003; 228:709–718.
15. Ward J, Naik KS, Guthrie JA, Wilson D, Robinson PJ. Hepatic lesion detection: comparison of MR imaging after the administration of superparamagnetic iron oxide with dual-phase CT by using alternative-free response receiver operator characteristic analysis. Radiology 1999; 210:459–466.
16. Ward J, Robinson PJ, Guthrie JA, et al. Liver metastases in candidates for hepatic resection: comparison of helical CT and gadolinium- and SPIO-enhanced MR imaging. Radiology 2005; 237:170–180.

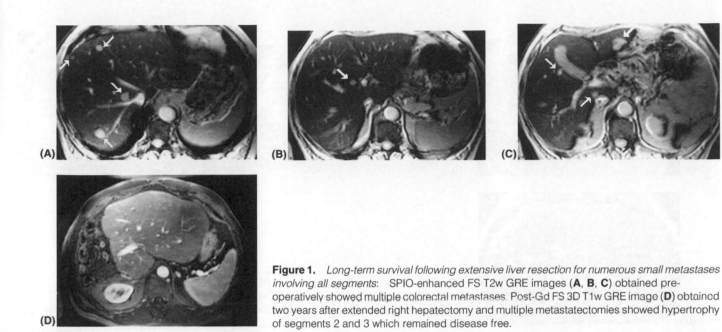

Figure 1. *Long-term survival following extensive liver resection for numerous small metastases involving all segments*: SPIO-enhanced FS T2w GRE images (**A**, **B**, **C**) obtained pre-operatively showed multiple colorectal metastases. Post-Gd FS 3D T1w GRE image (**D**) obtained two years after extended right hepatectomy and multiple metastatectomies showed hypertrophy of segments 2 and 3 which remained disease free.

Figure 2. *Colorectal metastases present on follow-up CT but missed on pre-operative imaging and IOUS*: SPIO-enhanced FS T2w GRE images (**A**, **B**) showed three large metastases. No other lesions were found at subsequent surgery with IOUS. The patient underwent extended right hepatectomy with local excision of the segment 3 metastasis. Histopathology of the resected specimen confirmed the pre-operative findings, but CT obtained four months after the surgery (**C**, **D**) showed multiple small metastases in a hypertrophied left lobe. In a second patient with a GIST tumor, SPIO-enhanced FS T2w GRE images (**E**, **F**) showed three lesions, one in segment 7/8, one in segment 2 (arrow) and one 5 mm metastasis in segment 3 (arrow). Surgery with IOUS confirmed the three lesions and identified one further small metastasis also in segment 2; the patient underwent multiple metastatectomies. Follow-up CT obtained five months after surgery (**G**) showed multiple small metastases which were not visible on pre-operative imaging or at surgery.

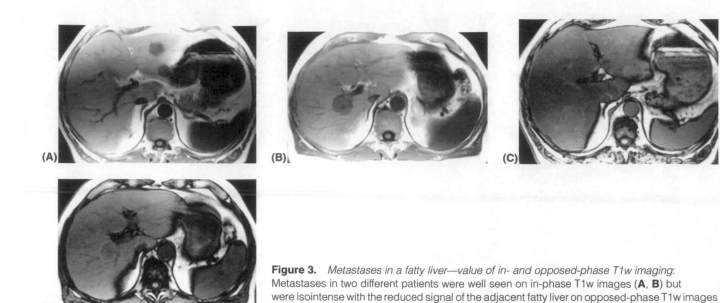

Figure 3. *Metastases in a fatty liver—value of in- and opposed-phase T1w imaging:* Metastases in two different patients were well seen on in-phase T1w images (**A**, **B**) but were isointense with the reduced signal of the adjacent fatty liver on opposed-phase T1w images (**C**, **D**).

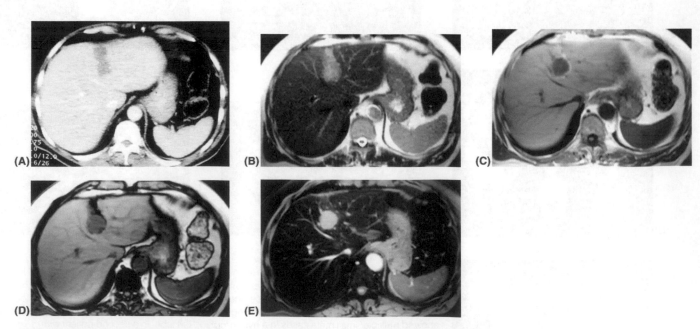

Figure 4. *Metastasis differentiated from focal fatty change with in- and opposed-phase T1w imaging:* CT (**A**) and T2w HASTE images (**B**) demonstrated a large metastasis in segment 4 which appeared to extend to the liver surface. In-phase (**C**) and opposed-phase (**D**) T1w images showed a centrally located metastasis with an adjacent focus of severe fatty change extending along the falciform ligament to the anterior liver surface. Superparamagnetic iron oxide-enhanced FS T2w GRE imaging (**E**) was confirmatory.

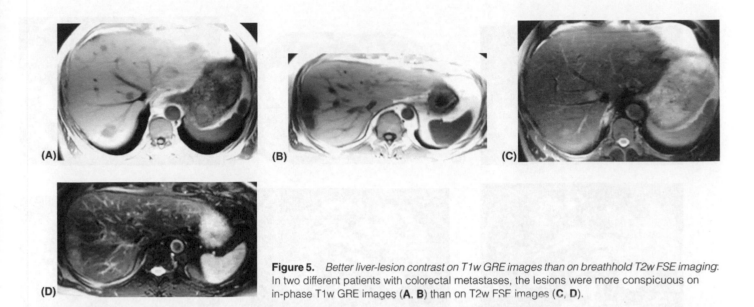

Figure 5. *Better liver-lesion contrast on T1w GRE images than on breathhold T2w FSE imaging:* In two different patients with colorectal metastases, the lesions were more conspicuous on in-phase T1w GRE images (**A**, **B**) than on T2w FSE images (**C**, **D**).

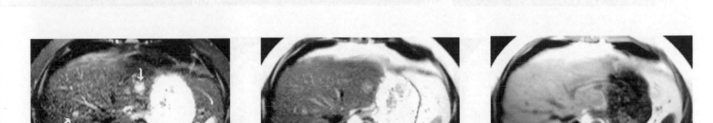

Figure 6. *Improved conspicuity of small metastases on STIR:* STIR image (**A**) illustrating strong lesion to liver contrast and improved conspicuity of two metastases (arrows) compared with T2w HASTE (**B**) and IPT1w GRE (**C**) images.

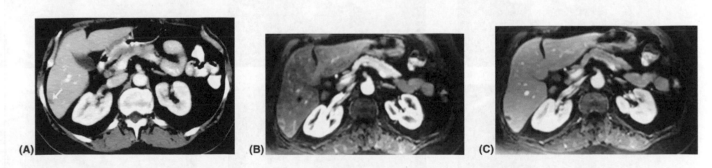

Figure 7. *Dynamic Gd-enhanced MR versus CT and unenhanced MR for lesion detection:* In a patient with colorectal cancer, a solitary lesion (arrow) was indeterminate on surveillance CT (**A**). Arterial (**B**) and portal (**C**) phase post-Gd FS 3D T1w GRE images confirmed the lesion to have the features of a metastasis. Portal phase post-Gd T1w imaging at a more cranial level (**D**) demonstrated a second metastasis (arrow) which was not visible on the corresponding unenhanced T2w FSE image (**E**) or CT (**F**). In second patient a small colorectal metastasis which was not visible on surveillance CT (**G**) was well seen (arrow) on portal phase post-Gd FS 3D T1w GRE imaging (**H**). In a third patient with pancreatic cancer small metastases just below the liver surface (arrows) were well seen on portal phase T1w GRE images (**I**) but were not visible on the corresponding IPT1w (**J**) or T2w FSE (**K**) images. (*Continued*)

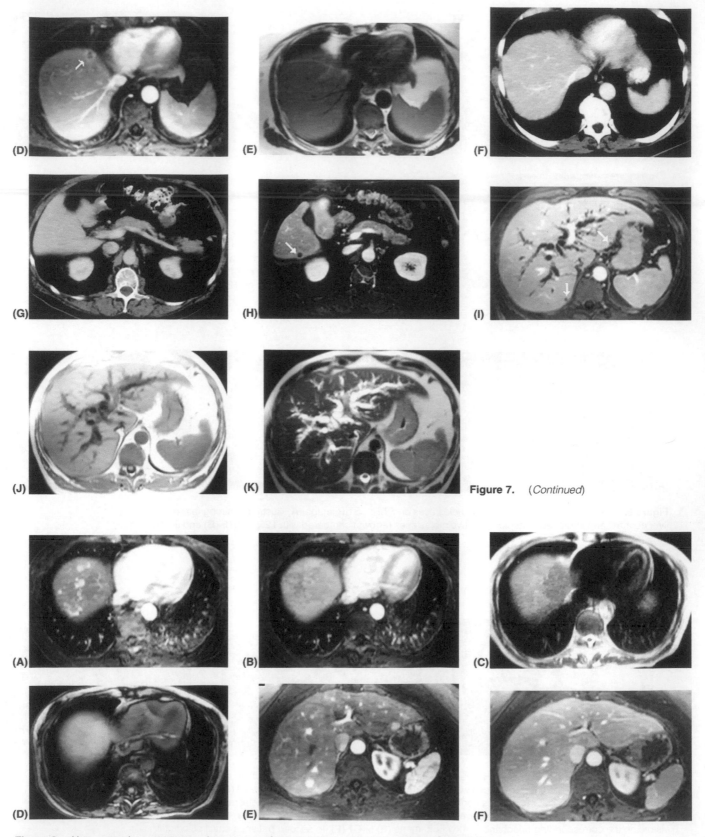

Figure 8. *Hypervascular metastases—importance of arterial phase post-Gd imaging*:   Arterial phase FS T1w 3D GRE imaging (**A**) showed multiple neuroendocrine metastases which were not visible on the corresponding portal phase (**B**) or unenhanced T2w FSE (**C**) and T1w (**D**) images. In a different patient with carcinoid disease, numerous small metastases were well seen at the post-Gd arterial phase (**E**) but were no longer visible by the portal phase (**F**).

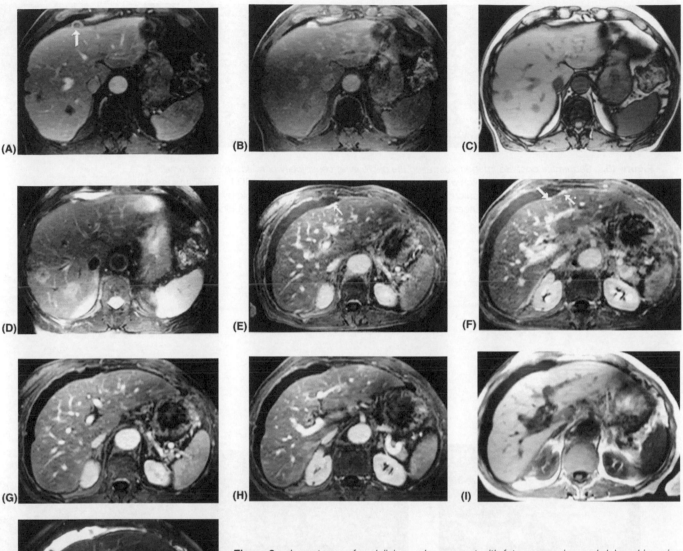

Figure 9.   *Importance of gadolinium enhancement with fat suppression and delayed imaging for depicting small deposits on the liver surface:*   In a patient with colorectal cancer a small surface deposit (arrow) was well shown on post-Gd FS 3D T1w GRE portal phase imaging (**A**) and showed pronounced and progressive enhancement on the corresponding delayed phase image (**B**). The lesion was barely visible on unenhanced T1w (**C**) and T2w FSE (**D**) images. In a second patient also with colorectal cancer, post-Gd FS 3D T1w GRE images obtained 10 minutes after injection (**E**, **F**) showed marked enhancement of peritoneal tumor deposits (arrows) which were not visible on the corresponding images obtained within the first 2 minutes after injection (**G**, **H**) or on unenhanced IPT1w (**I**) or T2w (**J**) images.

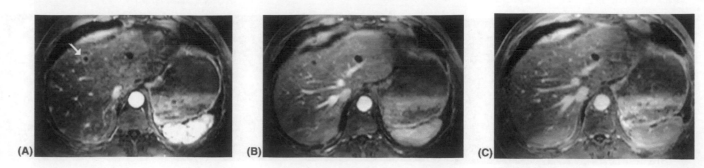

Figure 10. *Sequential post-Gd images illustrating the decreasing conspicuity of metastases over time:* A small colorectal metastasis (arrow) which was well shown on arterial phase post-Gd FS 3D Tw1 GRE images (**A**) was apparently smaller and less conspicuous by the portal phase (**B**) and barely visible by the equilibrium phase (**C**). Note the absence of enhancement on all phases in the simple cyst in the left lobe.

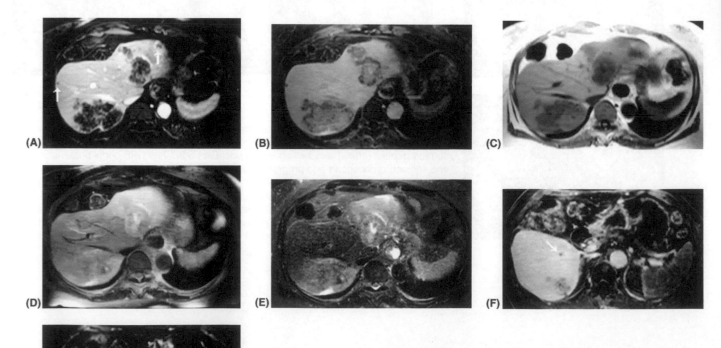

Figure 11. *Improved detection of small metastasis after gadobenate:* In a patient with multiple colorectal metastases there was a marked increase in lesion to liver contrast on post-gadobenate portal phase (**A**) and hepatocyte phase (**B**) FS 3D T1w GRE images compared with unenhanced IPT1 (**C**), T2w FSE (**D**) and STIR (**E**) images. Small metastases (arrows) in the right and left lobes were only visible after contrast. At a more caudal level a tiny additional lesion (arrow) which was well shown at the hepatocyte phase (**F**) was not visible on unenhanced images or on dynamic contrast enhanced images (**G**) obtained in the first two minutes after injection.

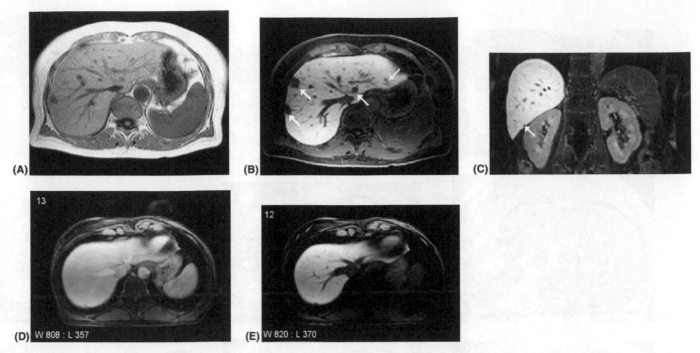

Figure 12. *Improved detection of small metastases after gadoxetic acid*:   Compared with unenhanced T1w imaging (**A**), axial and coronal hepatocyte-phase images (**B**, **C**) showed a marked improvement in lesion-to-liver contrast and several additional small lesions were found (arrows). Courtesy of Dr. Kuehn, Greifswald. In a different patient, high-resolution FS-3D T1w images at portal (**D**) and hepatocyte (**E**) phases clearly showed a small sub-capsular lesion with improved conspicuity on the delayed acquisition. Courtesy of Dr. W. Schima.

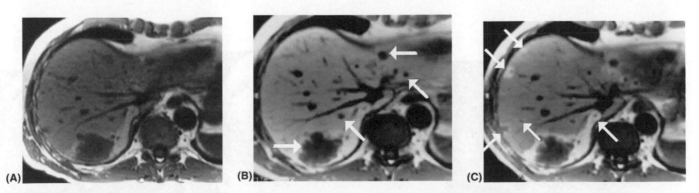

Figure 13. *Improved detection of small metastases after mangafodipir—value of 24-hour images*:   In a patient with colorectal cancer, compared with unenhanced T1w imaging (**A**), multiple metastases (arrows) were better seen with high lesion-to-liver contrast on 20 minute post-mangafodipir T1w images (**B**) when there was maximum enhancement of the background liver. However several additional small metastases (open arrows) were well seen on T1w images obtained 24 hours later (**C**) because retained contrast medium in the compressed liver tissue at the periphery of the lesions is particularly conspicuous against the normal signal of the background liver. Courtesy of Dr. J. Healy.

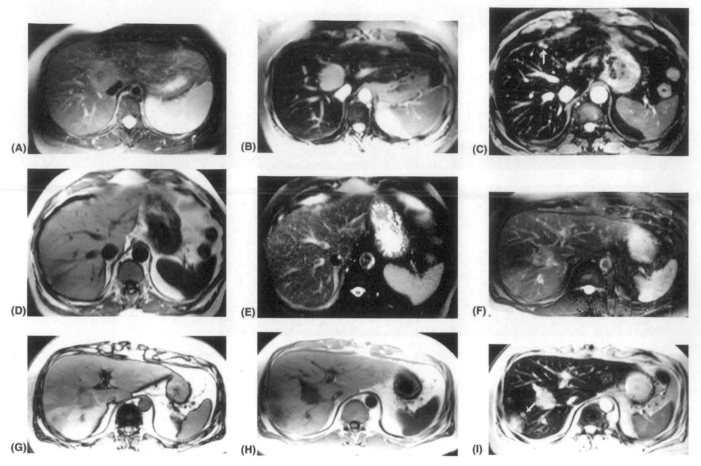

Figure 14. *Improved lesion conspicuity after SPIO in three patients with colorectal metastases:* Identical T2w FSE images obtained before (**A**) and after (**B**) injection of SPIO showed a dramatic improvement in lesion conspicuity after contrast. In a different patient, two small adjacent metastases were clearly shown with strong lesion-to-liver contrast on SPIO-enhanced FS T2w GRE (**C**); the lesions were barely visible on the corresponding unenhanced T1w (**D**) and T2w (**E**) images. In a third patient with colorectal metastases and a fatty liver, the tumors were poorly seen on unenhanced T2w FSE (**F**) and opposed-phase T1w images (**G**). Lesion-to-liver contrast was better on in-phase T1w images (**H**) but much improved on SPIO-enhanced T2w GRE images (**I**) which also showed an additional previously undetected small metastasis (arrow).

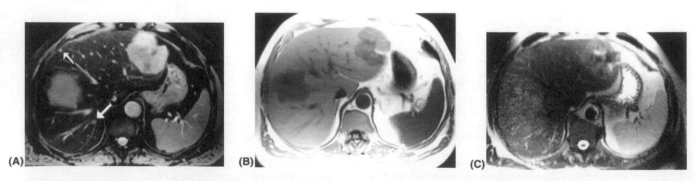

Figure 15. *Multiple metastases—improved detection with SPIO:* Several sub-cm colorectal metastases (arrows) were well shown on post-SPIO FS T2w GRE imaging (**A**); the lesions were not visible on the corresponding unenhanced T1w (**B**) and T2w (**C**) images. In a second patient with a solitary metastasis shown on surveillance CT (**D**), multiple additional lesions were visible on T1w (**E**) and T2w (**F**) GRE images obtained after SPIO. (*Continued*)

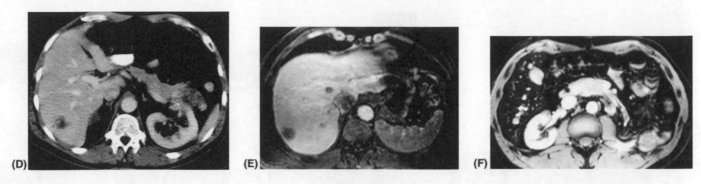

Figure 15. (*Continued*)

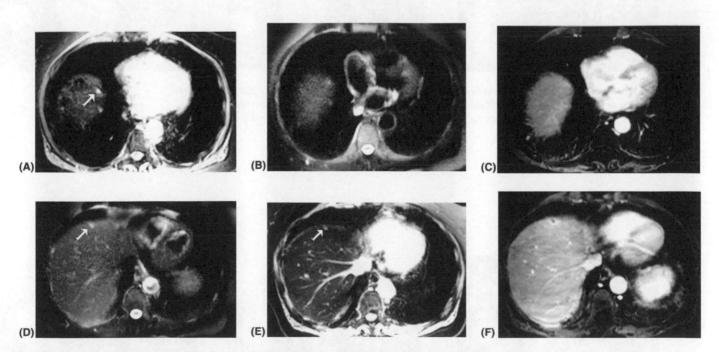

Figure 16. *Improved detection of small metastases after SPIO*:   A sub-cm colorectal metastasis (arrow) which was highly conspicuous on SPIO-enhanced FS T2w GRE imaging (**A**) was barely visible on the corresponding unenhanced HASTE (**B**) and post-Gd FS T1w 3D GRE (**C**) images. A second metastasis (arrow) in the same patient was visible on HASTE (**D**) and SPIO-enhanced FS T2w GRE (**E**) but was most conspicuous on post-Gd T1w images (**F**).

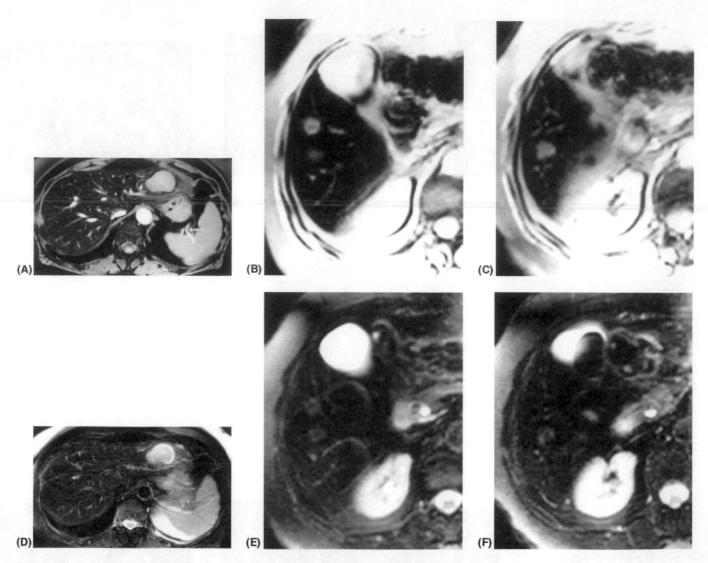

Figure 17. *Using an optimized GRE sequence with Superparamagnetic Iron Oxide for increasing lesion conspicuity and reducing ghosting artifact:* In three patients with colorectal metastases, lesion-to-liver contrast and motion artifact was substantially better on corresponding breathhold T2w GRE images (**A**, **B**, **C**) than on T2w FSE imaging (**D**, **E**, **F**).

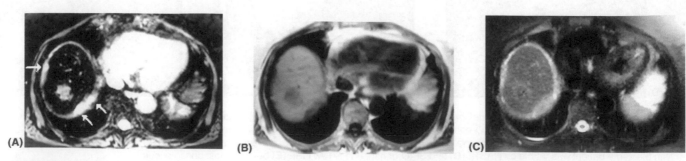

Figure 18. (*See facing page*)

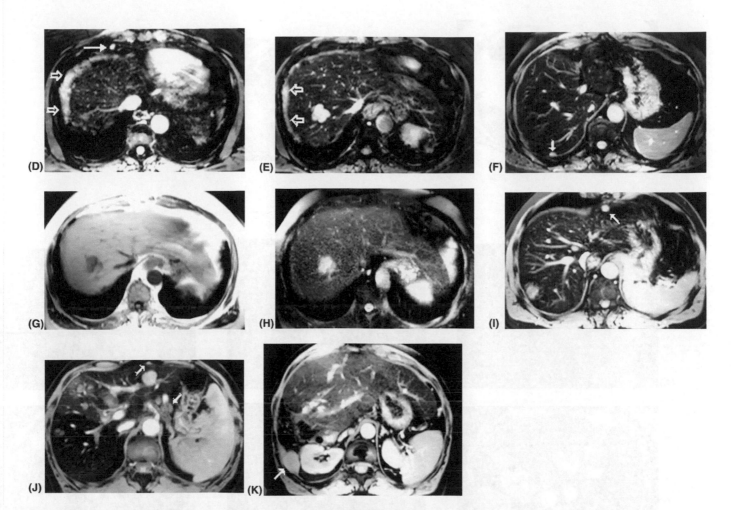

Figure 18. *Fat suppressed SPIO-enhanced T2w GRE images depicting upper abdominal extra-hepatic disease in patients with colorectal cancer.* Metastatic disease to the right sub-phrenic peritoneum (arrows) was more conspicuous on SPIO-enhanced FS T2w GRE (**A**) than on corresponding unenhanced T1w (**B**) and T2w (**C**) images. In a second patient, the high signal intensity of peritoneal disease (open arrows), lymphadenopathy (long arrow) and a small metastasis on the liver surface (short arrow) were well shown against the reduced signal intensity of the liver and the suppressed signal of intra-abdominal fat on post-SPIO FS T2w GRE images (**D, E, F**). The extra-hepatic disease was not visible on the corresponding unenhanced T1w (**G**) and T2w HASTE images (**H**). SPIO-enhanced FS T2w GRE images in three further patients (**I, J, K**) showed lymphadenopathy, surface metastasis and peritoneal disease in the right sub-hepatic space (arrows).

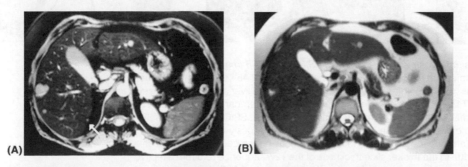

Figure 19. *Small surface lesions depicted with SPIO-enhanced FS T2w GRE:* A 5-mm surgically confirmed colorectal metastasis on the medial surface of the right lobe (arrow) was well shown on SPIO-enhanced FS T2w GRE images (**A**). The lesion was not visible on the corresponding unenhanced T2w images (**B**) and was visible but less conspicuous on in-phase T1w images (**C**). SPIO-enhanced FS T2w GRE imaging (**D**) in a second patient showed the enhanced conspicuity of a small surface lesions (arrow). (*Continued*)

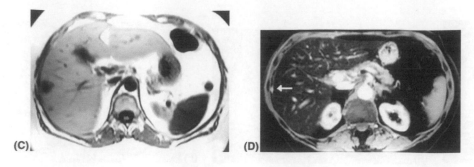

Figure 19. (*Continued*)

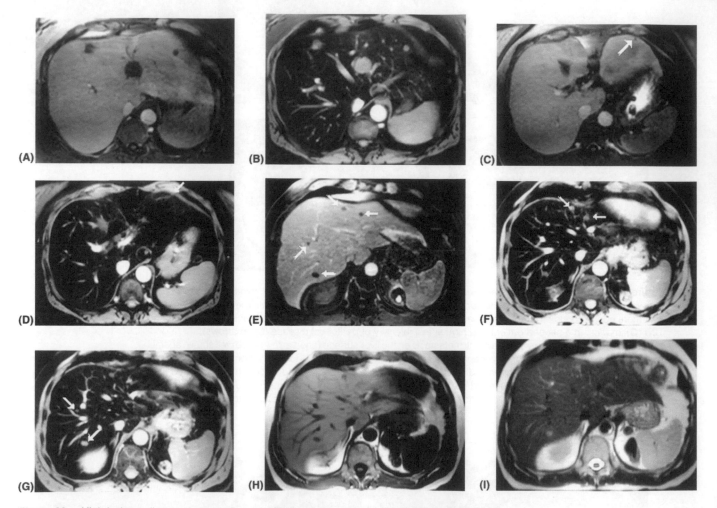

Figure 20. *High lesion-to-liver contrast on dynamic SPIO-enhanced FS 3D T1w GRE images*: Multiple colorectal metastases were highly conspicuous on FS 3D T1w GRE images obtained 45 seconds after bolus injection of ferucarbotran (**A**). The lesions were hypointense relative to the background liver and hepatic vessels which were isointense due to the weak T1 effect induced by a relatively low dose of ferucarbotran. The lesions were also well shown on FS T2w GRE images obtained 10 minutes after injection (**B**). SPIO-enhanced FS 3D T1w GRE image (**C**) obtained at a more caudal level than (**A**) clearly showed a previously undetected tiny metastasis just below the liver surface (arrow). The lesion was less conspicuous on the corresponding post-SPIO FS T2w GRE image (**D**) probably due to the thicker slice thickness of the T2w sequence (2.5 mm effective slice thickness for 3D T1w GRE versus 6 mm slice thickness for T2w GRE). In a second patient four colorectal metastases were well shown on SPIO-enhanced FS 3D T1w GRE (**E**) and T2w GRE images (**F**, **G**) (arrows) but only the two larger lesions were visible on the corresponding unenhanced T1w (**H**) and T2w (**I**) images. A further 5 mm metastasis (arrow) was clearly shown at a more caudal level on post-SPIO FS 3D T1w GRE imaging (**J**) and was visible but difficult to distinguish from adjacent vessels on post-SPIO FS T2w GRE imaging (**K**). (*Continued*)

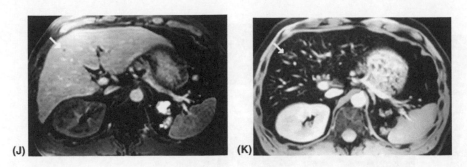

Figure 20. (*Continued*)

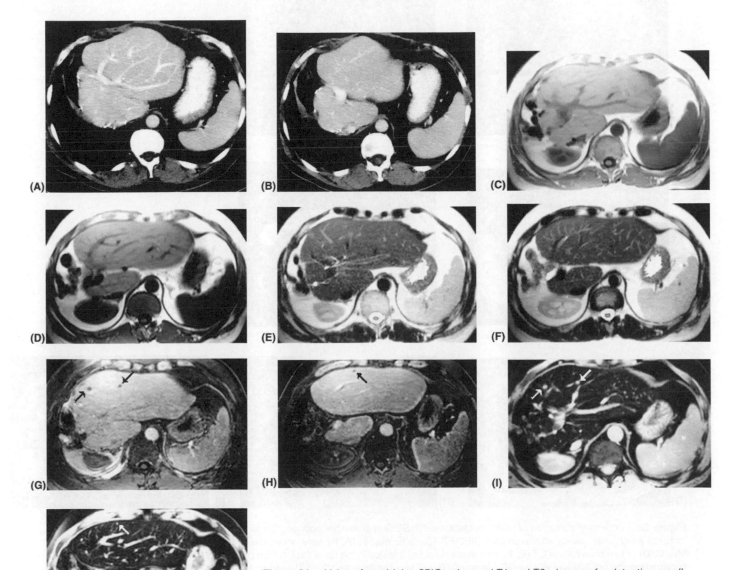

Figure 21. *Value of combining SPIO-enhanced T1 and T2w images for detecting small metastases:* In a patient with rising tumor markers after right hepatectomy for colorectal metastases, CT (**A**, **B**) and unenhanced T1w (**C**, **D**) and T2w (**E**, **F**) images showed no evidence of recurrent disease. However, multiple sub-cm lesions were well shown on the corresponding FS 3D T1w GRE (**G**, **H**) and FS T2w GRE (**I**, **J**) images obtained after ferucarbotran (arrows). Note the lesions are best distinguished from the adjacent vessels on the post-SPIO T1w images.

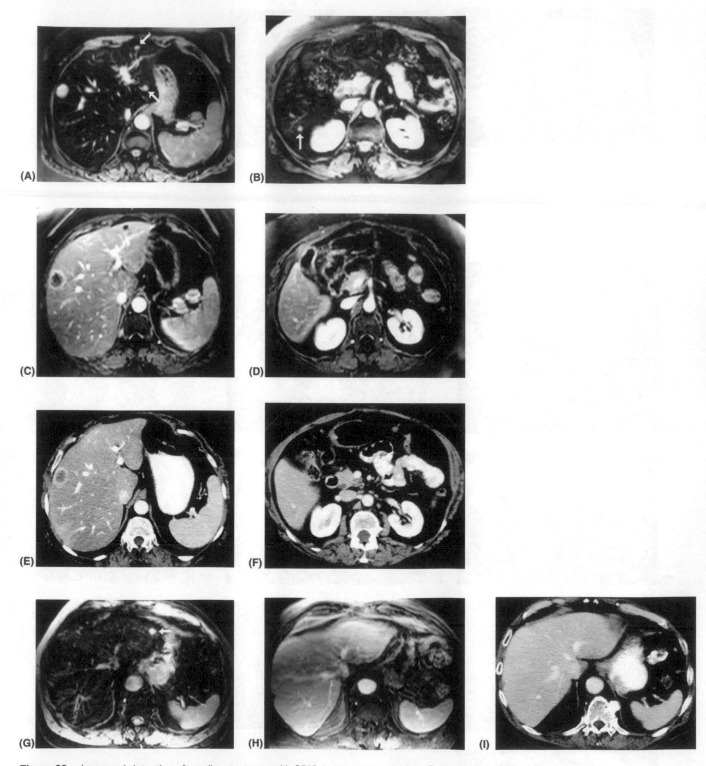

Figure 22. *Improved detection of small metastases with SPIO in colorectal cancer.* Small metastases (arrows) which were clearly shown on post-SPIO FS T2w GRE images (**A**, **B**) were not visible on Gd-enhanced MR (**C**, **D**) or thin slice helical CT (**E**, **F**). In a second patient a lesion in the tip of the left lobe (arrow) was highly conspicuous on post-SPIO FW T2w GRE imaging (**G**) but was not detected on post-Gd T1w MR (**H**) or on thin-slice CT images (**I**).

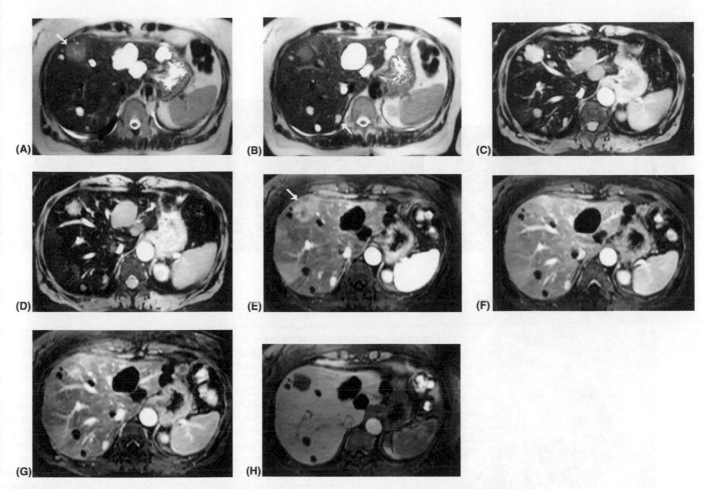

Figure 23. *Co-existent benign and malignant liver lesions in a surgical patient—lesions characterized with DGEI performed after SPIO-enhanced images for lesion detection:* Adjacent HASTE images (**A**, **B**) showed multiple well-defined markedly hyperintense lesions involving all liver segments as well as a moderately hyperintense lesion on the posterior aspect of segment 7 (arrow) and a lesion in segment 4 (arrow) which had much lower signal intensity than the other lesions. All the lesions were hypointense relative to the background liver on post-SPIO FS T2w GRE images (**C**, **D**). On sequential post-Gd T1w images (**E**, **F**, **G**) the enhancement in the segment 4 lesion was indicative of a metastasis (early heterogeneous enhancement which rapidly faded to isointensity followed by late central interstitial enhancement) but the segment 7 lesion showed the characteristic enhancement of a small hemangioma (rapid homogeneous and persistent enhancement which paralleled the enhancement of vessels at each post-contrast phase). The other lesions showed no enhancement, confirming simple cysts. Note also that unlike the metastasis and cysts, the hemangioma became invisible on early SPIO-enhanced 3D T1w FS GRE images (**H**) because its enhancement equalled that of the vessels which were virtually isointense with the background liver due to the weak T1 effect of SPIO.

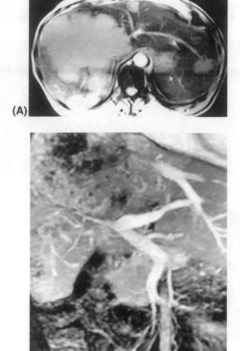

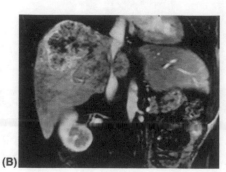

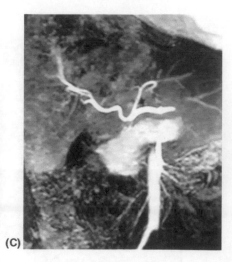

Figure 24. *Relationship of large tumor to major vessels delineated by dynamic post-Gd imaging following SPIO-enhanced imaging:*   Post-SPIO enhanced T2w GRE images (**A**) showed a large colorectal metastasis occupying most of the right lobe and several smaller lesions in the left lobe. Coronal oblique FS 3D T1w GRE imaging (**B**) obtained 20 minutes after injection of SPIO and 40 seconds after Gd injection clearly showed tumor encasing and narrowing the IVC. Arterial (**C**) and portal phase (**D**) post-Gd MIP images showed normal arterial anatomy, with tumor involving all three hepatic veins and the right portal vein and also abutting the proximal left main branch of the portal vein. The combination of high-resolution thin slice 3D imaging and more conspicuous vessel enhancement due to a synergistic increase in contrast between the Gd-enhanced vascular structures and the SPIO-enhanced background liver produced a high quality MIP image. The patient underwent an extended right hepatectomy with vascular reconstruction, and multiple metastatectomies from segments 2 and 3, and was alive and well more than 4 years after surgery.

CHAPTER 11

Characterization of Liver Metastases

After lymph nodes the liver is the most frequent site of metastatic spread of tumors and the commonest site of blood borne metastases. The presence of liver metastases alters the management of most patients with malignant disease and is probably the most frequent indication for liver MR. In patients presenting with clinical or biochemical evidence of liver disease, sonography is usually the first imaging investigation. CT is recommended in patients with unexpected or equivocal sonographic findings, and is also used for baseline staging and surveillance in patients with malignant disease. MRI is reserved for lesion characterization in patients with indeterminate lesions found on surveillance sonography or CT following treatment of a primary tumor, and also assessing the suitability of patients for hepatic resection. Accurate preoperative staging is essential to avoid fruitless surgery in patients with unresectable disease. The main objectives of MRI in this context are the detection and localization of all metastases, the correct characterization of co-existing benign lesions, and the demonstration of the anatomic relation of tumors to the main hepatic vessels.

Until recently, interest in surgical resection of liver metastases has largely focused on colorectal cancer and consequently, much experience in liver MRI relates to colorectal disease. This is because colorectal tumors are common, complete excision of the primary lesion is achieved in most patients, metastases are more likely to be localized to the liver, and hepatic resection has a proven impact on survival, with long-term cure in a proportion of cases. Further, the number, size and distribution of colorectal metastases are no longer regarded as limiting factors for surgery, providing that all tumors are removed with adequate clearance margins, and enough liver remains to sustain function during the post-operative period. Survival benefits of surgery are also well established in patients with neuroendocrine metastases and there is growing evidence to support the value of resection of localized metastases from some other primary tumors which show an indolent course.

Resection of hepatic metastases from other primary GI tract tumors (stromal, gastroesophageal and some pancreatic tumors) and from renal, breast, sarcoma and melanoma (particularly ocular) primaries, may be beneficial. Currently, only metachronous lesions, stable for a minimum of three months before surgery are considered; patients with unilobar disease up to a maximum of four lesions may be suitable although solitary lesions have a more favourable prognosis; anatomical limitations need to be clearly defined with a resection margin of at least 1 cm achievable, and there must be no evidence of lymphadenopathy or extrahepatic disease. Patients with widespread metastatic disease in bone, lungs or the central nervous system are not surgical candidates.

MR APPEARANCES OF LIVER METASTASES

Morphology

Liver metastases have a wide range of appearances on MR. They are usually multiple but they may be solitary or cluster to form conglomerate masses. Tumors range in size from under 1 mm to many cm. Metastases arising from the gastrointestinal tract which spread via the portal vein are usually few in number and of varying size, whereas tumors which arrive via the systemic circulation tend to be multiple and smaller than 2 cm at the time of presentation. Most lesions have a homogeneous internal architecture on unenhanced images and an ill-defined and irregular border, although occasionally the borders are sharp (most often in squamous cell and neuroendocrine tumors). Large colorectal metastases typically have a lobulated shape. Metastases from neuroendocrine tumors and poorly differentiated adenocarcinomas are usually multiple, widespread, and small. Metastases from breast cancer have particularly varied appearances. They maybe small, large or confluent, but are typically multiple and widespread.

Metastases on the liver surface are frequently seen in primaries that spread via the peritoneum—most commonly ovarian cancer, but also some gastrointestinal malignancies. To detect surface disease, particular attention should be given to the hepatic fissures, the right hemi-diaphragm and the liver capsule. Most peritoneal tumor deposits are best depicted on delayed FS post-Gd T1w images or on FS T2w GRE images after SPIO (see Chapter 10), but a minority of surface lesions are hypervascular and only visible in the arterial phase of post-Gd enhancement.

Tumor spread within the major portal veins and bile ducts is an uncommon but well recognized feature of colorectal metastases. Although vascular invasion is generally associated with a poor prognosis, macroscopic bile duct invasion appears to indicate a more indolent tumor and a favourable outcome following resection. Bile duct dilatation and tumor growth along the bile duct is best seen on heavily T2w thick slab SSFSE and thin-slice HASTE MRCP images while vascular invasion is most clearly depicted on portal phase post-Gd T1w images.

Signal Intensity on Unenhanced MR Images

Metastases have varied signal intensity (SI) characteristics. Most have longer T1 and T2 relaxation times than the surrounding liver due to a greater water content (T1 and T2 relaxation times at 1.5T for liver and metastases are approximately 500 msec and 40 msec for the liver; 900 msec and 80 msec for metastases) so they appear hypointense on unenhanced T1w and hyperintense on T2w images. Hypervascular metastases and tumors which have undergone colliquative necrosis may have a very high SI on T2w images and be indistinguishable from hemangiomas on unenhanced images, although most hyperintense metastases have irregular internal morphology and less distinct margins than hemangiomas.

Hypointensity on T2w images is occasionally seen with metastases. Some lesions have a low SI center surrounded by a moderately hyperintense rim on T2w images which histologically corresponds to viable tumor tissue surrounding a central area of coagulative necrosis. Desmoplastic reaction also lowers the SI of lesions on T2w images. Larger colorectal metastases often have a fibrous matrix resulting in a mixed low and high SI appearance on T2w images.

Hemorrhagic tumors and melanotic metastases may be hyperintense on T1w and have a mixed or low SI on T2w images, due to the paramagnetic properties of melanin and blood. T2w GRE acquisitions are useful for confirming hemorrhage by identifying hemosiderin which produces punctate areas of very low signal on this sequence. Amelanotic metastases from melanoma are moderately hypointense on T1w and moderately hyperintense on T2w images and so can be indistinguishable from other metastatic lesions. Metastases occasionally calcify causing a signal void on all sequences. Fat-containing metastases are rare and reflect the characteristics of the underlying tumor. If fat is present, tumors show a characteristic signal loss on opposed-phase T1w compared with in-phase T1w GRE images.

Metastases from mucin-producing primaries are often difficult to characterize an unenhanced MR and CT. They are typically hypo-attenuating on CT, exhibit little enhancement and may appear stable for long periods. On MRI they usually show marked homogeneous hyperintensity on T2w images and although they are most typically hypointense on T1w they maybe hyperintense due to a high protein content. The diagnosis usually becomes clear on dynamic post-Gd T1w imaging when a complete ring of enhancement is visible.

A rim of low SI on T1w and variable SI on T2w images is occasionally seen around the periphery of metastases. This feature corresponds histologically to local compression and atrophy of the liver parenchyma with a desmoplastic reaction which is thinner than the thick fibrous pseudocapsule seen in hepatocellular carcinoma.

Metastases in a diffusely fatty liver can be inconspicuous on OP T1w images because they have a SI similar to the decreased signal of the liver, but in such cases the lesions may be surrounded by a halo of non-fatty liver tissue, rendering them highly conspicuous. This finding is also seen with benign lesions but is usually less pronounced. With severe degrees of fatty change, the lesions may appear hyperintense on OP T1w and hypointense on IP T1w images (see also Chapter 7).

Contrast Enhancement Characteristics

Although the blood supply of metastases is derived almost totally from branches of the hepatic artery, their vascularity is usually similar to that of the primary tumor, so they exhibit variable enhancement patterns on post-Gd T1w images. Most metastases—typically those from colon, lung, prostate and bladder carcinoma—are hypovascular compared with liver parenchyma. Although these lesions are most conspicuous at the portal phase of enhancement when the liver is maximally enhanced, many exhibit a transient rim of enhancement which may only be visible at the arterial-dominant phase. This ring of enhancement indicates a well vascularised periphery surrounding a necrotic center, and is characteristic of metastases. Larger tumors usually enhance heterogeneously. Regardless of size, some metastases show incomplete progressive central enhancement with lesions appearing hyperintense relative to normal liver on delayed images. This pattern reflects slow diffusion of contrast into the extracellular space of the central part of the tumor which tends to be less well vascularised than the periphery. Transient perilesional enhancement ("corona enhancement") may also be seen in the liver tissue surrounding the tumor, more often with hypo- than with hypervascular metastases. This appearance is usually seen only on immediate post-Gd T1w images but occasionally it persists into the delayed phase. Pathologic correlations have shown variable combinations of inflammatory infiltration, sinusoidal congestion and desmoplastic reaction.

Many metastases show very little enhancement after gadolinium and some lesions are "isovascular" in that they have perfusion characteristics similar to normal liver, so are inconspicuous on post-Gd T1w images. Lesions which are visible on unenhanced images but "disappear" on post-Gd acquisitions should be regarded as metastases since this pattern is not observed with benign tumors. Lesions that are not visible on unenhanced images but become conspicuously hyperintense on post-SPIO images are also likely to be metastatic. Further, hypovascular lesions that become visible on post-Gd T1w images but are not detectable on unenhanced images are likely to be metastases. Small (<2 cm) hypovascular metastases most commonly show continual peripheral rim enhancement on arterial phase images with borders which become indistinct on subsequent acquisitions. Over time, these lesions appear to become smaller, and they may not be visible at all on later images due to diffusion of the contrast agent into the extracellular space of the lesions. Rarely, small hypovascular metastases show non-progressive rim enhancement in the early post-Gd images, but become inconspicuous by 10 minutes after injection. These lesions are usually inconspicuous on unenhanced T2w images.

Metastases which are most conspicuous during the arterial-dominant phase of enhancement are designated as "hypervascular." Hypervascular metastases most often arise in patients with primary carcinoid or islet cell tumors, renal cell cancer and melanoma. They occur less frequently in patients with pancreatic, breast, lung and colon primaries. Most show rapid washout of contrast, becoming isointense or slightly hypointense to the adjacent liver by the portal phase. Small hypervascular tumors which are only visible on immediate post-Gd images can be indistinguishable from benign hepatocellular lesions, but are easily distinguished after SPIO—metastases remain hyperintense and become more conspicuous on SPIO-enhanced T2w images, while small FNH and adenomas typically show SPIO uptake often becoming isointense or even hypointense to the surrounding liver.

Peripheral or central washout of contrast is indicative of malignancy and can be seen with both hyper- and hypovascular metastases, although peripheral washout tends to occur more often and be more striking with hypervascular lesions. Peripheral portal vein branches are often occluded by metastases, causing a wedge-shaped area of increased enhancement on post-Gd T1w images during the arterial phase of enhancement. Although these transient areas of increased SI (THIDs) also occur in the absence of tumors, this appearance should prompt a careful search for small lesions at the apex of the THID.

Although there is overlap in the MRI appearances of metastases from different primary tumors, some morphologic and enhancement characteristics favour specific pathologies. Colorectal metastases larger than 3 cm typically have a scalloped margin, a pronounced rim of arterial hypervascularity which persists on late acquisitions and progressively enhancing fibrous septae which produce a "cauliflower" appearance. Colon cancer tends to produce large solitary metastases which are frequently surrounded by small satellite lesions. Occasionally, metastases from breast cancer may look very similar to cholangiocarcinoma, appearing rather indistinct on unenhanced images and showing slowly progressive enhancement on post-Gd images. Pigmented metastases from malignant melanoma are hyperintense on T1w and have mixed signal on T2w images. Metastases from squamous cell carcinomas are commonly round, show central colliquative necrosis and continuous ring enhancement on post-Gd images. Neuroendocrine metastases are usually heterogeneously hyperintense on T2w and usually hypointense on T1w images, although larger lesions may show T1 hyperintensity, owing to their content of proteinaceous fluid. While neuroendocrine lesions smaller than 2 cm tend to show intense homogeneous enhancement on immediate post-Gd T1w images which fades to isointensity by the portal and delayed phases, larger metastases usually show diffuse heterogeneous enhancement, often with peripheral washout on delayed imaging.

DIFFERENTIAL DIAGNOSIS

In determining the appropriate management of patients who are at risk of developing liver metastases, the differentiation of malignant from benign lesions is of critical importance. Benign liver lesions are common in patients with established malignant disease, either alone or co-existing with metastases. Further, it is unsafe to assume that all malignant liver lesions in patients with a history of a primary tumor are metastases.

Distinguishing Liver Metastases from Benign Lesions

Benign liver tumors generally have SI and enhancement characteristics quite different from those of metastases and the vast majority are reliably characterized with MR, but a minority cause some difficulty in diagnosis (see also chapters 5, 6, and 7).

Metastases Versus Simple Cysts
Simple liver cysts are commonly present in patients referred for liver MR. They vary in size and number but are often under 1 cm. They are usually round, may be unilocular or multilocular, have a well-defined edge, show uniform marked hyperintensity on T2w and marked hypointensity on T1w images. A similar appearance is occasionally seen with some small hypervascular metastases, and with metastases after chemotherapy. On post-Gd T1w images, cysts show no enhancement, and relative to the adjacent liver they have an extremely low signal. Delayed imaging 5–10 minutes after injection is particularly helpful for differentiating cysts—which continue to show no enhancement—from hypovascular metastases which show some degree of gradual enhancement.

Metastases Versus Biliary Hamartomas (Von Meyenberg Complexes)
Biliary hamartomas are also commonly found as incidental benign liver lesions, occurring in about 3% of patients. They are developmental anomalies composed of clusters of malformed bile ducts embedded in dense connective tissue. They are always small (usually under 1 cm), and often located peripherally just below Glisson's capsule. They may be solitary or multiple, and round, ovoid or angular in shape. Many of these lesions have similar SI and enhancement characteristics to simple cysts, but others show a thin rim of enhancing tissue surrounding the lesion. This rim enhancement is non-progressive and is sustained on delayed images. With this typical appearance, biliary hamartomas should be distinguished from metastases which have a more progressive enhancement pattern. However, a small minority of biliary hamartomas are predominantly fibrous and exhibit MR characteristics indistinguishable from those of some small metastases. They can be inconspicuous on

non-contrast images, and show persistent or progressive enhancement after gadolinium. Their peripheral location may be a useful pointer, but in some cases the distinction from metastases cannot be made.

Metastases Versus Hemangiomas

Typical hemangiomas are well-defined with a homogeneous hyperintensity on T2w images which is more marked than that of most metastases. Larger hemangiomas are often inhomogeneous with a typical central scar which is more hyperintense on T2w and hypointense on T1w images than the rest of the lesion. On post-Gd T1w images, both metastases and hemangiomas may show peripheral enhancement with gradual centripetal in-filling to involve most or all of the lesion, but the early enhancement of hemangiomas is discontinuous and nodular, while with metastases the initial enhancement forms a continuous rim. With hemangiomas, the intensity of enhancement parallels that of normal vessels at each vascular phase, while the enhancement of metastases typically fades to hypointensity on delayed images. With small hemangiomas, enhancement is often rapid and homogeneous—similar to that of small hypervascular metastases—but distinction is made on delayed images, in which hemangiomas show persistent enhancement, while metastases rapidly fade to iso- or hypointensity.

Metastasis Versus Focal Nodular Hyperplasia

Focal Nodular Hyperplasia (FNH) is also a frequently found incidental lesion. Most FNHs are round or lobulated, iso- or slightly hypointense on T1w, and iso- or slightly hyperintense on T2w images. Larger lesions usually have a central stellate scar with a lower signal on T1w and a higher signal on T2w images than the rest of the lesion. On post-Gd T1w images, FNHs display intense arterial phase enhancement, fading close to isointensity by the portal venous phase. The central scar typically shows delayed enhancement and becomes hyperintense a few minutes after injection.

Most hypervascular metastases are highly conspicuous on unenhanced T1w and T2w images, but a minority are only visible on immediate post-Gd T1w images, mimicking small FHNs or adenomas. However, they behave quite differently with liver-specific contrast agents. Following injection of gadobenate, gadoxetic acid and mangafodipir, FNHs enhance about as much as liver parenchyma at the delayed hepatocyte phase. FNHs also show substantial signal loss after SPIO contrast, which accentuates the visibility of the central scar. Almost without exception, metastases show no intracellular concentration of liver-specific contrast agents.

Metastasis Versus Hepatic Adenoma

Unlike FNH, liver cell adenoma is a rare tumor. It is usually solitary, although a minority of patients have multiple lesions. The lesions may be asymptomatic and discovered incidentally, or they may present with symptoms of bleeding into the lesion. Distinction from metastasis is made on the following criteria:

1. Most patients are young women with a history of oral contraceptive use
2. Acute presentation with intra-lesional hemorrhage is typical of adenoma, but unusual with metastasis
3. Most adenomas have a substantial fat content resulting in decreased signal on opposed-phase T1w relative to in-phase T1w images; fat is very uncommon in metastases
4. Most adenomas have a SI similar to normal liver on in-phase T1w and T2w images; in the presence of hemorrhage they may show heterogenous hyperintensity on both T1w and T2w image
5. Adenomas often have a pseudocapsule composed of compressed adjacent liver tissue which is hypointense on T1w and T2w images—this is less common with metastases. The pseudocapsule is hypointense on immediate post-Gd T1w images but shows increasing enhancement on delayed images

6. The enhancement pattern on post-Gd T1w images is often non-specific, but the behaviour with liver-specific agents is distinctive. Unlike metastases, adenomas show some degree of uptake of mangafodipir, gadoxetic acid and SPIO (but probably not gadobenate) and the uptake of these agents is usually marked with small adenomas.

Metastases Versus Nodular Regenerative Hyperplasia

Nodular regenerative hyperplasia (NRH) is a reactive liver lesion which occurs in patients with a range of chronic non-hepatic disorders, including rheumatoid arthritis, myeloproliferative disorders and immune dysfunction from any cause. NRH is characterized by hyperplastic nodules with little or no fibrosis in the uninvolved liver parenchyma (see Fig. 70, chapter 8). The features distinguishing NRH from metastases are:

1. Like other benign hepatocellular lesions, the nodules of NRH are close to isointense with liver on unenhanced images
2. NRH nodules show signal loss comparable to normal liver after SPIO
3. Unlike FNH and hepatic adenomas, the lesions of NRH are iso-vascular in the arterial phase of enhancement, with perfusion characteristics similar to normal liver.

Metastases Versus Hepatic Abscesses

Differentiating metastases from abscesses may be difficult, and requires careful correlation of the imaging findings with clinical and biochemical data.

1. Developing abscesses may be indistinguishable in appearance from small metastases, but the central area of established abscesses shows marked hypo- and hyperintensity on T1w and T2w images respectively
2. A halo of less marked hypo- on T1w and hyperintensity on T2w images often surrounds the central fluid-filled area of abscesses, due to local liver edema
3. On post-Gd T1w images, the hyperaemic abscess wall usually shows intense enhancement which is non-progressive and maintained on later images, while metastases typically show rapid washout and become less conspicuous over time
4. With abscesses, there is no late enhancement in the fluid center, but some metastases show delayed central enhancement
5. Minor peri-lesional enhancement on early post-Gd T1w images, which gradually increases to become quite intense on delayed images, is indicative of abscesses rather than metastases, again reflecting a local inflammatory response in the adjacent liver.

Distinguishing Metastases from Primary Liver Malignancies

Metastasis Versus Peripheral Cholangiocarcinoma

Large solitary metastases may show similar morphology and SI to peripheral cholangiocarcinoma, and the contrast-enhancement characteristics overlap (see also chapter 6). Differentiating features include the following:

1. Most peripheral cholangiocarcinomas have a central fibrous component which is hypointense on T2w images—this is less common with metastases
2. The peripheral glandular component of cholangiocarcinoma shows more pronounced rim enhancement on immediate post-Gd T1w images, which typically fades by the portal phase and washes out on delayed images
3. Enhancement of the central fibrous component is slower, becoming most pronounced on delayed images
4. Capsular retraction adjacent to the tumor is rarely seen with untreated metastases, but is typical of peripherally-sited cholangiocarcinomas.

Metastasis Versus Hilar Cholangiocarcinoma

In patients with a history of malignancy who present with a tumor causing bile duct obstruction it can be difficult to make the distinction between metastasis and hilar cholangiocarcinoma (see also chapter 13):

1. Metastases are generally conspicuous on unenhanced images, while most hilar cholangiocarcinomas are relatively indistinct
2. Metastases exhibit a continuous rim of enhancement on early post-Gd T1w images, but hilar cholangiocarcinomas characteristically show slowly progressive enhancement
3. Portal vein occlusion with associated lobar atrophy and crowding of the bile ducts is a frequent and characteristic finding in cholangiocarcinoma, but rarely seen with metastases
4. Tumor spread along the major vessels is rarely seen with hilar cholangiocarcinomas, but occurs occasionally with metastases near the liver hilum.

Metastasis Versus Sporadic HCC

HCCs arising in the non-cirrhotic liver are usually large at presentation and most often solitary. Although multi-focal disease is rare, satellite lesions are common, so differentiation from metastasis is again required (see also chapter 6):

1. Alpha fetoprotein (AFP) levels are raised in over 50% of cases of sporadic HCC
2. HCCs are composed of nodules separated by fibrous stroma which produces a mosaic appearance, commonly with areas of hemorrhage, focal fat, calcification and necrosis, giving a heterogeneous SI on unenhanced T1w and T2w images
3. On post-Gd T1w images, these lesions typically show heterogeneous but marked arterial phase enhancement, followed by rapid washout
4. HCCs almost always have an enhancing capsule which is most conspicuous on equilibrium-phase images
5. Vascular invasion by sporadic HCCs occurs less frequently than with HCCs in cirrhosis, but is still more common than with metastases
6. Differentiating small (<2 cm) HCC's from hypervascular metastases is rarely problematic since they rarely, if ever, present at this stage in the non-cirrhotic liver. However, it is also important to seek evidence of unsuspected cirrhosis since this would change the balance of probabilities. In well-compensated cirrhosis, patients may be asymptomatic with only minor morphologic changes which are best shown on SPIO-enhanced T2w GRE images. Hepatic metastases are rare in advanced cirrhosis, so the discovery of one or more tumors in a patient with severely cirrhotic liver favours the diagnosis of HCC.

ILLUSTRATIVE FIGURES

REFERENCES

1. Bader TR, Semelka RD, Chiu VCY, et al. MRI of carcinoid tumors: spectrum of appearances in the gastrointestinal tract and liver. JMRI 2001; 14:261–269.
2. Berger JF, Laissy JP, Limot O, et al. Differentiation between multiple liver hemangiomas and liver metastases of gastrinomas: value of enhanced MRI. J Comput Assist Tomogr 1996; 20:349–355.
3. Danet IM, Semelka RC, Leonardou P, et al. Spectrum of MRI appearances of untreated metastases of the liver. Am J Roentgenol 2003; 181:809–817.
4. Harrison LE, Brennan MF, Newmann E, et al. Hepatic resection for noncolorectal, non-neuroendocrine metastases: a fifteen-year experience with 96 patients. Surgery 1997; 121:625–632.
5. Imam K, Bluemke DA. MR imaging in the evaluation of hepatic metastases. Magn Reson Imaging Clin N Am 2000; 8:741–756.
6. Jaeck D, Bachellier P, Guiget M, et al. Long-term survival following resection of colorectal hepatic metastases. Br J Surg 1997; 84:977–980.
7. Klatskin G, Conn HO. Neoplasms of the liver and intrahepatic bile ducts. Histopathology of the Liver. Oxford and New York: Oxford University press, 1993: 367–395.
8. Lodge JP, Ammori BJ, Prasad KR, et al. Ex vivo and in situ resection of inferior vena cava with hepatectomy for colorectal metastases. Ann Surg 2000; 231:471–479.
9. Luo TY, Itai Y, Egughi N, et al. Von Meyenberg complexes of the liver: imaging findings. J Comput Assist Tomogr 1998; 22:372–378.
10. Mahfouz AE, Hamm B, Wolf KJ. Peripheral washout: a sign of malignancy on dynamic gadolinium-enhanced MR images of focal liver lesions. Radiology 1994; 190:49–52.
11. Malafosse R, Penna Ch, Da Cunha A, et al. Surgical management of hepatic metastases from colorectal malignancies. Ann Oncol 2001; 12:887–894.
12. Miyazaki M, Itoh I, Nagakawa K, et al. Hepatic resection of liver metastases from gastric carcinoma. Am J Gastroenterol 1997; 92:490–493.
13. Miyazaki M, Ito H, Nakagawa K, et al. Aggressive surgical resection for hepatic metastases involving the inferior vena cava. Am J Surg 1999; 177:294–298.
14. Okano K, Yamamoto J, Kosuge T, et al. Fibrous pseudocapsule of metastatic liver tumors from colorectal carcinoma. Cancer 2000; 89:267–275.
15. Outwater E, Tomaszewski JE, Daly JM, Kressel HY. Hepatic colorectal metastases: correlation of MR imaging and pathologic appearance. Radiology 1991; 180:327–332.
16. Pedro MS, Semelka RC, Braga L. MR imaging of hepatic metastases. In: Semelka RC ed. MR Imaging of the Liver II: Diseases. Magn Reson Imaging Clin N Am 2002; 10:15–29.
17. Robinson PJ. Review: the characterization of tumors by MRI. Clin Radiol 1996; 51:649–761.
18. Robinson PJA. The Liver. In: Husband JE, Reznek RH, eds. Imaging in Oncology. Metastases, 2nd ed. London: Taylor & Francis, 2004:1059–1083.
19. Semelka RC, Braga L, Armao D, et al. Liver. In: Semelka RC, ed. Abdominal—Pelvic MRI. New York: Wiley-Liss, 2002:101–149.
20. Soyer P, Tidjani K, Laissy JP, Sibert A, Menu Y. Dynamic Gd-BOPTA-enhanced MR imaging of hepatic metastases from pancreatic neuroendocrine tumors. Euro J Radiol 1994; 18:180–184.
21. Stromyer FW, Ishak KG. Nodular transformation (nodular "regenerative" hyperplasia) of the liver: a clinicopathologic study of 30 cases. Hum Path 1981; 12:60–71.

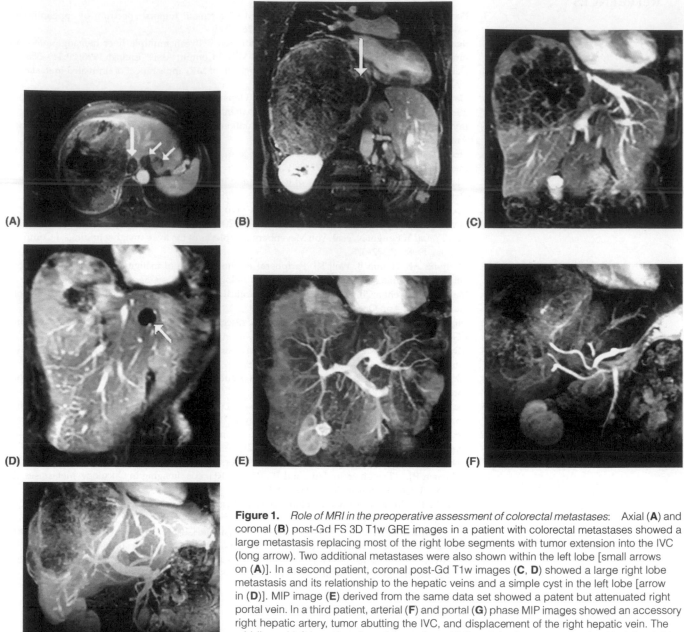

Figure 1. *Role of MRI in the preoperative assessment of colorectal metastases:* Axial (**A**) and coronal (**B**) post-Gd FS 3D T1w GRE images in a patient with colorectal metastases showed a large metastasis replacing most of the right lobe segments with tumor extension into the IVC (long arrow). Two additional metastases were also shown within the left lobe [small arrows on (**A**)]. In a second patient, coronal post-Gd T1w images (**C**, **D**) showed a large right lobe metastasis and its relationship to the hepatic veins and a simple cyst in the left lobe [arrow in (**D**)]. MIP image (**E**) derived from the same data set showed a patent but attenuated right portal vein. In a third patient, arterial (**F**) and portal (**G**) phase MIP images showed an accessory right hepatic artery, tumor abutting the IVC, and displacement of the right hepatic vein. The middle and left hepatic vein and the main and left portal veins were uninvolved but the right portal vein was obliterated by tumor. All three patients underwent successful surgical resection of the liver lesions.

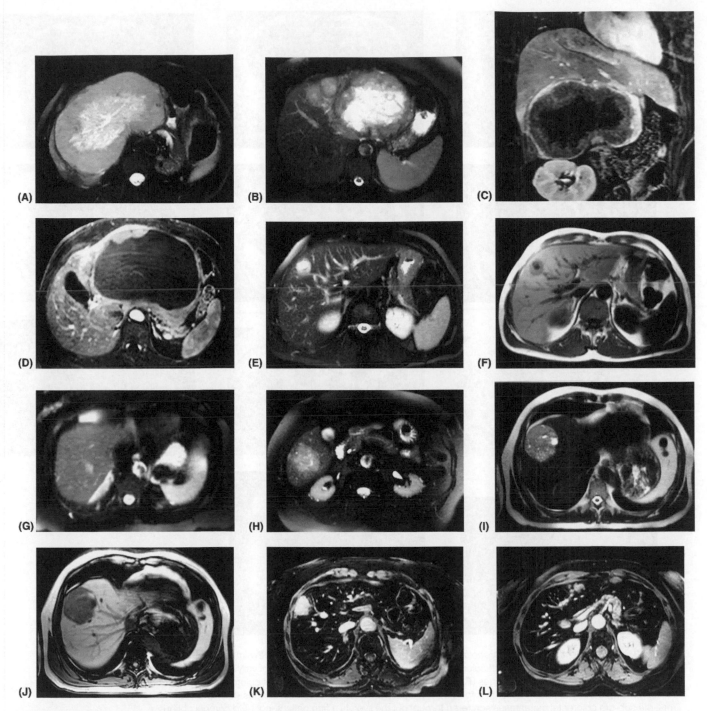

Figure 2. *Examples of surgically-treated metastases from non-colorectal primaries:* Axial HASTE (**A**, **B**), coronal (**C**) and axial (**D**) post-Gd FS 3D T1w GRE images in two different patients (**A**, **C** and **B**, **D**) with renal cell carcinomas showed large solitary metastases; in another patient axial HASTE (**E**) and IP T1w (**F**) images showed a solitary metastasis from a primary hemangiopericytoma; axial HASTE images (**G**, **H**) in a further patient with breast cancer showed two metastases; axial HASTE (**I**) and OP T1w (**J**) images showed a solitary metastasis in a patient with an ocular melanoma; post-SPIO T2w GRE images (**K**, **L**) in another patient with esophageal carcinoma showed two metastases with small satellite lesions; all patients underwent successful resection with prolonged survival.

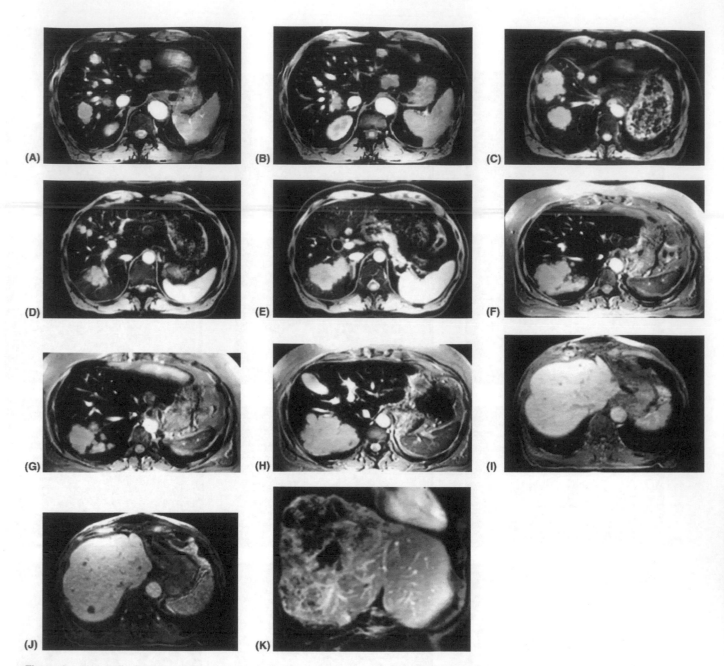

Figure 3. *Varied distribution and morphology of colorectal metastases:*   Post-SPIO T2w images in two different patients (**A**, **B** and **C**, **D**, **E**) with colorectal metastases showed multiple lesions of varying size involving all liver segments. Post-SPIO T2w images (**F**, **G**, **H**) in a third patient showed a cluster of colorectal metastases forming a single conglomerate mass. In a fourth patient post-SPIO FS 3D T1w GRE images (**I**, **J**) showed multiple sub-cm colorectal metastases scattered throughout the liver. In a fifth patient, post-Gd coronal oblique T1w imaging showed a large solitary tumor, subsequently resected.

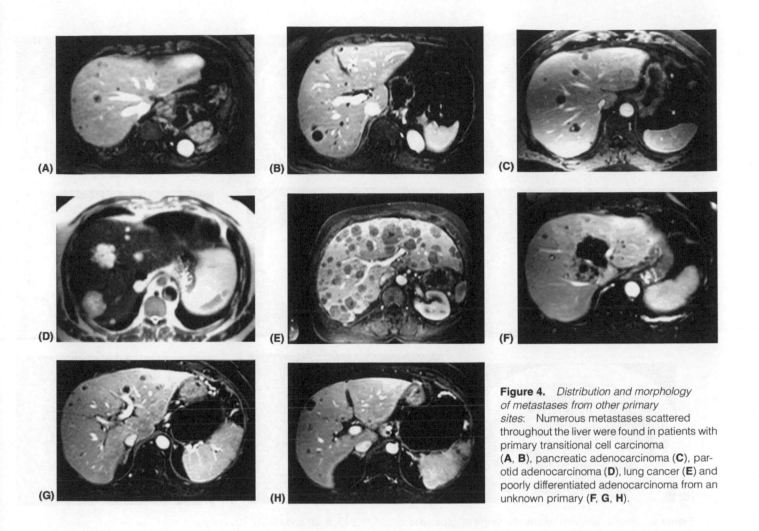

Figure 4. *Distribution and morphology of metastases from other primary sites:* Numerous metastases scattered throughout the liver were found in patients with primary transitional cell carcinoma (**A**, **B**), pancreatic adenocarcinoma (**C**), parotid adenocarcinoma (**D**), lung cancer (**E**) and poorly differentiated adenocarcinoma from an unknown primary (**F, G, H**).

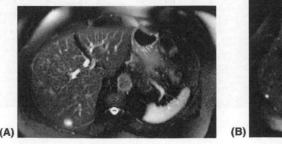
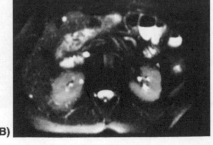

Figure 5. *Squamous cell and neuroendocrine metastases:* Metastases from primary squamous cell cancer of the anal verge (**A**) and a neuroendocrine tumor (**B**) showed well-defined margins and were markedly hypointense on HASTE images (**A**, **B**).

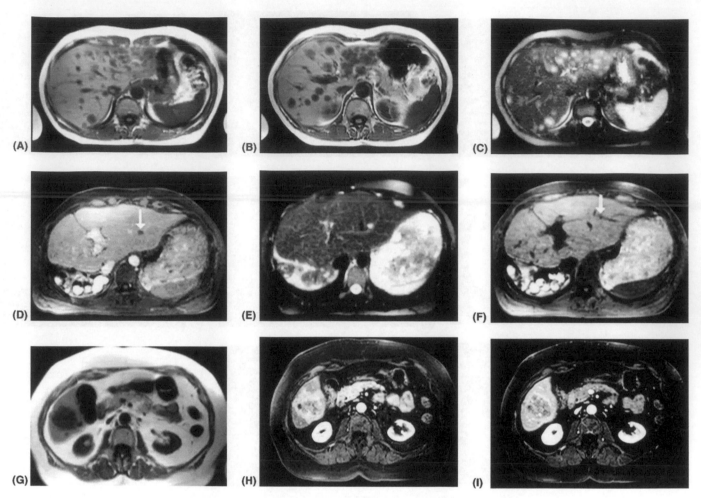

Figure 6. *Breast cancer metastases—range of appearances:* IP T1GRE (**A**, **B**) and HASTE (**C**) images showed numerous highly conspicuous lesions of varying size involving all liver segments. In a second patient, after right hepatectomy for a solitary breast metastasis, post-SPIO T1w 3D GRE imaging (**D**) showed a new single sub-cm metastasis (arrow) in the remnant liver; the lesion was hyperintense on HASTE (**E**) and hypointense on unenhanced T1w 3D GRE (**F**) images (arrow). In a third patient with two surgically confirmed metastases a 5 cm lesion was shown on IP T1w imaging (**G**); the lesion showed heterogeneous enhancement on post-Gd arterial phase (**H**) and portal phase (**I**) FS T1w GRE images.

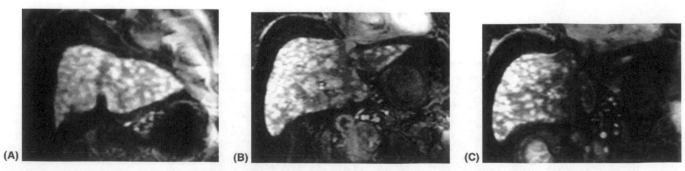

Figure 7. *Miliary metastases from pancreatic cancer.* Coronal oblique arterial phase post-Gd T1w images (**A**, **B**, **C**) showed numerous sub-cm hypervascular metastases throughout the liver.

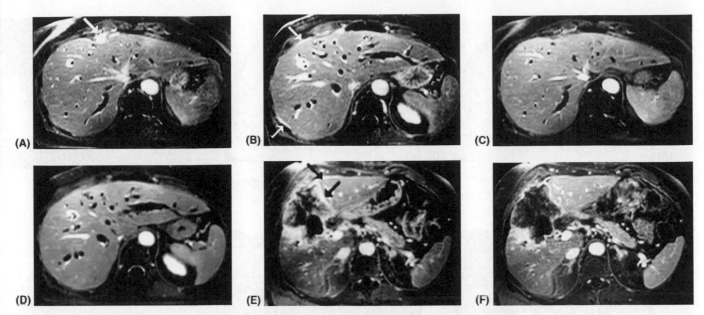

Figure 8. *Peritoneal spread—delayed post-Gd T1w imaging with fat suppression*: In two patients with gallbladder cancer and peritoneal tumor deposits, delayed post-Gd FS 3D T1w GRE images (**A**, **B**) showed marked enhancement of tumor deposits on the liver surface (arrows) which were not visible on the corresponding portal phase images (**C**, **D**). In a second patient with a large gallbladder tumor, extension over the liver surface and along the falciform ligament (arrows) was best shown on delayed post-Gd FS 3D T1w GRE images (**E**). The peritoneal disease was not visible at the portal phase of enhancement (**F**).

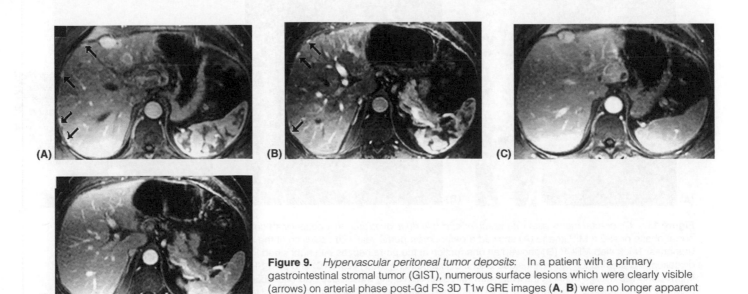

Figure 9. *Hypervascular peritoneal tumor deposits*: In a patient with a primary gastrointestinal stromal tumor (GIST), numerous surface lesions which were clearly visible (arrows) on arterial phase post-Gd FS 3D T1w GRE images (**A**, **B**) were no longer apparent by the portal phase acquisition (**C**, **D**).

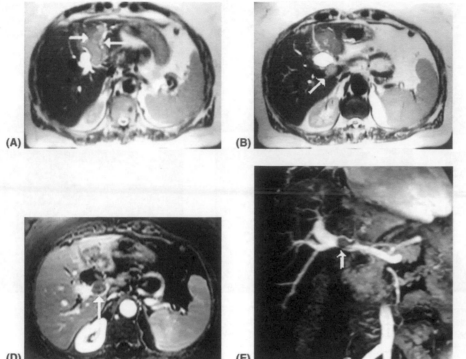

Figure 10. *Colorectal metastasis with vascular invasion:* In a patient with metastatic colorectal cancer HASTE (**A**, **B**) and portal phase post-Gd FS 3D T1w GRE images (**C**, **D**) showed an extensive soft tissue mass within the main and left portal veins (arrows); portal phase MIP image (**E**) showed a plug of tumor thrombus in the main portal vein (arrow) and complete occlusion of the left branch.

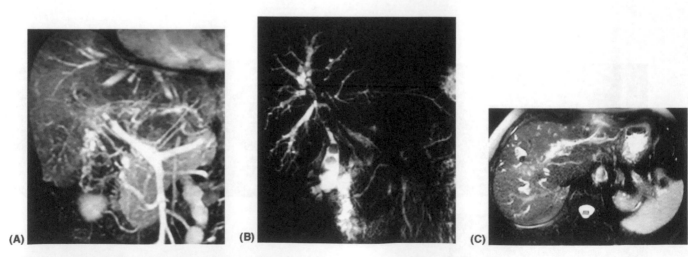

Figure 11. *Colorectal metastasis with vascular and bile duct invasion:* In a patient with colorectal cancer, portal phase post-Gd MIP image (**A**) showed a patent main portal vein with occlusion of the right and left branches. Thick-slab MRCP (**B**) showed an obstruction at the porta-hepatis with right sided intra-hepatic duct dilatation and attenuation of the left-sided ducts. Corresponding axial HASTE (**C**) and post-SPIO T2w GRE (**D**) images showed a large mass at the liver hilum with extension along the left duct. Coronal oblique portal phase post-Gd T1w images (**E**, **F**) showed the main tumor mass extending into the distal main portal vein and filling the right and left branches. (*Continued*)

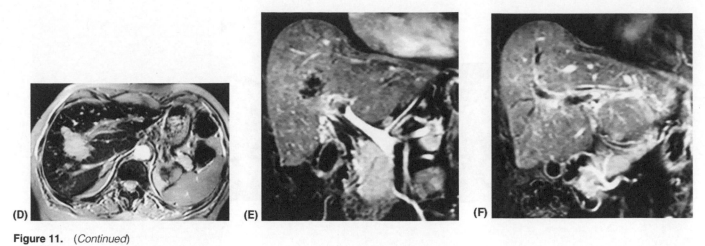

Figure 11. (*Continued*)

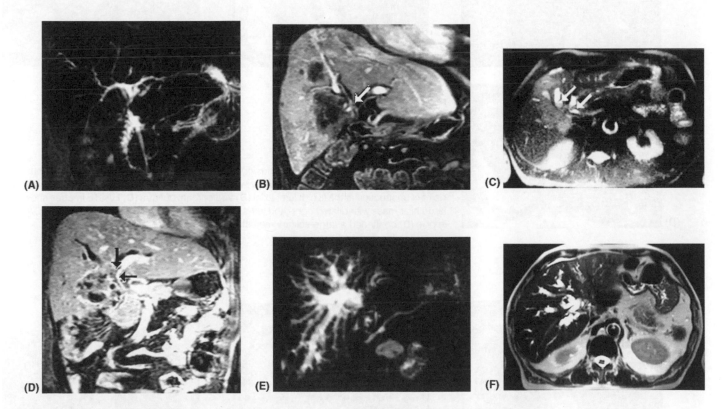

Figure 12. *Colorectal metastases with bile duct invasion:* In a patient with metastatic colorectal cancer, thick-slab MRCP (**A**) showed intrahepatic duct dilation with a point of obstruction at the liver hilum; coronal oblique portal phase post-Gd FS 3D T1w GRE imaging (**B**) showed a large metastasis obstructing the left-sided ducts and extending along the lumen of the right hepatic duct (arrow); axial HASTE imaging (**C**) also showed soft tissue filling defects within the ducts (arrows). In a second patient, coronal oblique portal phase FS 3D T1w GRE imaging (**D**) showed a large colorectal metastasis which had obliterated the gallbladder and extended along the proximal CBD (arrow). In a third patient, a thick-slab MRCP (**E**) showed grossly dilated right-sided ducts and absence of the left ducts; axial HASTE imaging (**F**) confirmed obliteration of the left-sided ducts, and the corresponding post-SPIO T2w GRE image (**G**) showed extensive tumor at the porta-hepatis with infiltration of the ducts in the left lobe; coronal oblique portal phase post-Gd FS 3D T1w GRE imaging (**H**) confirmed expansion of the left-sided ducts by tumor. (*Continued*)

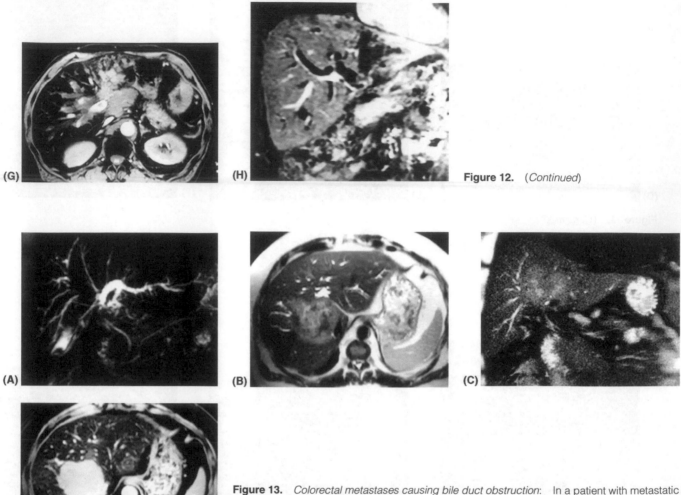

(G) **(H)** **Figure 12.** (*Continued*)

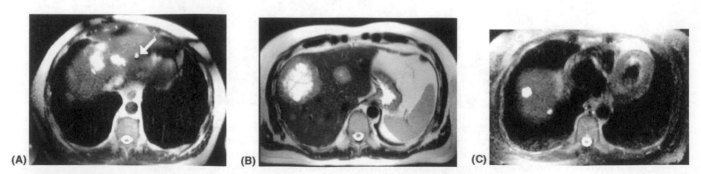

(A) **(B)** **(C)**

(D)

Figure 13. *Colorectal metastases causing bile duct obstruction:* In a patient with metastatic colorectal cancer, thick-slab MRCP (**A**) showed bilateral intrahepatic bile duct dilatation with the point of obstruction at the liver hilum; axial (**B**) and coronal oblique (**C**) HASTE images showed a large hilar mass with dilated right- and left-sided ducts; the corresponding post-SPIO T2w GRE image (**D**) confirmed a large solitary metastasis.

(A) **(B)** **(C)**

Figure 14. *Liver metastases with very high SI on T2w images:* Metastases in a patient with colorectal cancer were markedly hyperintense on HASTE imaging (**A**) but had less distinct margins than the simple cyst in segment 2 (arrow). In a second patient, a hyperintense renal cell metastasis had irregular internal morphology and indistinct margins on HASTE imaging (**B**). In a third patient with a carcinoid primary, hyperintense metastases were indistinguishable from hemangiomas on HASTE images (**C**, **D**) but on post-Gd T1w images (**E**, **F**) the lesions showed continuous rim enhancement with central progression (**G**), typical of metastases. (*Continued*)

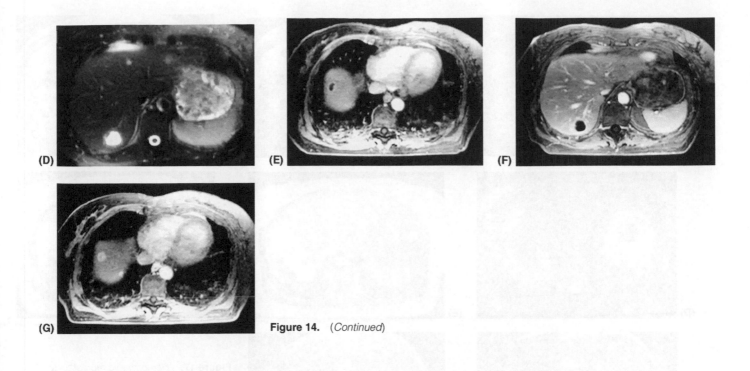

Figure 14. (*Continued*)

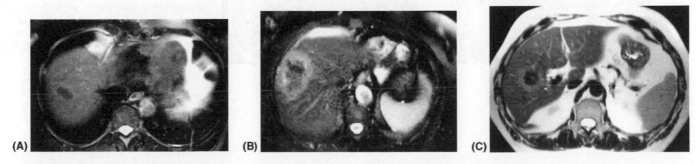

Figure 15. *Liver metastases with low SI on T2w images:* In three patients with colorectal metastases, HASTE images showed a small uniformly hypointense lesion (**A**) and two lesions (**B**, **C**) with a low SI center surrounded by a moderately hypointense ill-defined rim of tumor. In all cases histology confirmed metastases with central coagulative necrosis.

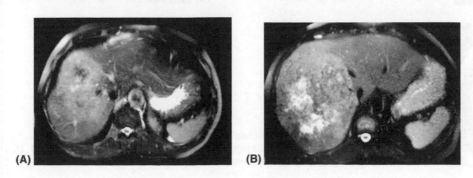

Figure 16. *Liver metastases with mixed SI on T2w images:* In two different patients, HASTE (**A, B**) images showed the typical appearance of large colorectal metastases, which often have a fibrous matrix and mixed low and high SI on T2w images.

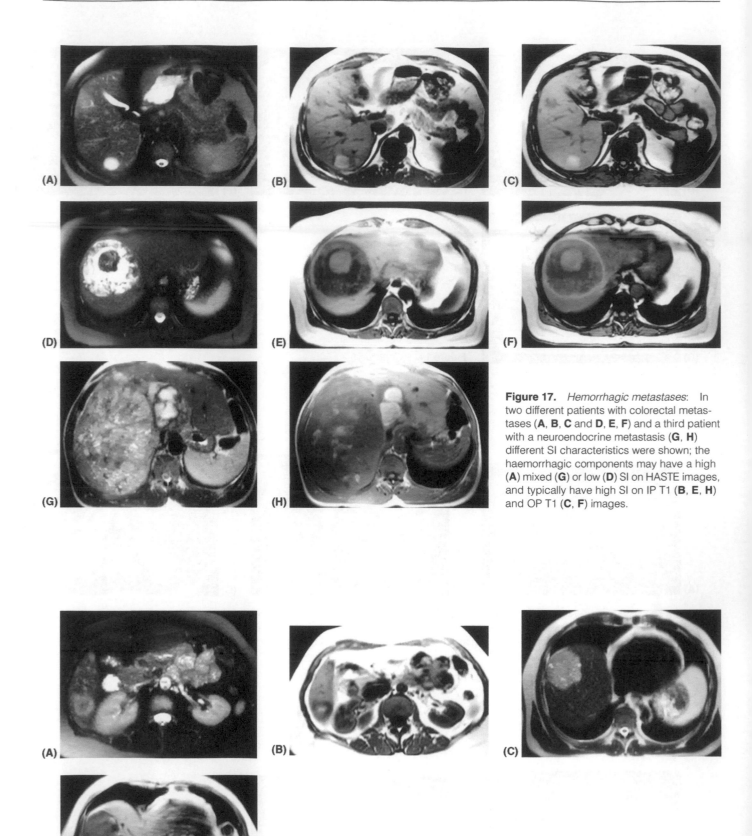

Figure 17. *Hemorrhagic metastases:* In two different patients with colorectal metastases (**A**, **B**, **C** and **D**, **E**, **F**) and a third patient with a neuroendocrine metastasis (**G**, **H**) different SI characteristics were shown; the haemorrhagic components may have a high (**A**) mixed (**G**) or low (**D**) SI on HASTE images, and typically have high SI on IP T1 (**B**, **E**, **H**) and OP T1 (**C**, **F**) images.

Figure 18. *Melanotic metastases:* In two different patients (**A**, **B** and **C**, **D**), melanin-containing metastases showed a mixed high and low SI on HASTE (**A**, **C**) and IP T1 (**B**, **D**) images reflecting the paramagnetic properties of melanin.

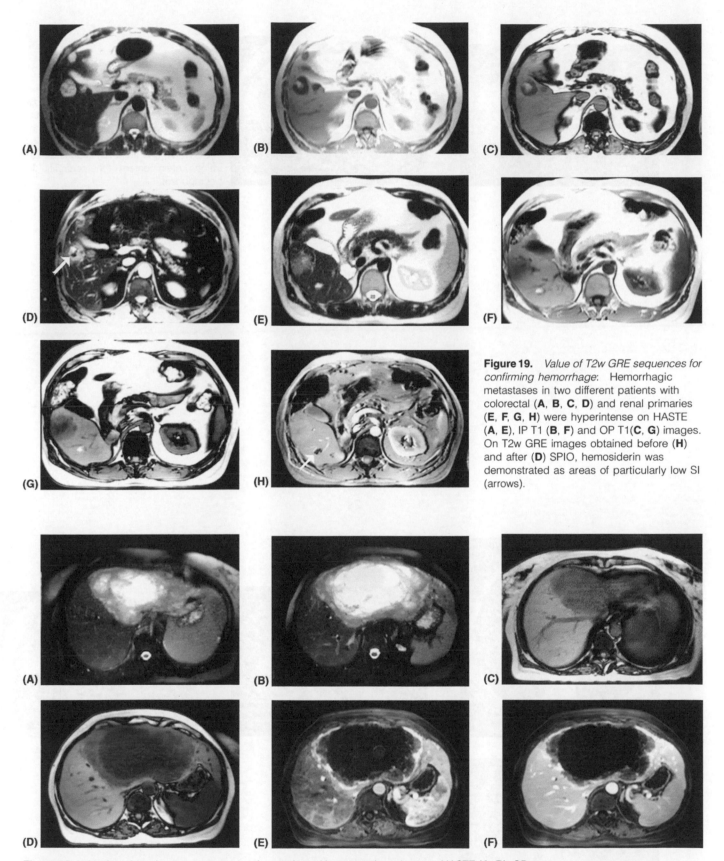

Figure 19. *Value of T2w GRE sequences for confirming hemorrhage*: Hemorrhagic metastases in two different patients with colorectal (**A**, **B**, **C**, **D**) and renal primaries (**E**, **F**, **G**, **H**) were hyperintense on HASTE (**A**, **E**), IP T1 (**B**, **F**) and OP T1(**C**, **G**) images. On T2w GRE images obtained before (**H**) and after (**D**) SPIO, hemosiderin was demonstrated as areas of particularly low SI (arrows).

Figure 20. *Amelanotic melanoma metastasis*: In a patient with metastatic melanoma, HASTE (**A**, **B**), OP T1 (**C**, **D**) and post-Gd arterial (**E**) and portal (**F**) phase FS 3D T1w GRE images showed a solitary malignant tumor with no evidence of melanin content; histopathology following hepatic resection showed an amelanotic tumor.

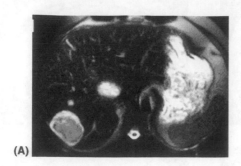
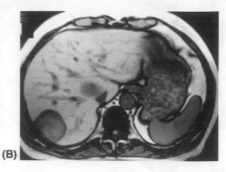

Figure 21.   *High SI on T1w images due to proteinaceous fluid*:   In a patient with metastases from a neuroendocrine tumor, the lesions showed mixed high and low SI on HASTE (**A**) and IP T1 (**B**) images due to the high protein content of the central fluid component.

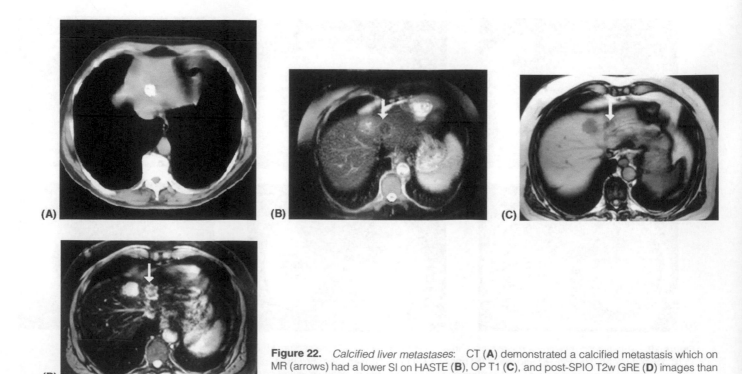

Figure 22.   *Calcified liver metastases*:   CT (**A**) demonstrated a calcified metastasis which on MR (arrows) had a lower SI on HASTE (**B**), OP T1 (**C**), and post-SPIO T2w GRE (**D**) images than the adjacent non-calcified metastasis.

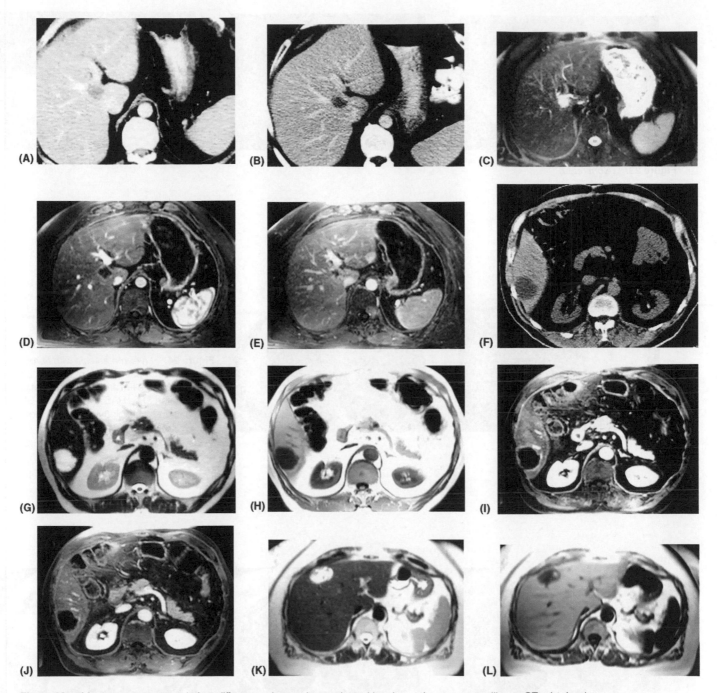

Figure 23. *Mucinous metastases in four different patients:*   In a patient with colorectal cancer, surveillance CTs obtained a year apart (**A**, **B**) showed a stable hypovascular lesion; the tumor was uniformly hyperintense on HASTE imaging (**C**) and indistinguishable from a hemangioma, but continuous rim enhancement on post-Gd portal phase (**D**) T1w images with progressive enhancement on delayed images (**E**) was indicative of metastasis. In a second patient unenhanced CT (**F**) showed a low attenuation lesion which was homogeneously hyperintense on HASTE (**G**) and hypointense on IP T1(**H**) images; the lesion showed an enhancing rim but no progression of the enhancement in portal (**I**) and delayed phase (**J**) post-Gd images. In a third patient HASTE (**K**) and IP T1GRE (**L**) images showed a largely cystic lesion with a hyperintense focus on the T1w image; a complete rim of enhancement on post-Gd arterial phase (**M**) T1w imaging indicated metastasis. In a fourth patient STIR imaging (**N**) showed a markedly hyperintense lesion which was more heterogeneous than the previous example; enhancement in the wall of the lesion was shown on post-Gd T1w images (**O**). Histology in all cases showed mucinous colorectal tumors. (*Continued*)

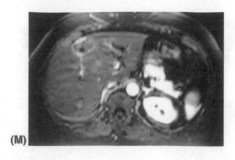
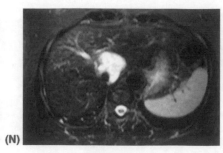
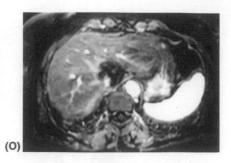

Figure 23. (*Continued*)

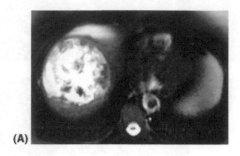
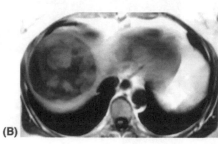

Figure 24. *Liver metastasis with fibrous capsule:* In a patient with metastatic colorectal cancer, the rim around a large metastasis showed high SI on HASTE (**A**) and low SI on IP T1 (**B**) images; histology confirmed the presence of a fibrotic capsule.

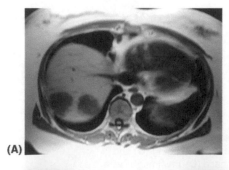
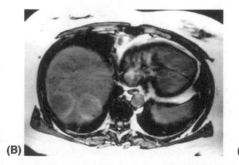
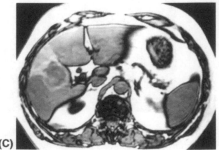
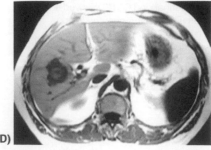

Figure 25. *Colorectal metastases in a fatty liver:* In a patient with colorectal cancer, two hypointense lesions were clearly shown on IP T1 imaging (**A**); the lesions were isointense with the low signal of fatty liver on OP T1 imaging (**B**) but were rendered highly conspicuous by a rim of compressed non-fatty liver tissue surrounding them. In a second patient the liver showed low SI on OP T1 (**C**) compared with IP T1 (**D**) images, and a bright rim of non-fatty liver tissue outlined the lesions in (**C**); note the wedge-shaped area of relative fatty sparing adjacent to the metastasis in (**C**), probably due to occlusion of a peripheral portal vein branch by the tumor.

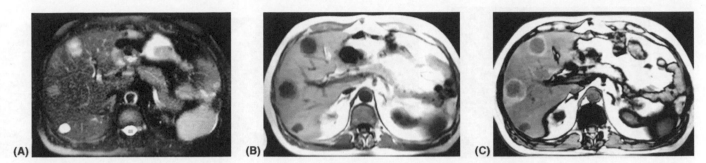

(A) (B) (C)

Figure 26. *Metastases and benign lesions in a fatty liver.* In a patient with colorectal cancer, HASTE imaging (**A**) showed two ill-defined and mildly hyperintense metastases in segments 4 and 8, and a well-defined markedly hyperintense cyst in segment 7; the liver showed normal SI on IP T1 (**B**) but low SI on OP T1 (**C**) images, indicating fatty change. A bright halo of non-fatty liver was seen around the metastases in (**C**) but was less pronounced around the cyst.

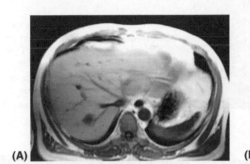

(A)

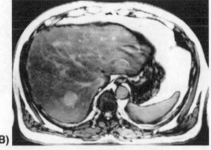

(B)

Figure 27. *Hyperintense metastases in a very fatty liver on OPT1w.* In a patient with colorectal cancer, a metastasis which was hypointense on IP T1 (**A**) appeared hyperintense on OP T1 (**B**) images, due to the marked drop in liver SI resulting from severe fatty infiltration.

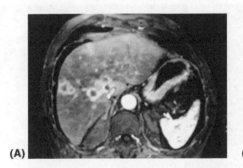

(A)

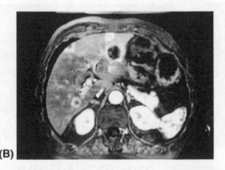

(B)

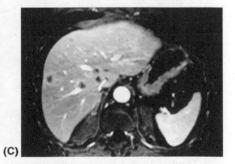

(C)

Figure 28. *Transient enhancement at the periphery of hypovascular metastases.* In two patients (**A**, **B**, **C**, **D**) and (**E**, **F**) with multiple colorectal metastases, post-Gd arterial phase FS 3D T1w GRE images (**A**, **B**, **E**) showed continuous peripheral rim enhancement which was no longer visible by the portal phase of enhancement (**C**, **D**, **F**). (*Continued*)

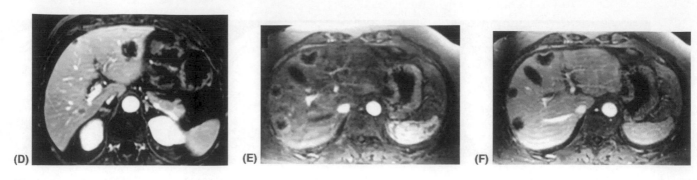

Figure 28. (*Continued*)

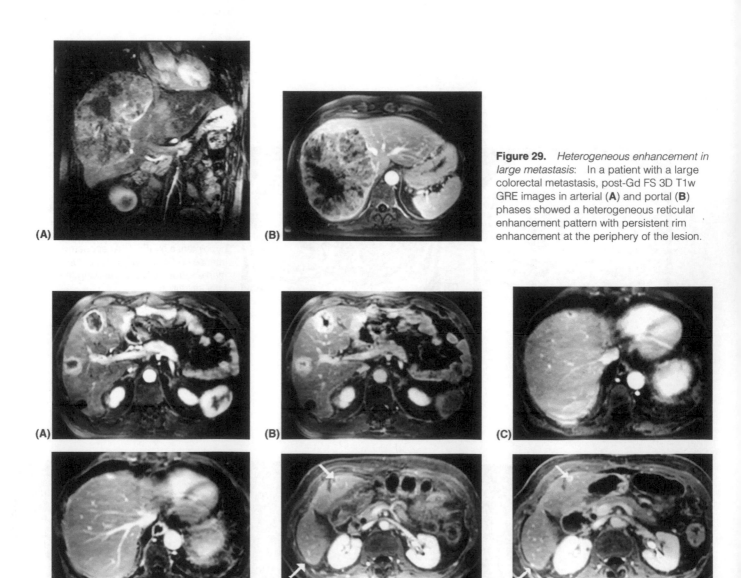

Figure 29. *Heterogeneous enhancement in large metastasis:* In a patient with a large colorectal metastasis, post-Gd FS 3D T1w GRE images in arterial (**A**) and portal (**B**) phases showed a heterogeneous reticular enhancement pattern with persistent rim enhancement at the periphery of the lesion.

Figure 30. *Progressive enhancement in metastases:* Post-Gd arterial (**A**, **C**) and delayed phase (**B**, **D**) images in two patients (**A**, **B** and **C**, **D**) with colorectal metastases showed continuous peripheral enhancement which progressed to involve most or all of the lesion over time; note delayed enhancement of the liver capsule (**D**), indicating peritoneal tumor infiltration. In a third patient with small neuroendocrine metastases (arrows) the same progressive enhancement was shown on post-Gd arterial (**E**) and delayed phase (**F**) images.

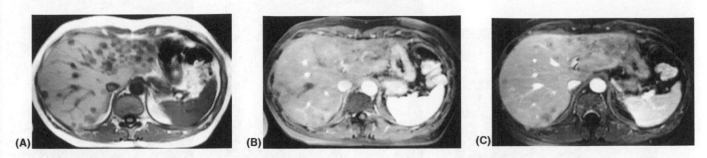

Figure 31. "*Isovascular*" *metastases*: In a patient with breast cancer, numerous breast metastases were highly conspicuous on IP T1imaging (**A**) but became much less apparent on post-Gd arterial (**B**) and portal phase (**C**) T1w images.

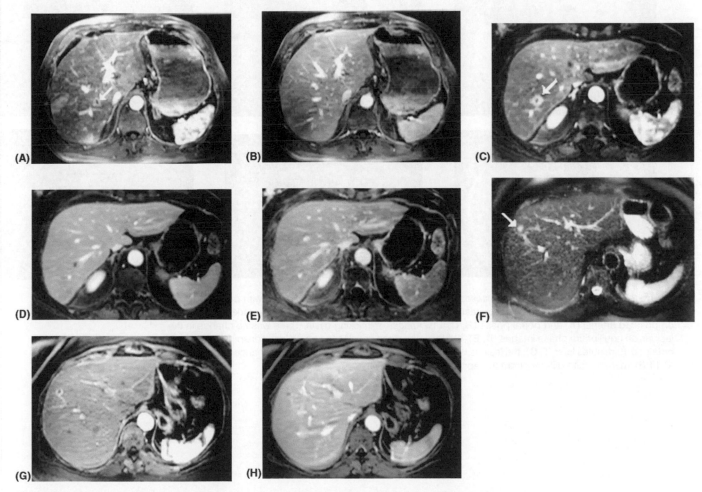

Figure 32. *Typical small hypovascular metastases*: A small colorectal metastasis (arrow) showed a complete rim of enhancement on post-Gd arterial phase FS 3D T1w GRE imaging (**A**); on the portal phase images (**B**) the lesion had a less distinct border and appeared smaller. In a second patient with metastatic breast cancer, a small lesion (arrow) was highly conspicuous on arterial phase post-Gd T1w images (**C**), apparently smaller and less distinct by the portal phase (**D**) and no longer visible on images obtained 5 minutes after injection (**E**). A small colorectal metastasis (arrow) in a third patient was well defined and hyperintense on HASTE imaging (**F**) but was indistinguishable from a hemangioma; the lesion showed continual peripheral rim enhancement on post-Gd arterial phase T1w images (**G**) which was no longer apparent by the portal phase (**H**) indicating metastasis. All cases were histologically confirmed.

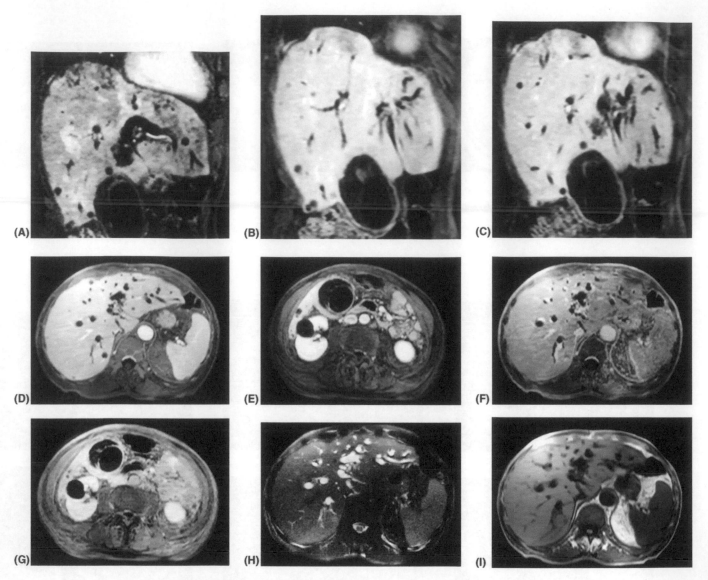

Figure 33. *Small hypovascular metastases with minimal enhancement:* In a patient with pancreatic adenocarcinoma, numerous small metastases showed minimal enhancement and were markedly hypointense on post-Gd arterial (**A**) and portal phase (**B**, **C**) T1w images, mimicking cysts. There was no change in the lesions on equilibrium phase images (**D**, **E**), but they appeared smaller and much less conspicuous on images obtained 10 minutes later (**F**, **G**); the lesions were inconspicuous on corresponding unenhanced HASTE (**H**) and IP T1 (**I**) images, quite different from the appearance of cysts.

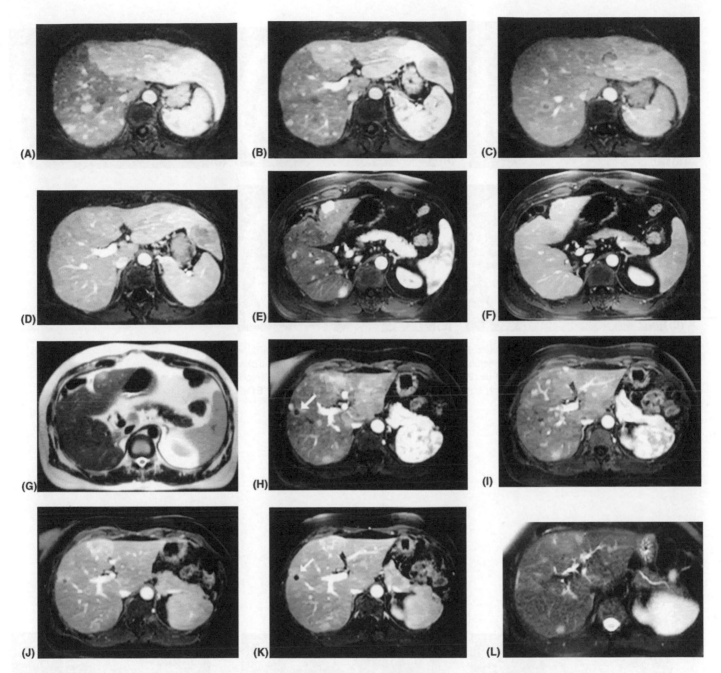

Figure 34. *Hypervascular metastases:* In a patient with a primary neuroendocrine tumor, post-Gd arterial phase T1w images (**A**, **B**) showed numerous hypervascular metastases which were no longer visible by the portal phase (**C**, **D**); note the marked arterial hyperperfusion of segments 2,3 and 4 indicating reduced portal venous inflow to the left lobe. In a second patient, metastases from renal cell carcinoma showed marked hyperintensity on arterial phase post-Gd T1w imaging (**E**) but became almost isointense by the portal phase (**F**); the lesions were barely visible on HASTE imaging (**G**). In a third patient, carcinoid metastases showed mixed vascularity; adjacent arterial (**H**, **I**) and portal phase (**J**, **K**) post-Gd T1w images showed numerous hypervascular lesions, some of which were only visible in the arterial phase, and a further hypovascular lesion (arrow) with characteristic continuous rim enhancement (**H**, **K**). The lesions were inconspicuous on corresponding HASTE images (**L**).

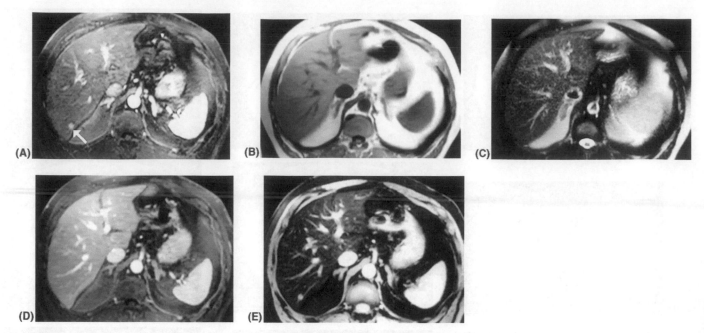

Figure 35. *Hypervascular metastases versus benign hepatocellular lesions—value of SPIO:*   In a patient with colorectal cancer, a small hypervascular lesion (arrow) was clearly shown on post-Gd arterial phase T1w images (**A**) but was isointense on unenhanced T1w (**B**), T2w (**C**) and portal phase (**D**) images, mimicking a benign hepatocellular lesion; the lesion was highly conspicuous on post-SPIO T2w GRE imaging (**E**) with no uptake of SPIO, indicating metastasis.

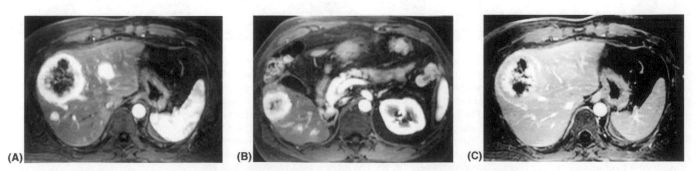

Figure 36. *Peripheral washout in liver metastases:*   In a patient with renal cell cancer, metastases showed marked arterial enhancement on immediate post-Gd T1w images (**A**, **B**). Peripheral washout was seen in the two larger lesions on 10 minute post-Gd T1w images (**C**, **D**); the smaller lesions were isointense and completely invisible by this phase. In a second patient, hypovascular pancreatic metastases with minimal enhancement on portal phase post-Gd T1w images (**E**) showed peripheral washout on the 10 minute post-Gd image (**F**). In a third patient with colorectal metastases, post-gadobenate portal phase T1w imaging (**G**) showed numerous hypovascular lesions; peripheral washout was apparent on the corresponding hepatocyte phase image (**H**) obtained 20 minutes after injection. (*Continued*)

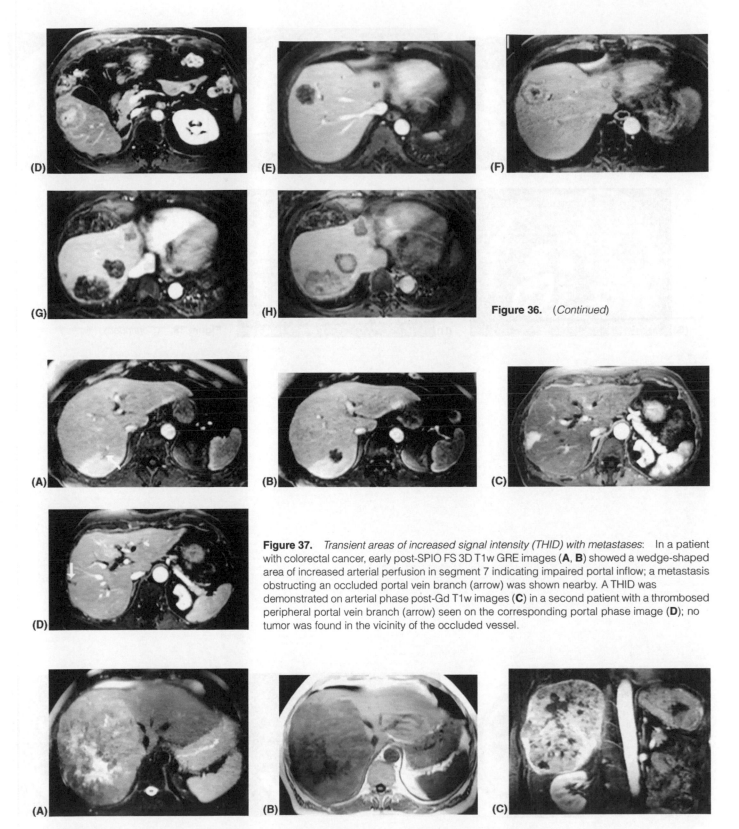

Figure 36. (*Continued*)

Figure 37. *Transient areas of increased signal intensity (THID) with metastases*:   In a patient with colorectal cancer, early post-SPIO FS 3D T1w GRE images (**A**, **B**) showed a wedge-shaped area of increased arterial perfusion in segment 7 indicating impaired portal inflow; a metastasis obstructing an occluded portal vein branch (arrow) was shown nearby. A THID was demonstrated on arterial phase post-Gd T1w images (**C**) in a second patient with a thrombosed peripheral portal vein branch (arrow) seen on the corresponding portal phase image (**D**); no tumor was found in the vicinity of the occluded vessel.

Figure 38. *Typical appearance of colorectal liver metastases*:   Colorectal metastases in two different patients (**A**, **B**, **C**, **D** and **E**, **F**, **G**, **H**) were heterogeneous and moderately hyperintense on HASTE images (**A**, **E**), moderately hypointense on IP T1images (**B**, **F**) and showed continuous peripheral rim enhancement on arterial phase post-Gd images (**C**, **G**). Equilibrium phase images (**D**, **H**) showed progressive enhancement of the fibrous septa in the lesions producing a characteristic "cauliflower" appearance. (*Continued*)

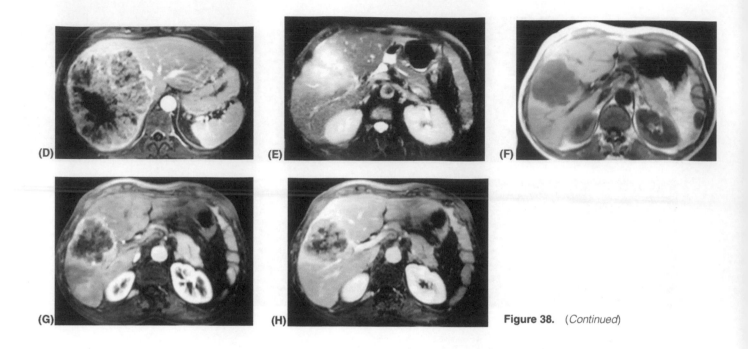

Figure 38. (*Continued*)

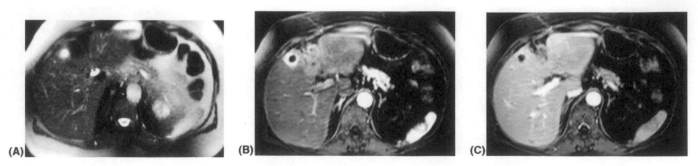

Figure 39. *Peripheral enhancement with metastases from squamous cell carcinoma:* In a patient with an anal verge carcinoma, HASTE imging (**A**) showed a lesion with a markedly hyperintense center due to colliquative necrosis, and a faintly hyperintense rim. The peripheral tissue showed pronounced and continuous enhancement on arterial phase post-Gd T1w images (**B**) which faded by the portal phase (**C**). There was minimal enhancement of the necrotic center.

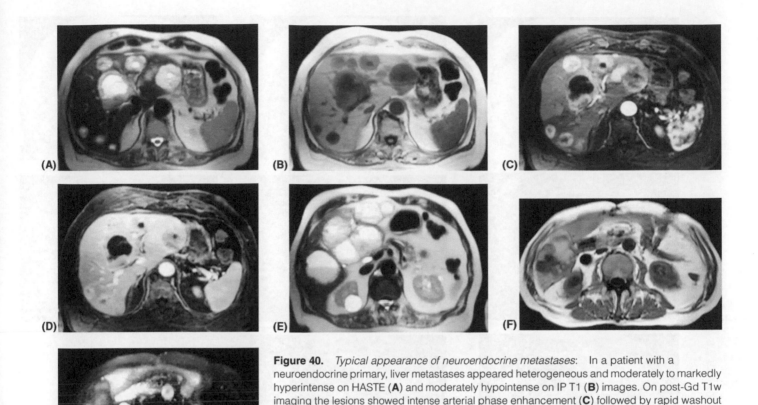

Figure 40. *Typical appearance of neuroendocrine metastases*: In a patient with a neuroendocrine primary, liver metastases appeared heterogeneous and moderately to markedly hyperintense on HASTE (**A**) and moderately hypointense on IP T1 (**B**) images. On post-Gd T1w imaging the lesions showed intense arterial phase enhancement (**C**) followed by rapid washout with some of the smaller lesions no longer visible by the portal phase (**D**); images obtained at a more caudal level in the same patient showed several lesions with a fluid level on HASTE (**E**) and layering of low SI material in the dependant portion of the metastases consistent with proteinaceous fluid. In a second patient, a neuroendocrine metastasis showed mixed high and low SI on IP T1 (**F**) and HASTE (**G**) images again indicating proteinaceous fluid contents.

Figure 41. *Metastases versus simple cysts in patients with known malignant disease*: In a patient with colorectal cancer, simple cysts (long arrows) were well defined and strongly hyperintense on HASTE imaging (**A**) while a metastasis (short arrow) was ill-defined and barely visible. On post-Gd T1w images the metastasis was moderately hypointense and more conspicuous in the portal phase (**B**) while the cysts showed no enhancement and had very low SI; images obtained 10 minutes after injection (**C**) showed progressive enhancement of the metastasis which became less conspicuous while the cysts remained highly hypointense.

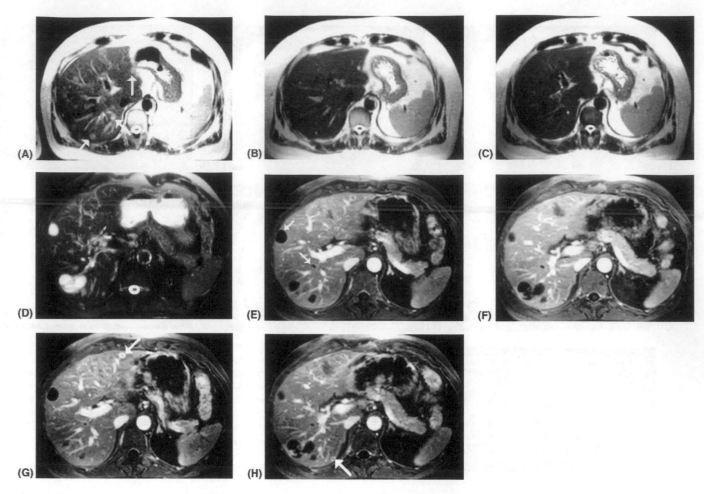

Figure 42. *Treated metastases mimicking simple cysts:*   Prior to treatment of colorectal metastases HASTE imaging (**A**) showed the lesions to be ill-defined and moderately hyperintense (arrows). After chemotherapy the lesions appeared smaller, well defined and markedly hyperintense on HASTE images (**B, C**) mimicking benign lesions. In a second patient with multiple cystic metastases following Glivec treatment for a metastatic GIST, numerous well-defined hyperintense lesions were shown on HASTE imaging (**D**); on post-Gd T1w images in portal (**E, F**) and delayed (**G, H**) phase images, some of the lesions showed minimal and non progressive enhancement (short arrows), while the larger confluent lesion in segment 7 showed progressive enhancement of internal septa. Characteristic continuous rim enhancement with progressive central enhancement was seen in other lesions (long arrows). Histopathology of the resected liver confirmed numerous cystic tumors containing gelatinous material and other more solid metastases with central necrosis.

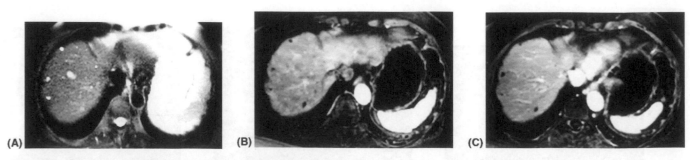

Figure 43. *Biliary hamartomas (von Meyenberg complexes):*   Multiple sub-capsular lesions in a patient with colon cancer resembled simple cysts on HASTE imaging (**A**), but showed a very faint rim of enhancement on post-Gd arterial phase T1w imaging (**B**) which persisted unchanged in the portal phase (**C**). In a second colorectal cancer patient small sub-capsular lesions were inconspicuous on HASTE (**D**) and IP T1 (**E**) images, showed early and persistent enhancement on arterial (**F**) and equilibrium phase (**G**) post-Gd T1w images, and were highly conspicuous on post-SPIO T2w images (**H, I**). The lesions were indistinguishable from small metastases on imaging criteria; histopathology of the resected liver confirmed von Meyenberg complexes. (*Continued*)

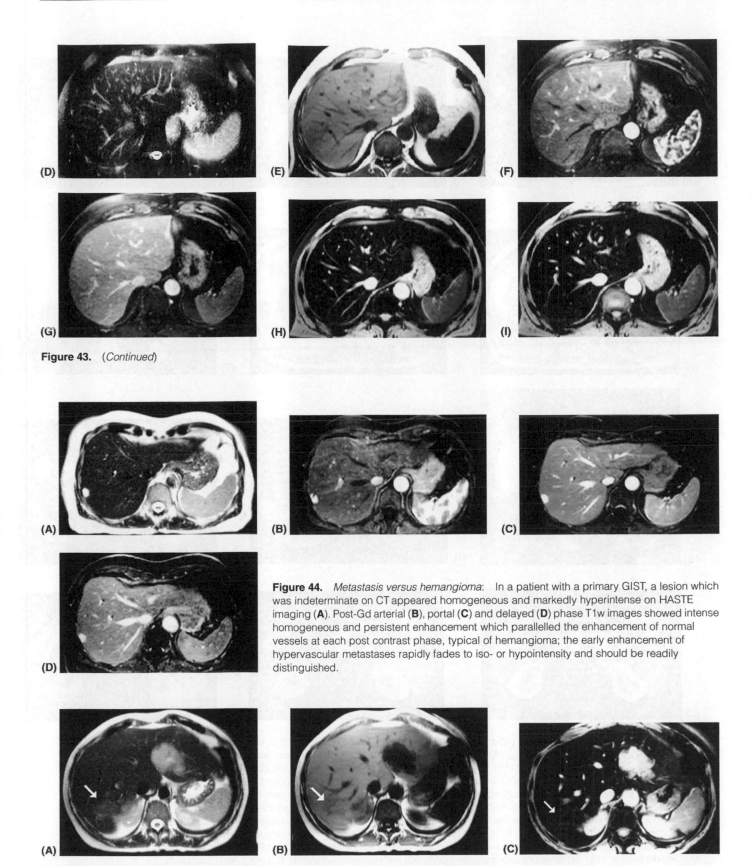

Figure 43. (*Continued*)

Figure 44. *Metastasis versus hemangioma*: In a patient with a primary GIST, a lesion which was indeterminate on CT appeared homogeneous and markedly hyperintense on HASTE imaging (**A**). Post-Gd arterial (**B**), portal (**C**) and delayed (**D**) phase T1w images showed intense homogeneous and persistent enhancement which parallelled the enhancement of normal vessels at each post contrast phase, typical of hemangioma; the early enhancement of hypervascular metastases rapidly fades to iso- or hypointensity and should be readily distinguished.

Figure 45. *Metastasis versus FNH*: In a patient with colorectal cancer, a metastasis in the left lobe was highly conspicuous on HASTE (**A**) IP T1 (**B**) and SPIO-enhanced T2w GRE (**C**) images; a second lesion in the right lobe (arrow) remained almost isointense with background liver on all sequences including post-SPIO, indicating FNH.

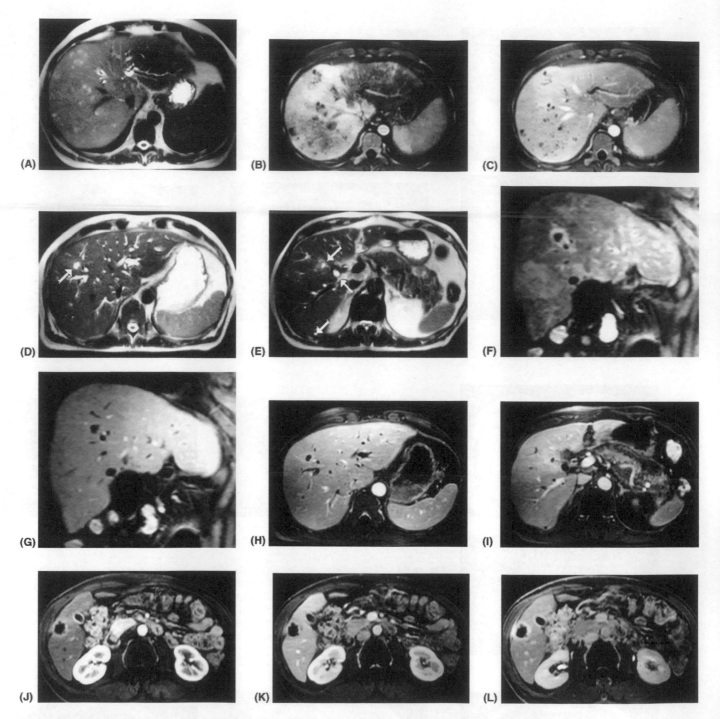

Figure 46. *Hepatic abscesses:* In a patient with a history of IV drug abuse and hepatitis C, who presented with severe acute pancreatitis, HASTE imaging (**A**) showed a large liver with numerous ill-defined moderately hyperintense lesions and increased SI throughout the right lobe consistent with edema. Arterial phase post-Gd T1w imaging (**B**) showed increased arterial flow to the right lobe due to an occluded right portal vein (not shown) and multiple hypovascular lesions which showed non-progressive enhancement, maintaining their appearance on equilibrium phase images (**C**). The features were consistent with multiple evolving liver abscesses which had not yet liquefied; biopsy confirmed liver edema and abscesses. In a different patient with cholangitic liver abscesses following stenting of a malignant stricture, HASTE images (**D, E**) showed several hyperintense lesions (arrows) surrounded by a peripheral halo of reduced signal; there was marked enhancement of the hyperaemic abscess wall on post-Gd T1w arterial phase imaging (**F**) and no "fill-in" of the lesions on subsequent portal (**G**) and equilibrium phase (**H, I**) images. In a third patient with RUQ pain and malaise following a trip to India, sonography identified a right lobe lesion interpreted as an inflammatory mass. Arterial (**J**), portal (**K**) and delayed phase (**L**) post-Gd T1w images showed a hypointense lesion with enhancement of the rim but not the center of the lesion, and intense delayed enhancement of the adjacent liver; the MRI findings were typical of liver abscess, and interval imaging showed a reduction in the size of the lesion.

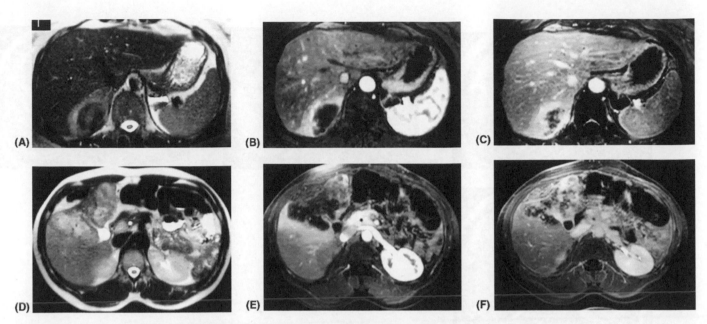

Figure 47.   *Metastasis versus peripheral cholangiocarcinoma:*   In a patient with no known primary tumor, CT showed a complex liver lesion; on HASTE imaging (**A**) the lesion showed a low SI center with a moderately hyperintense rim. Post-Gd arterial (**B**) and delayed phase (**C**) T1w images showed peripheral and central enhancement consistent with a metastatic lesion but histopathology following hepatic resection confirmed intrahepatic cholangiocarcinoma. In a different patient also with histologically confirmed peripheral cholangiocarcinoma, HASTE imaging (**D**) showed a large heterogeneous tumor with a central area of hypointensity associated with indrawing of the adjacent liver capsule. Post-Gd arterial (**E**) and delayed phase (**F**) T1w images showed early enhancement around the periphery of the lesion with progressive enhancement of the central fibrous component—a more typical MR appearance of peripheral cholangiocarcinoma.

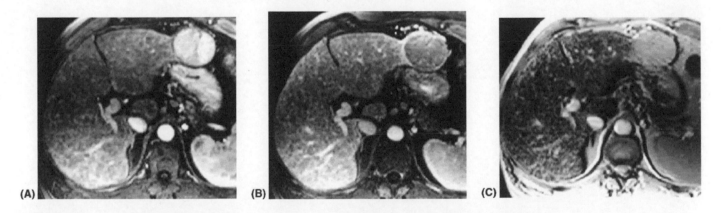

Figure 48.   *Unsuspected cirrhosis and HCC:*   In a patient with a history of colorectal cancer, surveillance CT showed a solitary largely exophytic liver lesion; post-Gd arterial (**A**) and equilibrium phase (**B**) T1w images showed a lesion with marked arterial phase enhancement and a well-defined capsule, typical of HCC. On post-SPIO T2w GRE imaging (**C**) the lesion showed no uptake of SPIO, and the liver architecture appeared nodular, suggesting cirrhosis; histopathology of the resection specimen confirmed HCC with underlying cirrhosis. In a different patient with no known primary malignancy, a 3.5 cm right lobe lesion initially found on sonography appeared hypointense on OP T1w imaging (**D**) and showed a thin rim of continuous peripheral enhancement on post-Gd T1w imaging (**E**) suggestive of metastatic disease—but note the slightly irregular contour of the liver surface as outlined by the fat-water artifact on OP T1w images (**D**); the patient was unfit for surgery and re-presented 18 months later with grossly elevated AFP levels, and OP T1w (**F**, **G**) images then showed an irregular liver contour, an expanded gallbladder fossa, and relative hypertrophy of the left lobe suggestive of cirrhosis; the original tumor had enlarged a little, but multiple tumor foci had developed elsewhere in the liver. MR appearances were typical of multi-focal HCC in a cirrhotic liver. (*Continued*)

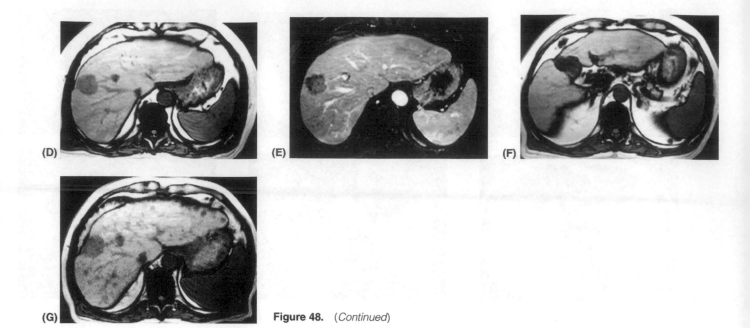

(D)   (E)   (F)

(G)   **Figure 48.**   (*Continued*)

CHAPTER 12

MRI of Liver Tumors After Treatment

W hile in the untreated patient we are concerned with the detection and recognition of disease, after treatment of focal liver lesions we must also be aware of the effects of different types of therapy on the residual liver itself. The treatment of benign liver tumors, if needed at all, is generally limited to surgical resection. With malignant tumors, local ablation using radiofrequency, laser, microwave, or cryo-probes may be used either as a definitive treatment or in combination with surgery. With more widespread disease, systemic chemotherapy is usually offered. Tumors with a rich arterial supply, particularly hepatocellular carcinoma and metastases from neuro-endocrine primaries, may be treated by trans-arterial chemo-embolization (TACE). It is now commonplace for patients to be treated with combinations of systemic chemotherapy, surgery, and ablation of focal lesions. Interpreting the imaging appearances of the treated liver then requires an appreciation of the various effects which treatment itself has on the residual parenchyma as well as the characteristics of residual tumor, the likely pattern of recurrent or new disease, and the discriminating features which allow us to distinguish the side-effects or local complications of treatment from new or continuing malignancy.

POST-OPERATIVE ANATOMY AND SURGICAL RESIDUES

The main anatomic changes of major resection, and the typical artifacts caused by clips, stents, and other residues of intervention have already been described and illustrated in chapter 4, so only a few additional points will be made here.

Types of Procedure

The extent of surgical liver resections is limited by the feasibility of preserving the biliary drainage, the venous outflow and the portal vein supply of the residual liver segments after removing that part of the liver containing the tumor(s). Integrity of the arterial supply is of less importance except in the case of liver transplantation, where there is little or no collateral supply to the biliary tree in the absence of arterial inflow. Traditional hepatic resections involve removal of the left lobe, the right lobe, or the lateral section of the left lobe (segments 2 and 3). Newer techniques allow more extensive resections, such as the removal of segments 4, 5, 6, 7, and 8 (right trisectionectomy) or removal of segments 2, 3, 4, 5, and 6 (left trisectionectomy). Part or the whole of segment 1 may also be removed with either of these procedures. Occasionally transverse resections of the right lobe are performed, retaining segments 7 and 8 or segments 5 and 6, while segments 6 and 7 may be removed en bloc (posterior sectionectomy). Newer techniques also allow non-segmental resections, and small tumors near the liver surface may be excised by taking a small wedge of liver tissue.

Interpreting Post-Operative Anatomy

After removal of part or the whole of the left lobe, the anatomic features of the right lobe are largely unchanged, and occupy their usual position in relation to the thoraco-abdominal wall and the inferior vena cava. When the right lobe is removed, the void is usually filled by the hepatic flexure of the colon, but the left lobe often hypertrophies in a rightward direction, so that the normal orientation of the left hepatic vein and its branches is altered. The presence of liver parenchyma on the right side of the falciform ligament will indicate preservation of segment 4, and the middle hepatic vein, when it is preserved, can be recognized as a large vein pointing in the same radial direction as the termination of the residual portal vein at the liver hilum. Excision of part or the whole of segment 1 is indicated by clip artifacts encircling the IVC. Resections of peripheral parenchymal tumors will usually leave the extrahepatic bile ducts intact (although the gallbladder is generally removed with right lobectomies since its arterial supply is from the right hepatic artery), but with more centrally placed tumors the hilar ducts may be excised and biliary continuity restored by bringing a jejunal loop to the cut surface of the liver for direct anastomosis with the residual duct or ducts. When interpreting the liver MRI of post-surgical patients, it is helpful to refer to the details of the operative procedure, since there are so many possible combinations of resections and anastomoses. Availability of an operative diagram provided by the surgeon is particularly useful.

"Normal" Surgical Residues

In addition to the clip artifacts already described, localized hematoma or collections of serous fluid or bile may remain along the resection margin, adjacent to the site of biliary anastomoses, or in the sub-phrenic or sub-hepatic spaces, particularly on the right. By a month or so after surgery, these collections typically show hypointensity on T1w and hyperintensity on T2w images. For the first few weeks after surgery, the walls of these fluid collections, like the cut surface of the liver itself, may show a thin rim of enhancement on post-Gd T1w imaging, probably caused by a mild inflammatory reaction or a layer of granulation tissue. This effect subsides within 3–6 months after surgery, by which time any residual fluid collections should be clearly shrinking.

The cut surface of the liver usually heals without fibrosis, but occasionally peripheral scars may develop at or close to the resection margin, probably due to occlusion of peripheral portal vein branches in the affected area. Occasionally, thrombosed portal vein branches may be visualized on post-operative imaging, typically accompanied by a "THID" with locally increased arterial perfusion. Perhaps as a result of the same mechanism, areas of focal fatty change or sparing within an otherwise fatty liver remnant may develop, particularly in patients undergoing post-operative chemotherapy. All of these benign features must be distinguished from residual or recurrent tumor (see below).

EFFECTS OF CHEMOTHERAPY

The imaging appearance of tumors is frequently altered by chemotherapy, but changes also often occur in the surrounding liver parenchyma.

EFFECTS OF CHEMOTHERAPY ON LIVER PARENCHYMA

Fatty Change

Fatty change is a common side-effect of systemic chemotherapy. Diffuse fatty change impairs the recognition of residual or recurrent disease on sonography and CT, but is readily recognized on chemical shift MRI. The degree of fatty change is variable, and partial or complete resolution may occur after cessation of chemotherapy. Fatty change may also be regional, patchy or focal, or localized areas of sparing may develop within an otherwise diffusely fatty liver. Again, differentiating focal fatty change or focal sparing from recurrent tumor may be difficult on CT and sonography, but in-phase and opposed-phase T1w MRI is usually decisive.

Fibrosis

Less commonly, patients undergoing systemic chemotherapy develop diffuse, regional, or patchy fibrosis. In our experience this feature is most often associated with the use of platinum-based drugs. In severe cases fibrosis is visible as a reticular pattern of hypointensity on unenhanced T1w imaging, hyperintensity on T2w images and delayed enhancement on post-Gd T1w imaging. However, the abnormality is most clearly shown on post-SPIO GRE T2w imaging, and in mild cases may only be visible after SPIO contrast. Like fatty change, this less frequent complication of chemotherapy can resolve after cessation of treatment.

Pseudocirrhosis

On very rare occasions the degree of fibrosis is much greater, producing shrinkage and distortion of the liver to give an appearance which is macroscopically indistinguishable from late stage cirrhosis. This "pseudo-cirrhosis" has been most often found in patients with liver metastases from breast cancer undergoing combination chemotherapy, but individual case reports also include patients with renal, bronchial, and pancreatic cancer, melanoma, and hematological malignancy. The mechanism for development of pseudo-cirrhosis remains uncertain. Histologic studies typically show dense fibrosis associated with residual tumor, sometimes described as desmoplastic reaction, but the absence of bridging fibrosis distinguishes this condition from true cirrhosis. Spread of tumor along the sinusoids has been shown histologically, and this mechanism could contribute to the portal hypertension which is seen in some cases. Histology indistinguishable from nodular regenerative hyperplasia has also been found in a high proportion of biopsies from these patients. Occasional cases have been found in which no residual tumor was detected histologically and rare case reports describe pseudo-cirrhosis in patients with metastatic breast cancer who have not received chemotherapy.

The imaging features of pseudo-cirrhosis are indistinguishable from those of true cirrhosis. Ascites, splenomegaly, and varices are not unusual. The liver appears small with a coarsely nodular architecture, and areas of capsular retraction. Nodules of relatively normal tissue are separated by bands of dense fibrosis which are hypointense on T1w, hyperintense on T2w and show delayed enhancement on post-Gd T1w imaging (see also chapter 8).

EFFECTS OF CHEMOTHERAPY ON TUMORS

Although some tumors remain unchanged in appearance during and after chemotherapy, the majority show changes in size, morphology, or in vascularity which are reflected in the MRI findings.

Size and Morphology

Change in size is the clearest indication of a response to treatment. As responding tumors become smaller, they often develop an irregular contour suggesting peri-lesional fibrosis. Capsular retraction is sometimes seen in association with superficial lesions. Metastases which were already small before treatment may become undetectable, and in such cases it is impossible to determine whether the lesions have been sterilized or whether they remain viable but below the limits of imaging resolution. Following cessation of therapy, fibrotic scars may persist at the site of previous metastases, but again it is impossible on imaging criteria to determine the growth potential of the residues.

Signal Intensity Changes

As tumors shrink in response to treatment, they become less hyperintense on T2w imaging, and when fibrotic scars develop the signal intensity on T2 may be less than that of the surrounding liver, so the lesions appear hypointense on both T1w and T2w images. Larger lesions also show shrinkage and peri-lesional fibrosis in response to chemotherapy, but usually remain hyperintense on T2w and hypointense on T1w images. A further feature of response to treatment is reduction in vascularity which on MRI is shown as diminished enhancement on post-Gd T1w images. With small lesions which were already hypovascular, the loss of peripheral rim enhancement, together with colliquative necrosis of the center of the lesion, can result in an appearance which is indistinguishable from that of a simple cyst. In rare cases, peripheral vascularity increases, so the lesions develop an appearance similar to that of hemangiomas—marked hyperintensity on T2w images with nodular, peripheral, and centripetal enhancement on post-Gd T1w imaging; however, the progression of enhancement of hemangiomas is more consistently parallel with the major vessels. Central colliquative necrosis is fairly common in untreated metastases, and develops in other lesions as a result of treatment. Occasionally the central necrosis may be accompanied by hemorrhage, although this is less frequently seen with systemic chemotherapy than with local therapies. Metastases from neuro-endocrine tumors are particularly prone to central colliquative necrosis, and also often develop quite marked peri-lesional fibrosis.

THERMAL ABLATION

While radiofrequency ablation (RFA) is now the most widely practised technique, similar results and similar appearances have been achieved with microwave and cryo-ablation. The imaging appearances following percutaneous ethanol injection are essentially similar, although intra-lesional hemorrhage appears to be less common with this technique.

Following thermal ablation, imaging is used to confirm the extent of the destructive lesion which has been produced, to seek evidence of residual disease, and then later to detect recurrence and to look for new sites of disease.

Tumor Response

The essential aim of ablation is to produce coagulative necrosis throughout the lesion, and in a rim of surrounding liver parenchyma. Successfully treated lesions are shown on MRI as areas of hypointensity on both T1w and T2w images. Rim enhancement on post-Gd T1w imaging is commonly seen during the first few weeks after ablation and is explained by inflammatory reaction with granulation tissue at the interface between viable and necrosed tissue. Peripheral enhancement which appears nodular, or more than about 2 mm in thickness, is suggestive of residual or recurrent tumor in the wall of the lesion. Central hemorrhage is fairly common, producing patchy or uniform hyperintensity on unenhanced T1w imaging and may be either hyper- or hypointense on T2w images. A minority of lesions undergo colliquative rather than coagulative necrosis, so their residues resemble cysts. Sites of successful ablation either persist unchanged or become smaller during follow up.

Residual and Recurrent Tumor

With appropriate patient selection and operative technique, recurrence at the site of ablation is relatively uncommon. The majority of recurrences develop in untreated areas of the liver, or extra-hepatically.

Residual disease is indicated by the presence of nodular areas of hyperintensity on T2w images, rim enhancement on post-Gd T1w imaging later than three months after treatment, nodular or peripheral enhancement, or growth of the lesion.

TRANSARTERIAL CHEMO-EMBOLIZATION

The aim of TACE is to destroy malignant tumors by obliterating or depleting their arterial blood supply and simultaneously delivering an ablative dose of cytotoxic chemotherapy into the tumor. This approach is often preferred to thermal ablation for tumors which have a rich arterial supply, including neuro-endocrine metastases and, most commonly, hepatocellular carcinoma in cirrhosis.

Tumor Response

The imaging features of successful treatment, and of residual or recurrent disease, are essentially similar to those seen after RFA. Coagulative necrosis in successfully sterilized lesions produces hypointensity on both T1w and T2w images. Larger lesions often have a central area of colliquative necrosis producing watery signal characteristics. A thin peripheral rim of enhancement on post-Gd T1w images commonly remains for a few weeks after treatment. Central hemorrhage occurs occasionally, but is less common than with RFA. In some cases the treated lesions become isointense on T2w images.

Residual and Recurrent Tumor

Persistent or recurrent disease at the sites of treated lesions is indicated by increase in size, by nodular or peripheral areas of hyperintensity on T2w imaging, and by nodular enhancement on post-Gd T1w images. Unlike thermal ablation, where local recurrences develop in the wall of the treated area, recurrence after TACE may be anywhere within the lesion. Recurrences after TACE are more likely in patients with multiple tumors, with lesions close to the liver surface, or with large tumors. Alpha-fetoprotein (AFP) levels provide a useful indicator for monitoring HCC patients post-therapy, since 80–90% of patients show a marked fall in AFP after successful treatment, with any subsequent rise being suggestive of recurrence.

DIFFERENTIAL DIAGNOSIS

Distinguishing between the effects of systemic or local therapy, and residual or recurrent disease can be problematic.

Post-Operative Residues or Tumor?

Like recurrent tumor, residues of old hematoma or small collections of bile or serous fluid may appear as hypointense areas on T1w imaging, even many months after surgery. Their signal intensity on T2w images is variable, but hematomas typically become hypointense after a few weeks, bile, and serous fluid remains markedly hyperintense, while recurrent tumor typically shows a moderately hyperintense signal. Enhancement on post-Gd T1w imaging is not seen with post-operative residues, except for a thin rim around the lesion in the first few weeks after surgery. Post-operative residues usually become smaller on consecutive examinations—growth indicates tumor recurrence.

Fat or Tumor?

Irregularities in the portal vein supply to areas of the liver along the resection line may be responsible for the occasional development of focal fatty change at the site of surgery, which can produce local hypoattenuating areas on CT, mimicking recurrent tumor. These lesions usually show isointensity on T2w imaging, and the change in signal between in-phase and opposed-phase T1w imaging is decisive. Further confirmation, if needed, can be obtained using liver specific contrast agents, which show normal uptake in the fatty areas.

Cyst or Tumor?

This distinction is rarely problematic when pre-operative imaging is available for correlation, since cysts in the liver remnant will always be visible on the pre-operative series. Occasionally, post-operative hypertrophy of the residual liver distorts the anatomy such that the position of the cyst may appear quite different from the pre-operative imaging. Although successful chemotherapy may render small metastases necrotic and avascular—and so indistinguishable from cysts—we have seen no cases in which new metastases first appeared in this cystic form, even in patients undergoing post-operative chemotherapy.

Venous Thrombosis or Tumor?

Occasionally, small branches of the portal veins or hepatic veins, usually near the liver surface, become thrombosed after either systemic or local treatment of liver tumors. This typically produces an area of heterogeneous but abnormal attenuation on CT which may be suspicious for recurrent tumor. The MR appearance is usually of hypointensity on T1w and hyper-, hypo- or isointensity on T2w images. Post-Gd T1w imaging shows increased enhancement in the arterial phase in a heterogeneous distribution with an ill-defined margin. A key feature is visualization of unenhanced tubular structures which represent the thrombosed vessels. The liver parenchyma in the area affected by local venous thrombosis may undergo fatty change. Local fibrosis, sometimes with capsular retraction, can develop and this should be recognized by its delayed enhancement on post-Gd T1w imaging.

Bile Duct Stenosis or Tumor?

The development of obstructive jaundice with dilated intrahepatic ducts in patients who have previously undergone hepatic resection usually indicates recurrent tumor. However, the possibility of benign stricture of the bile duct has to be considered, particularly in patients who have undergone biliary reconstruction, eg., with trisectionectomies for metastases or hilar cholangiocarcinoma. The presence of stones in the upstream (obstructed) ducts is usually indicative of a benign stricture. Recurrent tumor will typically be visible as a mass at the neo-hilum, often extending into the lumen of the ducts. The absence of an obstructing mass effectively excludes recurrent metastasis, but recurrent cholangiocarcinoma can be extremely difficult to differentiate from fibrotic stricture of the bile duct, particularly in patients with pre-existing primary sclerosing cholangitis.

RECURRENT DISEASE

Experimental evidence suggests that the trophic factors which stimulate hypertrophy of residual liver segments after major resections also increase the growth rate of microscopic metastases which may remain in the liver residue. Not surprisingly, the most frequent pattern for recurrent disease is the appearance of new lesions in the remaining liver. Recurrent tumor developing along the line of resection is less common, although not rare. Following extended liver resections in which biliary drainage has been diverted by joining the duct or ducts from the residual segments to a roux loop, there is a propensity for recurrent tumor to obstruct and invade the ducts (see above). Extra-hepatic sites of recurrence which can also be detected during liver MRI include lymph nodes in the hepatic hilar, celiac axis and inferior mediastinal groups, as well as new lesions in the adjacent soft tissues or abdominal wall.

ILLUSTRATIVE FIGURES

Post-operative anatomy and surgical residues—Figures 1–6
Effects of chemotherapy on the liver—Figures 7–12
Tumor response to chemotherapy—Figures 13–18
Post-ablation changes—Figures 19–27
Effects of TACE—Figures 28–37
Differential diagnosis—recurrence or therapy effects?—Figures 38–47
Sites of tumor recurrence—Figures 48–53

REFERENCES

1. Fusai G, Davidson BR. Management of colorectal liver metastases. Colorectal Dis 2003; 5:2–23.
2. Braga L, Semelka RC, Pedro MS, et al. Post-treatment malignant liver lesions: MR imaging. Magn Reson Clin N Am 2002; 10:53–73.

3. Nascimento AB, Mitchell DG, Rubin R, et al. Diffuse desmoplastic breast carcinoma metastases to the liver simulating cirrhosis at MR imaging: report of two cases. Radiology 2001; 221:117–121.
4. Semelka RC, Worawattanakul S, Noone TC, et al. Chemotherapy-treated liver metastases mimicking hemangiomas on MR images. Abdom Imaging 1999; 24:378–382.
5. Aliberti C, Soriani M, Tilli M, et al. Radiofrequency ablation of liver malignancies: MRI for evaluation of response. J Chemother 2004; 16:79–81.
6. Kosari K, Gomes M, Hunter D, et al. Local, intrahepatic, and systemic recurrence patterns after radiofrequency ablation of hepatic malignancies. J Gastrointest Surg 2002; 6:255–263.
7. Kubota K, Hisa N, Nishikawa T, et al. Evaluation of hepatocellular carcinoma after treatment with transcatheter arterial chemoembolization: comparison of Lipodol-CT, power Doppler sonography, and dynamic MRI. Abdom Imaging 2001; 26:184–190.
8. De Santis M, Torricelli P, Cristani A, et al. MRI of hepatocellular carcinoma before and after transcatheter chemoembolization. J Comput Assist Tomogr 1993; 17:901–908.

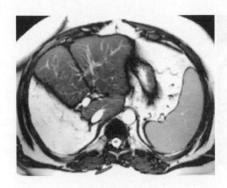

Figure 1. *Right hemihepatectomy:* Post-operative true FISP image showed the residual segments; the presence of the falciform ligament indicates that segment 4 has not been removed.

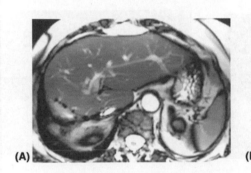 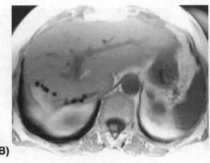

(A)   (B)

Figure 2. *Right trisectionectomy:* True FISP (**A**) and T1w (**B**) images showed residual segments 1, 2, and 3 only. Note the line of clip artifacts along the resection margin.

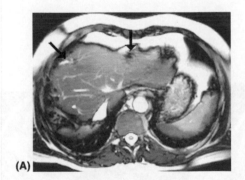 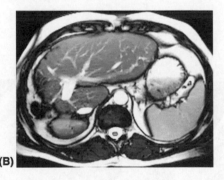

(A)   (B)

Figure 3. *Right trisectionectomy:* True FISP images at two levels (**A, B**) showed residual segments 1, 2, and 3; note also the irregularities on the anterior surface of the liver (arrows) where local excision of superficial metastases was also carried out.

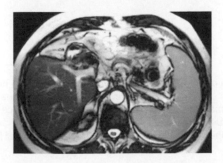

Figure 4. *Left trisectionectomy:* True FISP image showed the residual segments 6 and 7. Note biliary diversion via a Roux loop at the neo-hilum of the liver.

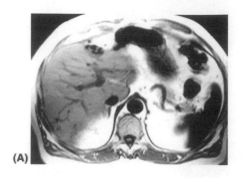

(A)

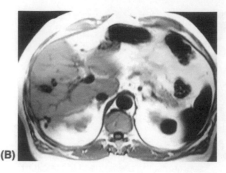

(B)

Figure 5. *Non-segmental resections*: T1w images at two levels (**A**, **B**) showed residual anatomy after excision of segments 2, 3 and the anterior part of segment 4, also excision of parts of segments 5, 6, and 7, highlighted by clip artifacts.

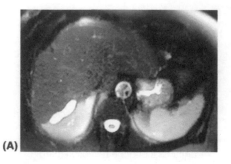

(A)

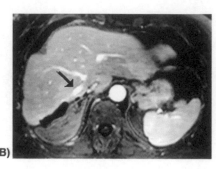

(B)

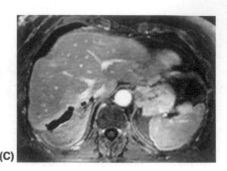

(C)

Figure 6. *Posterior sectionectomy*: Three months after resection of segments 6 and 7 for colorectal metastases, HASTE (**A**) and post-Gd T1w images in portal (**B**) and delayed (**C**) phases showed the line of resection with a localized fluid collection adjacent. Note the right hepatic vein was still present [arrow in (**B**)] and the fluid collection showed a thin rim of faint enhancement on the delayed image, a normal finding in the first few months after surgery.

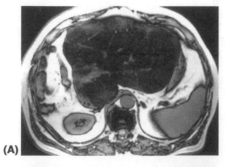

(A)

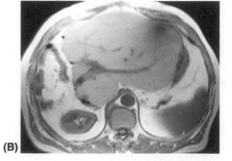

(B)

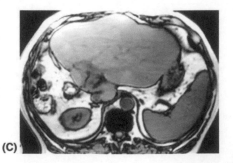

(C)

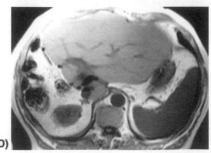

(D)

Figure 7. *Resolution of fatty change*: In a patient undergoing chemotherapy following right trisectionectomy for colorectal metastases, the liver remnant showed grossly reduced signal on opposed-phase T1w (**A**) compared with normal signal on in-phase T1w (**B**) imaging, indicating gross fatty change. Two years later, after a further resection and following cessation of chemotherapy, opposed-phase (**C**) and in-phase (**D**) T1w imaging showed the liver signal had returned almost to normal.

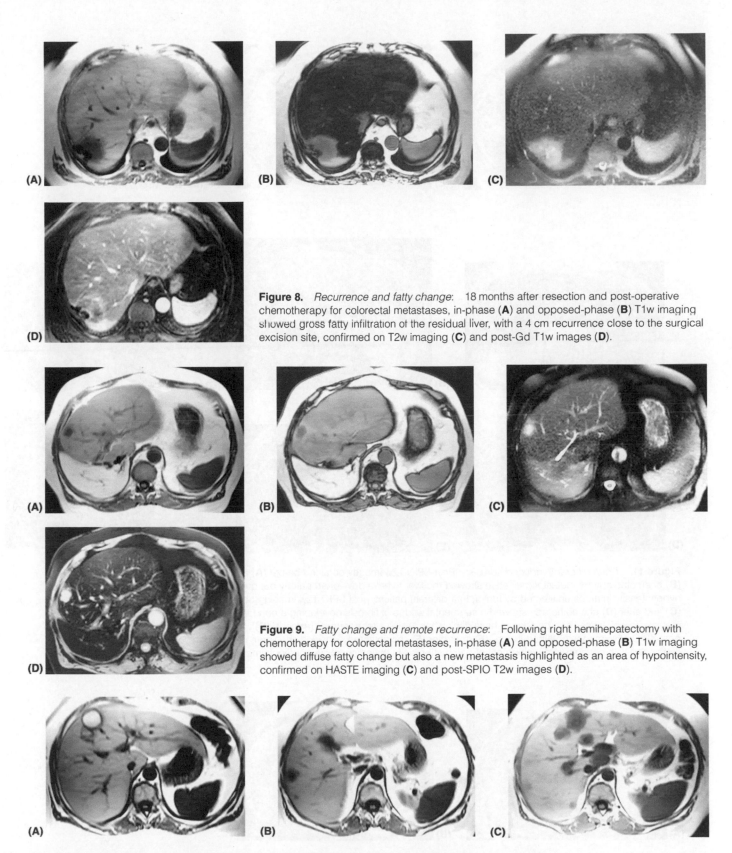

Figure 8. *Recurrence and fatty change*:   18 months after resection and post-operative chemotherapy for colorectal metastases, in-phase (**A**) and opposed-phase (**B**) T1w imaging showed gross fatty infiltration of the residual liver, with a 4 cm recurrence close to the surgical excision site, confirmed on T2w imaging (**C**) and post-Gd T1w images (**D**).

Figure 9. *Fatty change and remote recurrence*:   Following right hemihepatectomy with chemotherapy for colorectal metastases, in-phase (**A**) and opposed-phase (**B**) T1w imaging showed diffuse fatty change but also a new metastasis highlighted as an area of hypointensity, confirmed on HASTE imaging (**C**) and post-SPIO T2w images (**D**).

Figure 10. *Fatty change and progressive disease*:   In a patient with untreated colorectal metastases, initial in-phase T1w images (**A**, **B**) showed several lesions with the largest showing a haemorrhagic center. Repeat imaging after five months chemotherapy showed no evidence of hemorrhage, but the lesions were larger with many new lesions having developed (**C**, **D**). Opposed-phase T1w imaging also showed quite severe fatty change (**E**). (*Continued*)

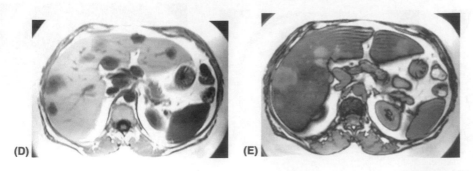

Figure 10. (*Continued*)

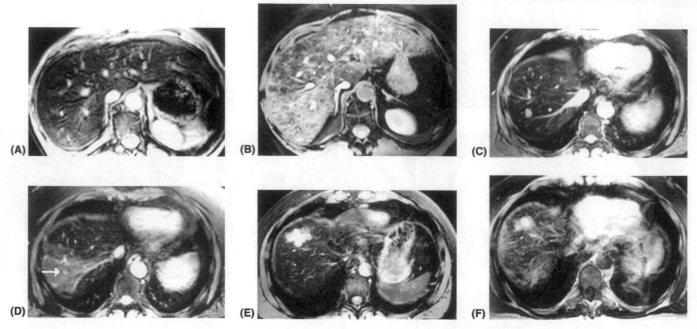

Figure 11. *Chemotherapy-induced fibrosis*:   Post-SPIO T2w images obtained before (**A**) and after (**B**) chemotherapy for metastatic disease showed the liver to have developed patchy but quite marked hyperintensity in areas unaffected by tumor. In a different patient, post-SPIO T2w imaging obtained before (**C**) and after (**D**) chemotherapy showed a segmental wedge of fibrosis developing around the site of a small metastasis which itself can be seen to have diminished in size after treatment [arrow in (**D**)]. In a third patient, post-SPIO T2w images obtained before (**E**) and after (**F**) chemotherapy, showed shrinkage of the right lobe metastasis with concurrent development of patchy fibrosis in the adjacent liver parenchyma.

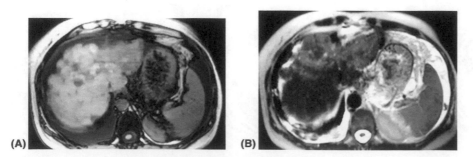

Figure 12. *Pseudo-cirrhosis*:   A patient with previously treated breast cancer presented with abnormal liver function. T1w (**A**) and HASTE (**B**) imaging showed a small nodular liver with moderate ascites and mild splenomegaly. Post-Gd T1w images in axial (**C**) and coronal (**D**) planes confirmed diffuse nodular change with fibrosis and esophageal varices [arrows in (**D**)]. Metastatic breast cancer was confirmed on laparoscopic biopsy. (*Continued*)

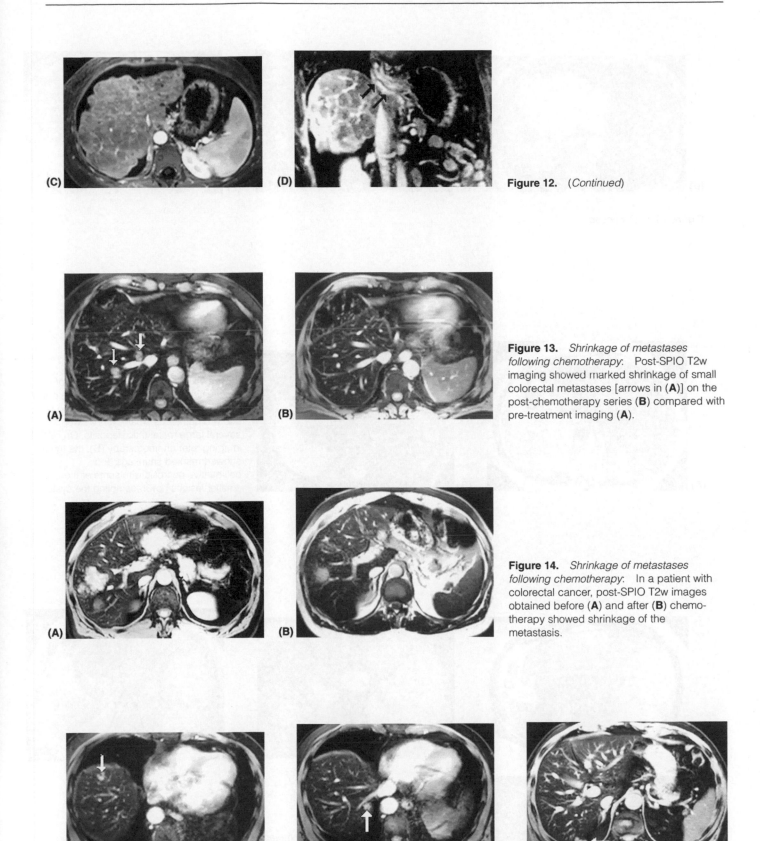

Figure 12. (*Continued*)

Figure 13. *Shrinkage of metastases following chemotherapy*: Post-SPIO T2w imaging showed marked shrinkage of small colorectal metastases [arrows in (**A**)] on the post-chemotherapy series (**B**) compared with pre-treatment imaging (**A**).

Figure 14. *Shrinkage of metastases following chemotherapy*: In a patient with colorectal cancer, post-SPIO T2w images obtained before (**A**) and after (**B**) chemotherapy showed shrinkage of the metastasis.

Figure 15. *Shrinkage of tumors after chemotherapy*: In a patient with numerous small colorectal metastases, post-SPIO T2w images (**A–C**) obtained before treatment showed several lesions of 1–2 cm size (arrows). On repeat imaging following completion of chemotherapy (**D–F**), the lesions were visible only as tiny scars. (*Continued*)

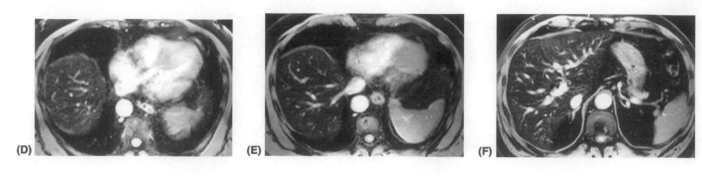

Figure 15. (*Continued*)

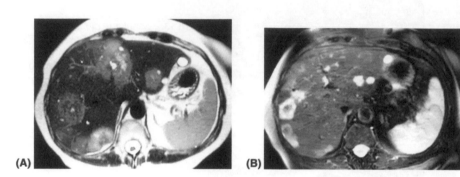

Figure 16. *Shrinkage and necrosis of metastases after chemotherapy.* In a patient with colorectal cancer, HASTE imaging (**A**) showed numerous small cysts as well as several large metastatic deposits. On HASTE imaging after chemotherapy (**B**), the tumors showed marked shrinkage and colliquative necrosis with some of the smaller lesions now resembling the cysts.

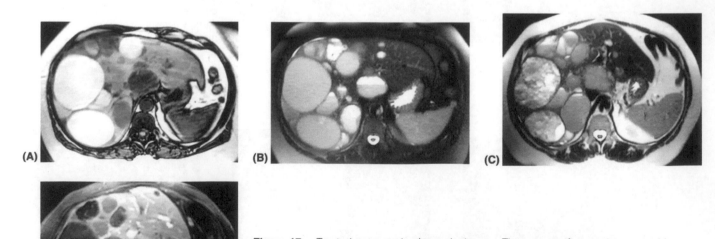

Figure 17. *Treated neuro-endocrine metastases:* Three years after starting octreotide treatment for neuro-endocrine metastases, post-T1w images (**A**) showed numerous well-defined lesions with signal intensity varying from markedly hyperintense to hypointense, indicating variable hemorrhage components. Concurrent HASTE imaging (**B**) also showed variable fluid content, with fluid/fluid levels in some of the lesions. After a further six months' treatment, repeat HASTE imaging (**C**) showed heterogeneous debris within most of the larger lesions and post-Gd T1w imaging (**D**) confirmed an avascular appearance to the lesion walls.

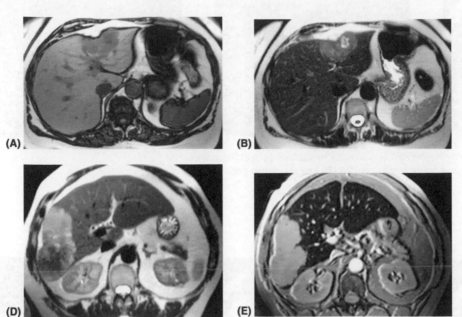

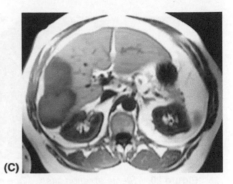

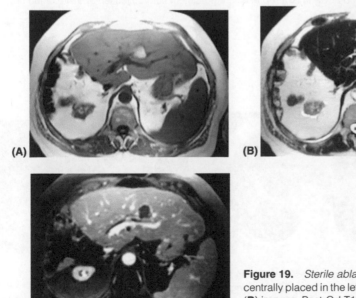

Figure 18. *Capsular retraction developing over a lesion:* A patient with colorectal metastasis in the anterior aspect of the left lobe developed pronounced local capsular retraction after chemotherapy, shown on T1w (**A**) and HASTE (**B**) images. Similar but less marked retraction occurred in another patient with colorectal metastasis in the right lobe, shown on T1w (**C**), HASTE (**D**) and post-SPIO T2w (**E**) images.

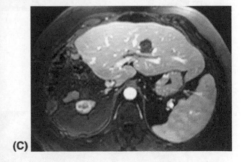

Figure 19. *Sterile ablation site:* Five months after right trisectionectomy with RFA of a lesion centrally placed in the left lobe, the ablation site remained hyperintense on both T1w (**A**) and T2w (**B**) images. Post-Gd T1w imaging showed no portal phase enhancement (**C**) with a thin rim of faint enhancement on delayed imaging (**D**).

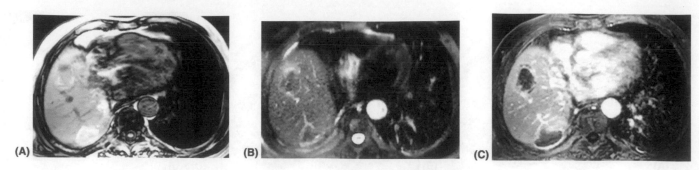

Figure 20. *Sterile ablation sites*: One month after RFA of colorectal metastases, the ablation sites showed patchy hyperintensity on T1w (**A**) and hypointensity on T2w (**B**) images. A thin peripheral rim of enhancement was shown on post-Gd T1w imaging (**C**).

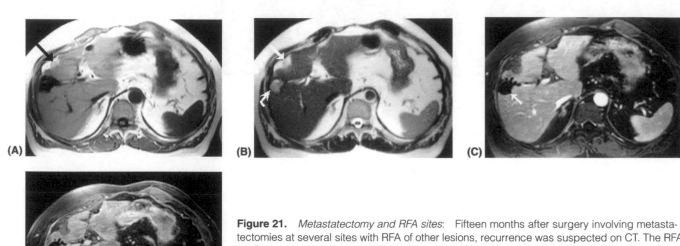

Figure 21. *Metastatectomy and RFA sites*: Fifteen months after surgery involving metasta-tectomies at several sites with RFA of other lesions, recurrence was suspected on CT. The RFA site [arrows in (**A**, **B**)] appeared isointense on both T1w (**A**) and T2w (b) images, and showed no enhancement on post-Gd T1w images on portal (**C**) and delayed (**D**) phases. Clip artifacts mark the position of metastatectomies from the anterior aspects of segments 3 and 5 [arrows in (**C**, **D**)], again with no enhancement to indicate recurrent tumor. The area of hyperintensity on the T2w image [curved arrow in (**B**)] represents a persistent fluid collection at a site of tumor excision.

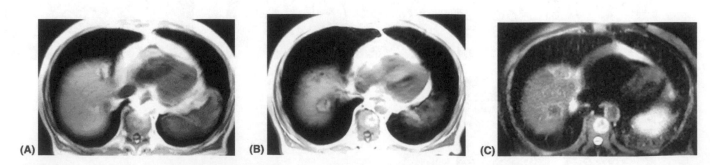

Figure 22. *Evolution of RFA sites*: One month after RFA of several metastases the lesion sites showed heterogeneous hyperintensity on T1w imaging (**A**, **B**), heterogeneous signal on T2w imaging (**C**) and no enhancement on post-Gd T1w images (**D**, **E**). At repeat MRI 4 months later, post-Gd T1w images (**F**, **G**) showed the lesions to have diminished in size. (*Continued*)

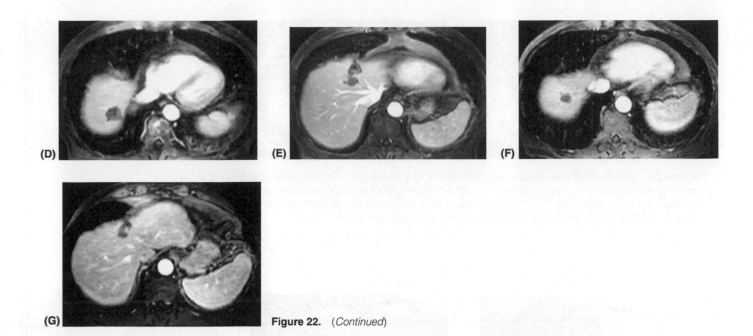

(D)   **(E)**   **(F)**

(G)   **Figure 22.**   (*Continued*)

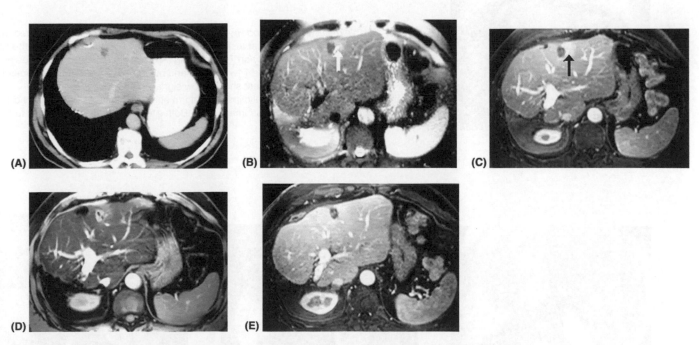

(A)   **(B)**   **(C)**

(D)   **(E)**

Figure 23.   *Metastatectomy and ablation sites*:   14 months after right trisectionectomy with excision and RFA of two lesions near the anterior surface of the left lobe, CT (**A**) showed a circumscribed hypo-attenuating area separate from the surgical clips on the anterior liver surface. This lesion appeared hypointense on both T2w (**B**) and post-Gd T1w (**C**) images, but an adjacent area [arrows in (**B**, **C**)] showed hyperintensity on T2w and increased enhancement on the post-Gd T1w images. On post-SPIO T2w images (**D**) the suspicious area showed normal uptake of contrast, suggesting local branch portal vein occlusion. Post-Gd T1w images obtained 6 months later (**E**) showed the abnormal vascularity had diminished, with no signs of recurrent tumor.

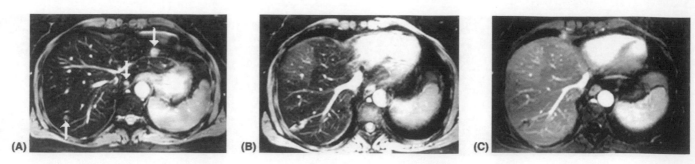

Figure 24.   *Extended left hemihepatectomy with RFA of right lobe lesion*:   Pre-operative post-SPIO T2w imaging (**A**) showed metastases in segments 1, 2 and 7 (arrows). More lesions were present at other levels in the left lobe. Following excision of the left lobe and segment 1, post-SPIO T2w (**B**) and post-Gd T1w (**C**) imaging showed a stable RFA ablation defect at the site of the small right lobe lesion.

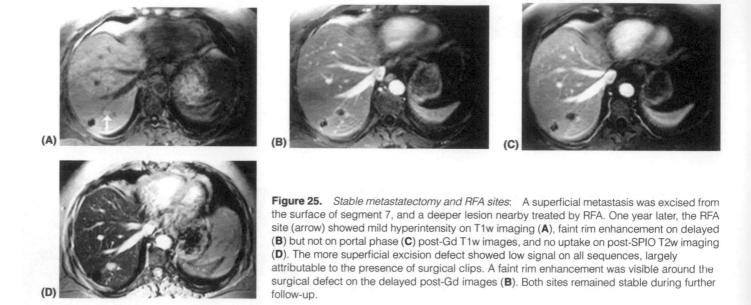

Figure 25.   *Stable metastatectomy and RFA sites*:   A superficial metastasis was excised from the surface of segment 7, and a deeper lesion nearby treated by RFA. One year later, the RFA site (arrow) showed mild hyperintensity on T1w imaging (**A**), faint rim enhancement on delayed (**B**) but not on portal phase (**C**) post-Gd T1w images, and no uptake on post-SPIO T2w imaging (**D**). The more superficial excision defect showed low signal on all sequences, largely attributable to the presence of surgical clips. A faint rim enhancement was visible around the surgical defect on the delayed post-Gd images (**B**). Both sites remained stable during further follow-up.

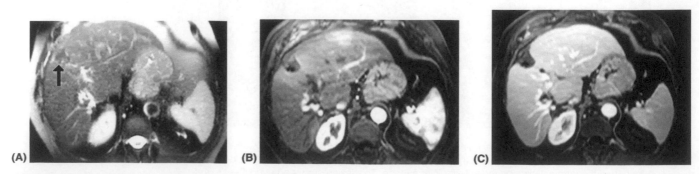

Figure 26.   *Sterile RFA site, recurrence elsewhere*:   Seven months after RFA for metastasis, the treated area (arrow) showed hypointensity on T2w imaging (**A**) and no early or delayed enhancement on post-Gd T1w images (**B**, **C**). However, sections at a more cranial level (**C**, **D**, **E**) showed typical appearances of a new metastasis. (*Continued*)

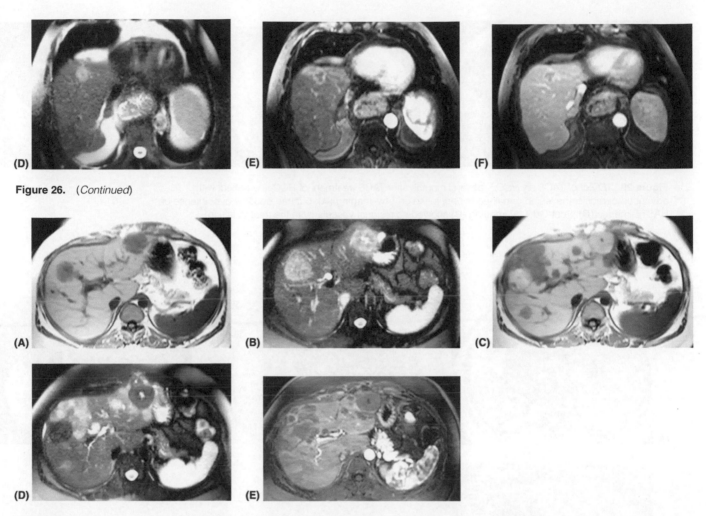

Figure 26. (*Continued*)

Figure 27. *Recurrent metastases after RFA:* Two metastases of 3–4 cm size were shown on pre-treatment T1w (**A**) and T2w (**B**) images. Three months after RFA, the treated lesions showed mild hyperintensity on T1w (**C**) and hypointensity on T2w (**D**) images except for the small fluid focus at the center of the left lobe lesion. No enhancement was shown in the treated lesions on post-Gd T1w imaging (**E**), but numerous new metastases had developed in the untreated part of the liver.

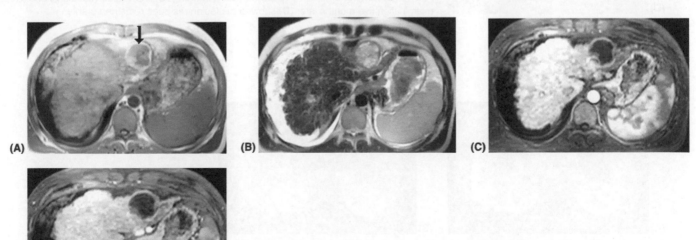

Figure 28. *Effect of TACE on HCC:* Three months after TACE therapy of a 4 cm HCC in a patient with late stage cirrhosis, the lesion (arrow) showed a well-defined margin with mixed signal intensity on T1w (**A**) and heterogeneous hyperintensity on HASTE (**B**) images. Post-Gd T1w images in arterial (**C**) and portal (**D**) phases showed no hypervascularity in the wall of the lesion. Subsequent explant histology confirmed extensive necrosis within the mass.

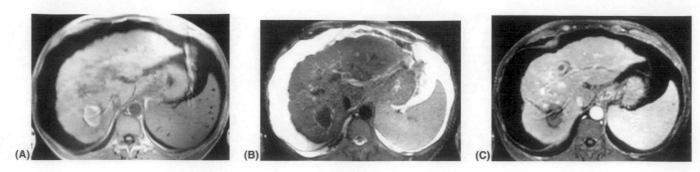

Figure 29.   *Effect of TACE on HCC:*   Several months after TACE treatment of HCC in a patient with advanced cirrhosis, the lesion remained hyperintense on T1w imaging (**A**), but had become hypointense on HASTE images (**B**). Post-Gd T1w imaging (**C**) showed no residual vascularity in the treated lesion.

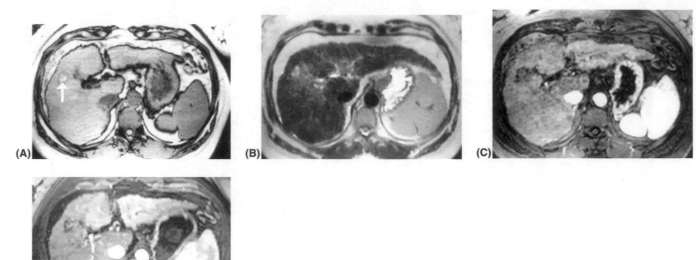

Figure 30.   *Stable HCC after TACE:*   Eight months after TACE for HCC in a patient with cirrhosis the treated lesion (arrow) appeared heterogeneously hyperintense on both T1w (**A**) and HASTE (**B**) imaging. Post-Gd T1w arterial phase imaging (**C**) showed no vascularity and a repeat examination five months later (**D**) showed the lesion residues remained stable.

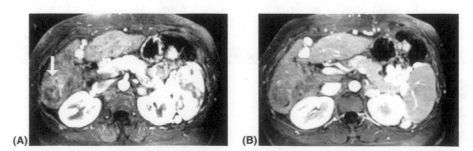

Figure 31.   *HCC pre and post-TACE treatment:*   In a patient with advanced cirrhosis, post-Gd T1w imaging in arterial (**A**) and portal (**B**) phases showed a 4 cm HCC in segment 5 with low grade patchy arterial enhancement [arrow in (**A**)]. Eight months after TACE therapy, arterial (**C**) and portal (**D**) phase post-Gd T1w images showed the lesion to be a little smaller, uniformly hypointense with no peripheral vascularity. However, a new small lesion had developed in segment 1 [arrow in (**D**)]. (*Continued*)

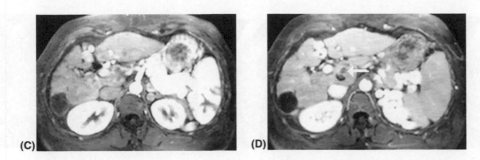

Figure 31. (*Continued*)

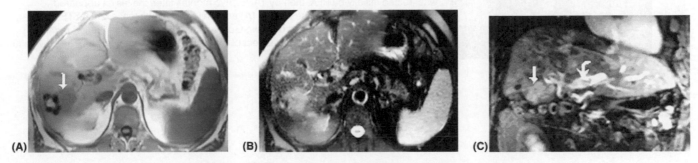

Figure 32. *Recurrent HCC following resection:* Four months after resection of HCC from the right lobe, T1w imaging (**A**) showed a hypointense recurrent mass (arrow) adjacent to a small haemorrhagic collection surrounded by clip artifacts. HASTE imaging (**B**) confirmed a moderately hyperintense recurrence and post-Gd T1w imaging in arterial phase (**C**) illustrated moderate hypervascularity in the recurrent tumor (straight arrow) with extension into the right portal branch, and extending partway along the left portal branch (curved arrow).

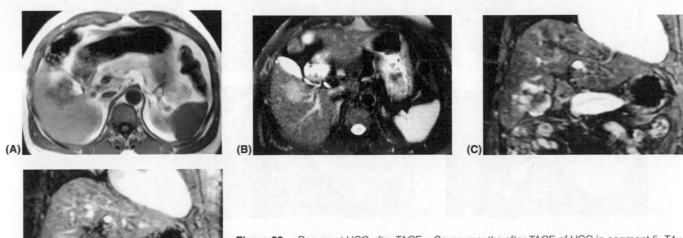

Figure 33. *Recurrent HCC after TACE:* Seven months after TACE of HCC in segment 5, T1w imaging showed an ill-defined hypointense lesion associated with subcapsular hematoma producing local hyperintensity (**A**). HASTE imaging (**B**) confirmed a moderately hyperintense mass at the site of previous treatment. Post-Gd coronal T1w images in arterial (**C**) and venous (**D**) phases confirmed recurrent hypervascular tumor nodules surrounding the avascular area of coagulative necrosis.

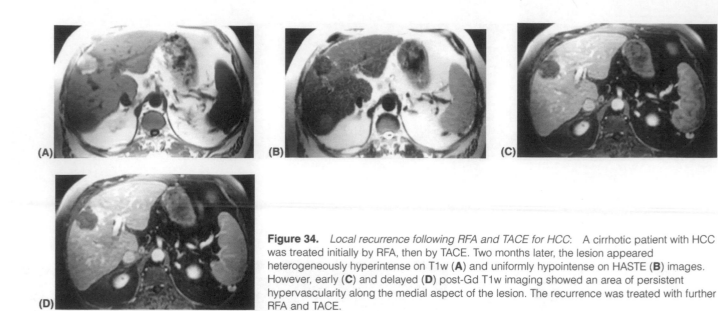

Figure 34.   *Local recurrence following RFA and TACE for HCC:*   A cirrhotic patient with HCC was treated initially by RFA, then by TACE. Two months later, the lesion appeared heterogeneously hyperintense on T1w (**A**) and uniformly hypointense on HASTE (**B**) images. However, early (**C**) and delayed (**D**) post-Gd T1w imaging showed an area of persistent hypervascularity along the medial aspect of the lesion. The recurrence was treated with further RFA and TACE.

Figure 35.   *Effect of TACE on HCC:*   Several months after TACE for HCC in a cirrhotic patient, T1w imaging (**A**) showed the lesion to have a hyperintense center with an ill-defined hypointense halo around it. On HASTE imaging (**B**) the center of the lesion appeared hypointense with a faintly hyperintense halo. Post-Gd T1w imaging in arterial (**C**) and portal (**D**) phases showed the center of the lesion to be avascular, but the surrounding area showed patchy hypervascularity. Post-SPIO T2w images (**E**) confirmed recurrent tumor surrounding the hypointense center of the treated lesion.

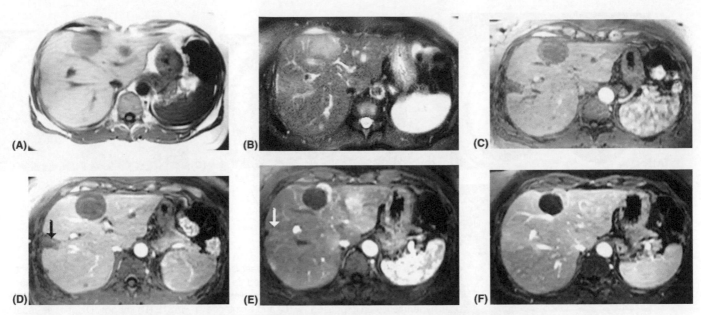

Figure 36. *Recurrence following TACE:* A patient with multiple carcinoid metastases underwent several TACE procedures. At initial follow-up, the treated areas appeared hypointense on T1w (**A**) and mildly hyperintense on HASTE (**B**) imaging, with no evidence of residual tumor shown on arterial (**C**) or portal (**D**) phase post-Gd T1w images. One year later, post-Gd T1w images in arterial (**E**) and portal (**F**) phases showed local hypervascular tumor recurrence in the wall of one of the treated areas. Note the resolution of the successfully treated lesion in segment 8 [arrows in (**D, E**)].

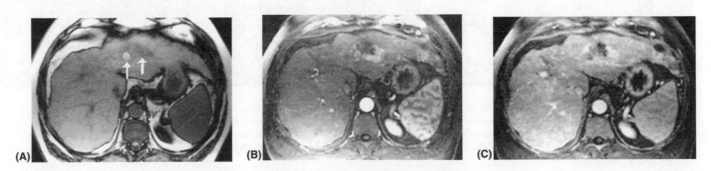

Figure 37. *Recurrent HCC following TACE:* One month following initial TACE for HCC, T1w imaging (**A**) showed areas of hyper- and hypointensity in the left lobe lesion (arrows). Post-Gd T1w imaging in arterial (**B**) and portal (**C**) phases confirmed residual hypervascular tumor around the previous ablation site.

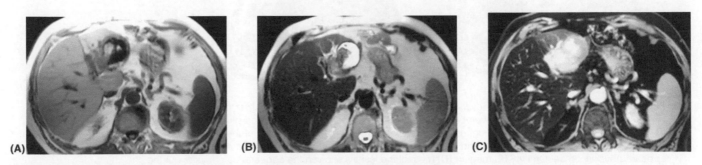

Figure 38. *RFA changes or recurrent metastasis?:* Several months after RFA treatment of a colorectal metastasis in the left lobe, T1w (**A**), HASTE (**B**) and post-SPIO T2w (**C**) imaging showed a cystic area at the site of previous ablation together with an irregular solid component. Histology of the excised specimen confirmed recurrent tumor.

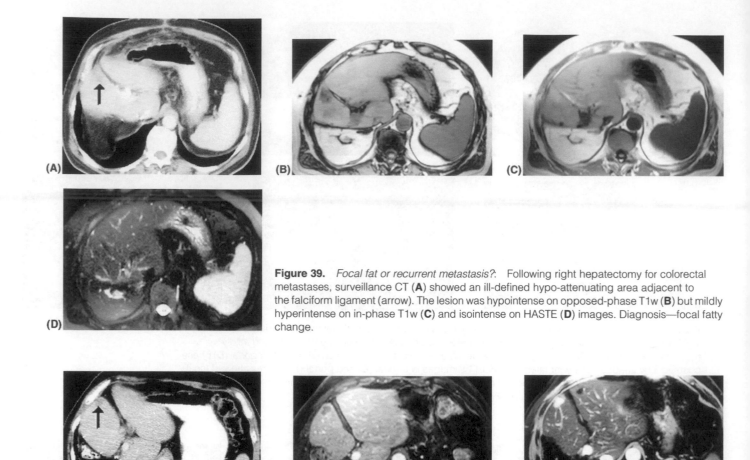

Figure 39. *Focal fat or recurrent metastasis?.* Following right hepatectomy for colorectal metastases, surveillance CT (**A**) showed an ill-defined hypo-attenuating area adjacent to the falciform ligament (arrow). The lesion was hypointense on opposed-phase T1w (**B**) but mildly hyperintense on in-phase T1w (**C**) and isointense on HASTE (**D**) images. Diagnosis—focal fatty change.

Figure 40. *Focal fat or recurrent metastasis?.* Following right hepatectomy for colorectal metastases, surveillance CT (**A**) showed a hypointense lesion adjacent to the falciform ligament (arrow). Chemical shift imaging (not illustrated) showed no evidence of fatty change, but post-Gd T1w images (**B**) showed the lesion to have an enhancing rim and post-SPIO T2w imaging (**C**) confirmed the lesion to be non-functioning. Diagnosis—recurrent metastasis.

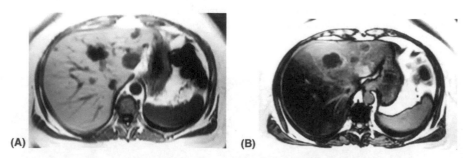

Figure 41. *Recurrent metastases or cysts?.* Following chemotherapy for colorectal liver metastases, in-phase T1w imaging (**A**) showed several hypointense lesions in the left lobe. Opposed-phase T1w imaging (**B**) showed marked fatty change throughout the liver, worse in the right lobe; several of the left lobe lesions showed a rim of focal fatty sparing around them, while the lesion on the posterior surface of segment 2 appeared hyperintense. On HASTE imaging (**C**) most of the lesions showed the appearance of cysts, but the segment 2 lesion (arrow) showed only minimal hyperintensity. Post-Gd T1w imaging (**D**) confirmed multiple cysts with no vascularity, and a single metastasis in the posterior aspect of segment 2, subsequently excised at surgery. Histology of several of the cystic lesions excised in the same specimen confirmed simple liver cysts. (*Continued*)

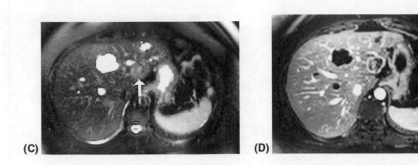

(C)   **(D)**   **Figure 41.**   (*Continued*)

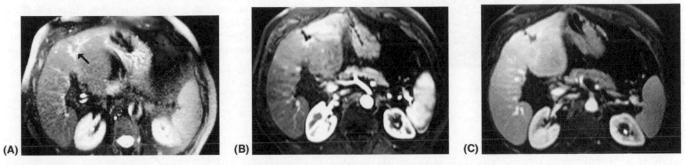

(A)   **(B)**   **(C)**

Figure 42.   *Venous occlusion or recurrence?.*   Following RFA for colorectal metastases, recurrence was suspected on surveillance CT. HASTE imaging (**A**) showed an area of hyperintensity with a branching structure (arrow). Post-Gd arterial (**B**) and portal (**C**) phase T1w images showed an avascular branching structure indicative of peripheral portal vein branch thrombosis, associated with a "THID" in the adjacent liver parenchyma.

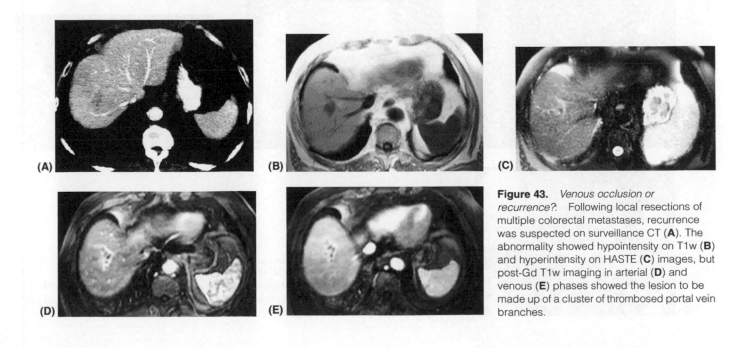

(A)   **(B)**   **(C)**

(D)   **(E)**   **Figure 43.**   *Venous occlusion or recurrence?.*   Following local resections of multiple colorectal metastases, recurrence was suspected on surveillance CT (**A**). The abnormality showed hypointensity on T1w (**B**) and hyperintensity on HASTE (**C**) images, but post-Gd T1w imaging in arterial (**D**) and venous (**E**) phases showed the lesion to be made up of a cluster of thrombosed portal vein branches.

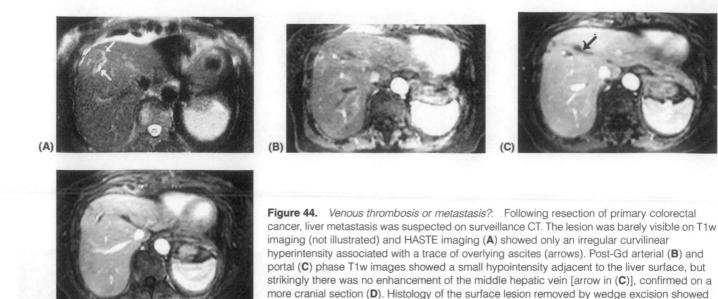

Figure 44.   *Venous thrombosis or metastasis?*.   Following resection of primary colorectal cancer, liver metastasis was suspected on surveillance CT. The lesion was barely visible on T1w imaging (not illustrated) and HASTE imaging (**A**) showed only an irregular curvilinear hyperintensity associated with a trace of overlying ascites (arrows). Post-Gd arterial (**B**) and portal (**C**) phase T1w images showed a small hypointensity adjacent to the liver surface, but strikingly there was no enhancement of the middle hepatic vein [arrow in (**C**)], confirmed on a more cranial section (**D**). Histology of the surface lesion removed by wedge excision showed focal fibrosis but no malignancy.

Figure 45.   *Recurrent tumor or bile duct stenosis?*.   Two years after hemihepatectomy for tumor, MRCP (**A**) and HASTE imaging (**B**) showed obstruction of the residual intrahepatic ducts by a stone associated with a stricture at the neo-hilum, but no evidence of recurrence (confirmed on follow up); in a different patient with previous liver resection for trauma, MRCP (**C**) and post-Gd MIP (**D**) images showed similar anatomic distortion but no tumor.

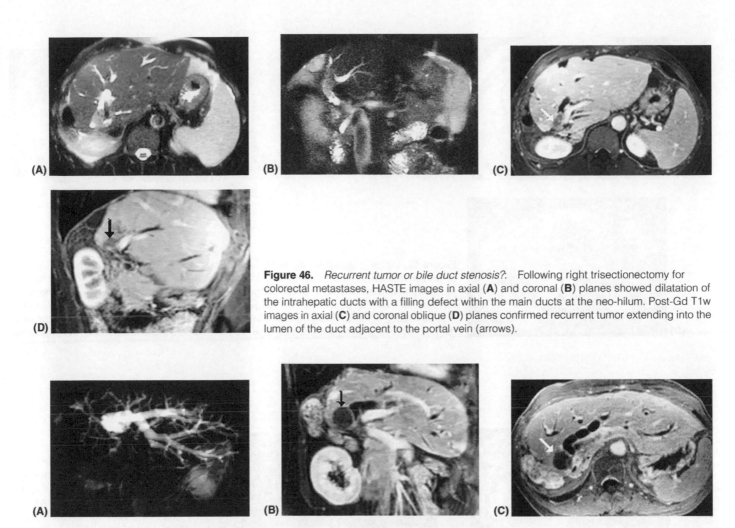

Figure 46. *Recurrent tumor or bile duct stenosis?*: Following right trisectionectomy for colorectal metastases, HASTE images in axial (**A**) and coronal (**B**) planes showed dilatation of the intrahepatic ducts with a filling defect within the main ducts at the neo-hilum. Post-Gd T1w images in axial (**C**) and coronal oblique (**D**) planes confirmed recurrent tumor extending into the lumen of the duct adjacent to the portal vein (arrows).

Figure 47. *Recurrent tumor or bile duct stenosis?*: Following right trisectionectomy for colorectal metastases, MRCP (**A**) showed dilatation of the intrahepatic ducts; post-Gd T1w images in coronal (**B**) and axial (**C**) planes confirmed obstruction of the residual ducts by recurrent tumor at the neo-hilum (arrows).

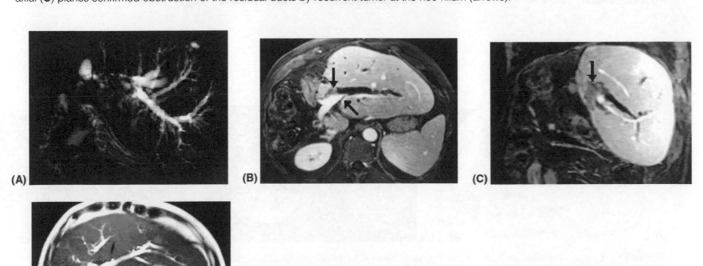

Figure 48. *Recurrence close to the resection line* Following right trisectionectomy for colorectal metastases, this patient developed dilatation of the intrahepatic ducts shown on MRCP (**A**) with the impression of intraductal filling defects. Post-Gd T1w images in axial (**B**) and coronal (**C**) planes confirmed recurrent tumor obstructing the main residual ducts and also narrowing the residual portal vein branch (arrows). A similar recurrence was shown on HASTE imaging in a different patient (**D**).

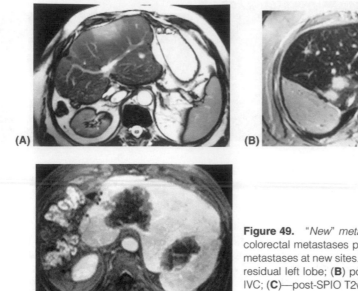

(A)

(B)

(C)

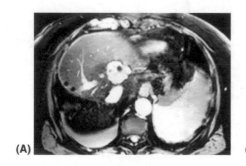

(D)

Figure 49. *"New" metastases following hepatic lobectomy:* In four different patients with colorectal metastases previously treated by excision, follow up imaging showed recurrent metastases at new sites. (**A**) true FISP image showed a new lesion on the anterior surface of the residual left lobe; (**B**) post-SPIO T2w image showed two new lesions just antero-lateral to the IVC; (**C**)—post-SPIO T2w imaging showed a centrally placed lesion within a residual right lobe; (**D**) post-Gd T1w imaging showed two large recurrent tumors in the residual left lobe segments.

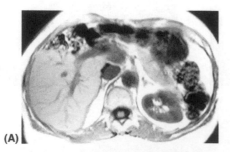

(A)

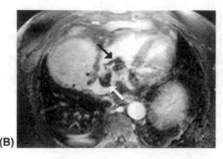

(B)

Figure 50. *Recurrence with vascular invasion:* 18 months after right trisectionectomy followed by chemotherapy for colorectal metastases, post-SPIO T2w imaging (**A**) showed a recurrent mass just anterior to the inferior vena cava; post-Gd T1w imaging at a more cranial level (**B**) showed extension of tumor into the suprahepatic cava and right atrium (arrows).

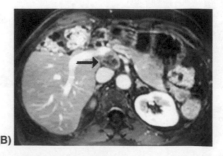

(A)

(B)

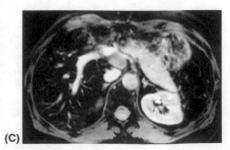

(C)

Figure 51. *Lymph node recurrences:* Following extended left hepatectomy for colorectal metastases, T1w (**A**), post-Gd T1w (**B**) and post-SPIO T2w (**C**) imaging showed a typical appearance of metastasis to a porto-caval lymph node [arrow in (**B**)]; in a different patient also with colorectal metastases, SPIO T2w images obtained before (**D**) and after (**E**) chemotherapy showed not only a marked increase in the extent of the liver metastases but also the development of new lymph node metastases in the porto-caval and celiac groups [arrows in (**E**)]. In a patient with cirrhosis and HCC previously treated by TACE, post-Gd T1w imaging in arterial (**F**) and portal (**G**) phases showed a hypervascular deposit in the porto-caval node [arrow in (**F**)]. (*Continued*)

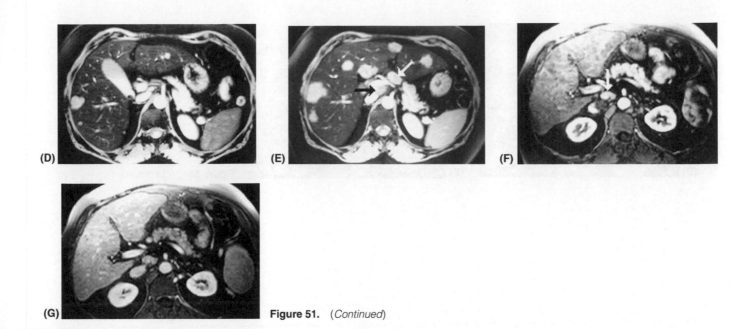

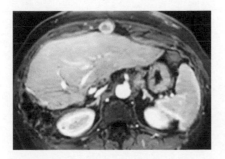

Figure 51. (*Continued*)

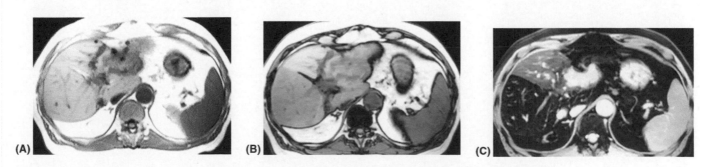

Figure 52. *Abdominal wall recurrence:* Following right hepatectomy for colorectal metastases, post-Gd T1w imaging showed a tumor nodule anterior to the liver surface and in line with the surgical scar.

Figure 53. *Fibrotic recurrence, portal vein involvement, regional fatty change:* In a patient previously treated for colorectal metastases by right hepatectomy with left lobe metastatectomy, in-phase T1w imaging (**A**) showed an ill-defined hypointense mass affecting the posterior surface of residual segment 2, along with several clip artifacts in the same area. Opposed-phase T1w imaging (**B**) showed diffuse fatty change in segments 1 and 4, with relative sparing of the part of segment 2 which was not affected by tumor. Post-SPIO T2w imaging (**C**) showed the crescent-shaped mass of tumor in segment 2, together with a peripheral wedge-shaped area of reduced contrast uptake in segment 4 indicating reduced portal inflow, confirmed on the coronal post-Gd MIP image (**D**) showing malignant obstruction of the left main portal vein branch (arrow). A coronal post-Gd T1w image in a more anterior position (**E**) illustrated the marked arterial hyperperfusion of segments 2 and 3 resulting from segmental occlusion of the portal vein. (*Continued*)

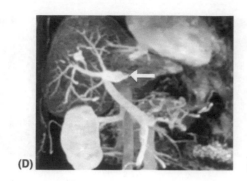

(D)

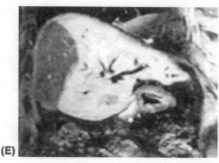

(E)

Figure 53. (*Continued*)

CHAPTER 13

Hilar Cholangiocarcinoma and Its Mimics

C holangiocarcinoma is a malignant tumor arising in biliary epithelium. Although there are differences in the morphology and growth patterns of tumors arising in different parts of the biliary tree, all cholangiocarcinomas have biological similarities based on their origin from the epithelial surface of the bile ducts. The incidence of bile duct malignancy appears to be increasing in Western countries where it is now approximately equal to hepatocellular carcinoma as a cause of death. The majority of cases occur in older patients.

ASSOCIATIONS

Although most cases are sporadic, a significant minority of cases occur in patients with primary sclerosing cholangitis (PSC). The lifetime risk of cholangiocarcinoma in patients with PSC is said to be about 10%. Chronic inflammatory disease of the gallbladder and chronic choledocholithiasis predispose to malignant change, as do adenomas and papillomas of the biliary tree. Patients with Caroli's disease and those with choledochal cysts have a small but well-established risk of developing cholangiocarcinoma. In Southeast Asia, common risk factors also include infestation with liver flukes (*Clonorchis* and *Opisthorchis*) and chronic typhoid carrier state.

ANATOMIC CLASSIFICATION

About 10% of cholangiocarcinomas arise within the liver substance and are described as peripheral or intrahepatic. These usually present with local pain, fever, weight loss, or other systemic features, rather than jaundice—they are discussed further in chapter 6. Of the more common cholangiocarcinomas, the majority are hilar or perihilar (Klatskin tumors) and the rest are extrahepatic in location. However, some hilar tumors extend into the liver parenchyma, and peripheral tumors may spread to reach the hilum so this anatomic distinction is indistinct in some cases. Further, in a small proportion of cases, cholangiocarcinomas are multifocal in origin.

MORPHOLOGY AND MODES OF SPREAD

Almost all of these lesions are adenocarcinomas. The typical glandular epithelium is interspersed with a varying proportion of fibrous tissue. Hilar and extrahepatic tumors typically provoke a florid fibrotic reaction, while intrahepatic masses are mostly glandular with a less prominent fibrous component. Least commonly seen in Western practice, but more frequently in Southeast Asia, is the intraductal papillary type of tumor which presents as an obstructing plug of tumor tissue within the lumen of the ducts, often with considerable mucin production, similar to the intraductal mucin-producing tumors of the pancreas. Both intrahepatic and extrahepatic tumors show a strong tendency to spread along the duct walls while perineural and perilymphatic permeation are commonly found near the tumor margins. Intrahepatic tumors also spread by local metastasis which may be found as satellite lesions on imaging. Metastases to local and regional lymph nodes are common and transcoelomic spread produces peritoneal nodules. The intraductal papillary tumors spread primarily along the lumen of the ducts, so these patients tend to present with biliary obstruction at an early stage.

CLINICAL PRESENTATION

Most patients present with progressively increasing obstructive jaundice which is usually, but not always, painless. General malaise and weight loss are not uncommon, but acute cholangitis is a rare manifestation of cholangiocarcinoma prior to diagnostic or therapeutic interventions. In patients with pre-existing biliary tract disease—particularly PSC—diagnosis of cholangiocarcinoma is more difficult (see below).

TREATMENT

Surgical excision offers the only curative treatment but is successful in only a minority of cases. Liver transplantation is usually associated with rapid recurrence of disease and is not recommended at present. Trials of chemotherapy are continuing and for non-resectable patients, biliary tract stenting is used for palliation. Because surgical resection is the preferred treatment, pre-operative imaging to show the full extent of disease is of critical importance.

OBJECTIVES OF IMAGING

The presence of biliary duct dilatation should be established by ultrasonography, which will also indicate the level of obstruction, and may give a clear enough demonstration of the ducts to exclude gallstones as the cause of obstruction. The presence of a mass lesion, nodal involvement, and vascular invasion will be detectable in some cases, but small tumors are often undetectable at sonography. Peripheral cholangiocarcinomas usually appear as non-specific mass lesions on sonography and CT (see Chapter 6 for details). Hilar and extrahepatic tumors are more difficult to identify.

Computed tomography shows the approximate level of obstruction and will usually indicate the presence of an intrahepatic mass, although the edges of the tumor are usually unclear. Multiple phases of imaging give an indication of vascular involvement and lymph node disease may also be shown. Ascites and peritoneal deposits are rarely found at presentation, although a common feature of recurrence in the later stages of disease. The best indication of tumor extent is shown on images obtained about 10 minutes after contrast injection when prolonged retention of contrast is seen in the fibrous component of the tumor, but even so the full extent of tumor is not as readily shown on CT as on MRI. Small hilar or ductal tumors may be extremely difficult to show with CT, although thin slice techniques with multi-format reconstruction have had some success.

For bile duct lesions arising in or close to the head of the pancreas, endoscopic ultrasonography may be helpful in localizing the tumor, identifying lymph nodes and assessing vascular invasion, and biopsy samples may be obtainable. Contrast angiography may be needed in patients who are ineligible for MRI. The role of PET remains to be developed—currently its most useful contribution may be in detecting distant metastatic disease or recurrence after surgery.

The traditional approach to the diagnosis of cholangiocarcinoma also includes direct visualization of the biliary tree by ERCP or by percutaneous transhepatic cholangiography. Because the introduction of radiographic contrast into an obstructed biliary tree substantially increases the risk of cholangitis, external biliary drainage or stenting is often carried out at the same procedure. The presence of a stent, or an internal/external drain, itself appears to cause local inflammatory effects in the bile duct and/or in the pancreatic head, which make the interpretation of staging MRI more difficult.

The optimum approach is to obtain MRI before interventional procedures, even if it is expected that pre-operative biliary drainage would be indicated.

MRI TECHNIQUES

Thick slab MRCP is used to show the presence and level of obstruction. In addition to showing the anatomy of the involved ducts, it is important to examine the intraluminal contents to establish the presence of tumor nodules or stones within the ducts, so thin slice acquisitions are needed. 3D dynamic gadolinium-enhanced T1w imaging is used to identify the tumors and their local extent, including vascular invasion and lymph node disease. Arterial and venous phases are needed to look at local vascular anatomy, but it is critically important also to obtain delayed images about 10 minutes after contrast injection. After this delay, the fibrotic areas of tumor which appear relatively avascular in the early dynamic imaging, typically show their maximal enhancement. Only on these delayed images is the full extent of the tumor apparent in many cases. Even on delayed imaging however, the margins of intrahepatic extension from hilar tumors can be difficult to define and in these cases, and also in peripheral cholangiocarcinomas, T2w imaging after SPIO contrast allows the edge of the tumor to be visualized, and is also helpful in identifying satellite nodules and intrahepatic metastases elsewhere.

APPEARANCES ON MRI

Peripheral lesions are discussed in chapter 6. Central tumors tend to present earlier with duct obstruction and are usually smaller at the time of diagnosis. Their margins are typically very ill-defined and there is little or no contrast with the adjacent liver on unenhanced images. The characteristic feature is the presence of multiple dilated ducts, all converging and tapering fairly abruptly at the site of the obstructing mass. The tumors are hypovascular in arterial and portal phases with gadolinium, but like peripheral tumors, central lesions show delayed enhancement which persists. Delayed images show the full extent of the tumor, but intrahepatic extension is best seen after SPIO contrast, as are satellite lesions and intrahepatic metastases, which are not uncommon.

With hilar, perihilar, and distal cholangiocarcinomas, vascular involvement is a common and characteristic feature. The tumor may involve the main portal vein or its intrahepatic divisions. Encasement of the main left or right portal divisions is typical, and commonly results in atrophy of the affected lobe, more often the left than right. Venous obstruction leads to arterial hyper-perfusion of the affected segments, which may be persistent when chronic duct obstruction causes local fibrosis. A halo of hyper-perfused liver parenchyma may also be shown surrounding the tumor (corona enhancement). Distinction between reactive hyper-perfusion in peri-tumoral liver tissue, and an enhancing rim of active tumor, may be impossible on post-Gd images, but SPIO contrast uptake is less influenced by the perfusion changes and this distinction can be made on post-SPIO T2w imaging. The combination of lobar atrophy with dilated ducts and arterial hyper-perfusion points strongly towards to hilar cholangiocarcinoma, even when the tumor itself is small and difficult to define.

Unlike HCC, cholangiocarcinomas rarely spread along the lumen of the hepatic and portal vein branches, but spread along the ducts—usually in the wall, less commonly in the lumen—is common. With endoluminal papillary tumors, vascular changes are much less likely to occur. The major imaging features are of duct dilatation with intraluminal filling defects which may expand the ducts locally as well as producing upstream dilatation. Intraductal tumors, being formed largely of glandular tissue, show more marked enhancement with gadolinium than the typically fibrous hilar tumors.

Extrahepatic or distal cholangiocarcinomas usually present as a small mass causing common duct obstruction. As with hilar tumors, vascular involvement is common but in some cases the only evidence of tumor may be localized thickening of the wall of the bile duct. Tumors may occasionally arise in the cystic duct and when the gallbladder is involved, the distinction between cholangiocarcinoma and gallbladder cancer may be difficult (see below). Bile duct tumors arising within or adjacent to the head of the pancreas may be impossible to differentiate from pancreatic cancer on imaging or even at the time of surgery, but histological differentiation is usually possible.

Prolonged enhancement of a thickened duct wall is suggestive of infiltrative cholangiocarcinoma, but may be difficult to distinguish from the inflammatory reaction produced by placement of a stent. One helpful feature in such cases is that the acute inflammatory reaction around stents tends to enhance early and fade on delayed images whereas fibrotic strictures and tumors show slower and more prolonged enhancement.

Involvement of the hepatic arteries by tumor is an occasional finding, but is not usually a bar to surgical treatment. Lymph node metastasis is a common feature with the usual sites being between the IVC and main portal vein, along the gastro-hepatic ligament and adjacent to the head of pancreas. A significant proportion of patients who have otherwise resectable tumors are found at laparoscopy or surgery to be harbouring small peritoneal deposits. These are often impossible to detect pre-operatively, but if delayed post-contrast images show areas of peritoneal thickening either over the liver capsule or on the adjacent peritoneal surfaces, metastatic spread here is very likely.

DIFFERENTIAL DIAGNOSIS

Metastases may occasionally present with hilar obstruction when the differential diagnosis from cholangiocarcinoma will require biopsy or resection histology. Although it is not rare for metastases to obstruct intrahepatic bile ducts either locally or centrally, it is exceptional for metastatic tumor to invade the lumen of the ducts, so intraluminal tumor points towards cholangiocarcinoma. Conversely, cholangiocarcinoma often constricts or occludes the portal vein branches but uncommonly extends into the vessel lumen, and so the presence of intra-luminal tumor points towards metastatic disease.

Carcinoma of the gallbladder typically produces a heterogeneous tumor causing hilar obstruction which may be indistinguishable from hilar cholangiocarcinoma extending into the adjacent liver. The biology of these tumors, their modes of spread and the surgical options are sufficiently similar for their differentiation to be of only minor significance. More problematic is the distinction between hilar cholangiocarcinoma or gallbladder cancer and a Mirizzi syndrome—with stones in the gallbladder neck or cystic duct causing obstruction of the bile ducts at the liver hilum—which is occasionally associated with an inflammatory mass which may mimic a tumor. Early enhancement favours an inflammatory lesion but the appearances may overlap even at surgery, and histology may be needed to confirm the diagnosis.

When the biliary tract is affected by non-Hodgkin's lymphoma, it is usually in the form of enlarged nodes at the liver hilum which are typically associated with extensive nodal disease elsewhere in the abdomen. However, in occasional cases a solitary lymphoma may involve the bile duct and produce appearances very similar to those of a hilar cholangiocarcinoma.

Probably the most difficult differential diagnosis is that from benign strictures in patients with PSC. In patients with known PSC, a search for cholangiocarcinoma is often triggered by a worsening of symptoms, the development of new features such as weight loss or ascites, or a deterioration in liver function. In many such patients MRCP will show a dominant stricture and post-gadolinium imaging will usually reveal a localized mass. In some cases no mass can be found and localized thickening of the wall of the duct may be the only indication of a cholangiocarcinoma. However, a fibrous stricture may produce identical appearances and the distinction can only be made at histology. In other cases, imaging indicates widespread ductal disease but fails to localize a dominant stricture or tumor mass. In some such patients who have undergone liver transplantation, pathology of the explant specimen has revealed microscopic deposits of cholangiocarcinoma.

ILLUSTRATIVE FIGURES

Intraductal cholangiocarcinoma—Figures 1–3
Distal (extrahepatic) cholangiocarcinoma—Figures 4–9
Hilar cholangiocarcinoma—Figures 10–18
Effects of stenting—Figures 19–20
Cholangiocarcinoma with lymph node/peritoneal metastasis—Figures 21–25
Differentials—colorectal metastasis—Figures 26–27
Differentials—NHL, cystadenocarcinoma—Figures 28–29
Differentials—gallbladder cancer, Mirizzi—Figures 30–36
Differentials—PSC with strictures—Figures 37–43

REFERENCES

1. Khan SA, Davidson BR, Goldin R, et al. Guidelines for the diagnosis and treatment of cholangiocarcinoma: consensus document. Gut 2002; 51:1–9.
2. Lim JH. Cholangiocarcinoma: morphologic classification according to growth pattern and imaging findings. AJR Am J Roentgenol 2003; 181:819–827.

3. Lee WJ, Lim HK, Jang KM, et al. Radiologic spectrum of cholangiocarcinoma: emphasis on unusual manifestations and differential diagnoses. Radiographics 2001; 2:S97–S116.

4. Lee MG, Park KB, Shin YM, et al. Preoperative evaluation of hilar cholangiocarcinoma with contrast-enhanced three-dimensional fast imaging with steady-state precession magnetic resonance angiography: comparison with intraarterial digital subtraction angiography. World J Surg 2003; 27:278–283.

5. Guthrie JA, Ward J, Robinson PJ. Hilar cholangiocarcinomas: T2-weighted spin-echo and gadolinium-enhanced FLASH MR imaging. Radiology 1996; 201:347–351.

6. Altehoefer C, Ghanem N, Furtwangler A, et al. Breathhold unenhanced and gadolinium-enhanced magnetic resonance tomography and magnetic resonance cholangiography in hilar cholangiocarcinoma. Int J Colorectal Dis 2001; 16:188–192.

7. Lopera JE, Soto JA, Munera F. Malignant hilar and perihilar biliary obstruction: use of MR cholangiography to define the extent of biliary ductal involvement and plan percutaneous interventions. Radiology 2001; 220:90–96.

8. Zidi SH, Prat F, Le Guen O, Rondeau Y, Pelletier G. Performance characteristics of magnetic resonance cholangiography in the staging of malignant hilar strictures. Gut 2000; 46:103–106.

9. Manfredi R, Masselli G, Maresca G, et al. MR imaging and MRCP of hilar cholangiocarcinoma. Abdom Imaging 2003; 28:319–325.

10. Kim M-J, Michell DG, Ito K, Outwater EK. Biliary dilatation: differentiation of benign from malignant causes—value of adding conventional MR imaging to MR cholangiopancreatography. Radiology 2000; 214:173–181.

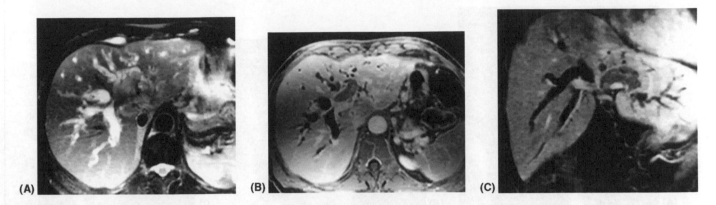

Figure 1. *Intraductal cholangiocarcinoma of papillary type*: Axial HASTE image (**A**) showed bi-lobar duct dilatation with intraluminal filling defects within the left lobe ducts. Axial (**B**) and RAO coronal (**C**) post-Gd T1w images showed intraluminal tumor occupying the main left hepatic duct and some of its branches with bi-lobar obstruction.

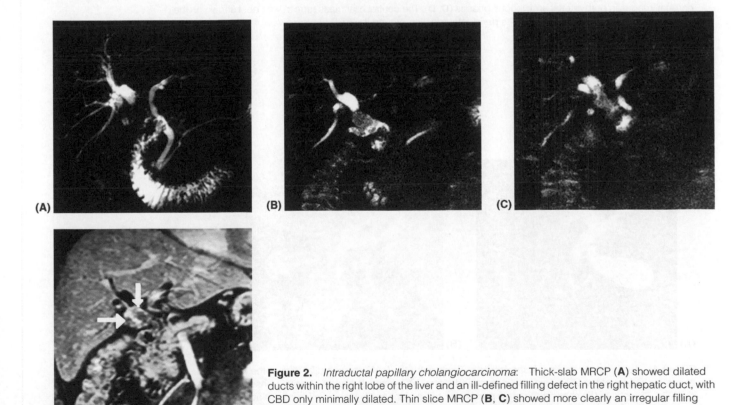

Figure 2. *Intraductal papillary cholangiocarcinoma*: Thick-slab MRCP (**A**) showed dilated ducts within the right lobe of the liver and an ill-defined filling defect in the right hepatic duct, with CBD only minimally dilated. Thin slice MRCP (**B**, **C**) showed more clearly an irregular filling defect within the ducts. RAO coronal post-Gd T1w image (**D**) confirmed a rounded tumor mass at the liver hilum showing patchy enhancement (arrows).

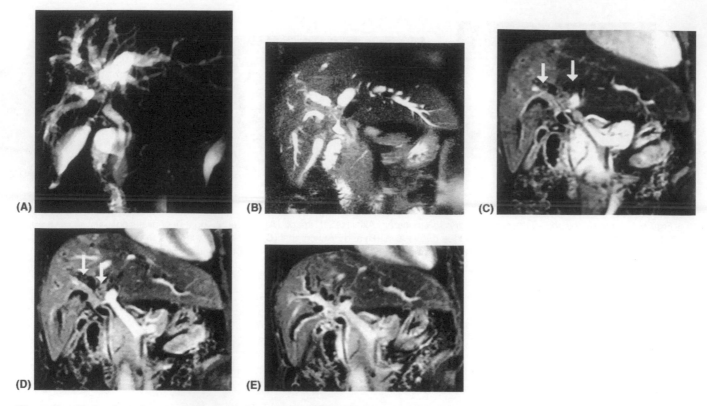

Figure 3. *Cholangiocarcinoma with intraluminal extension*: MRCP (**A**) showed a hilar stricture involving left and right hepatic ducts, CHD and cystic duct, with a lower CBD of normal caliber. Coronal HASTE image (**B**) showed the extensive peri-hilar mass infiltrating between the major ducts causing multiple strictures (Bismuth type IV). Tumor nodules within the lumen of ducts (arrows) close to the hilum were visible on post-Gd T1w coronal images in both arterial and venous phases (**C**, **D**). The central hilar mass (arrow) was best shown on the delayed image (**E**) which also highlights periductal reaction around the CBD.

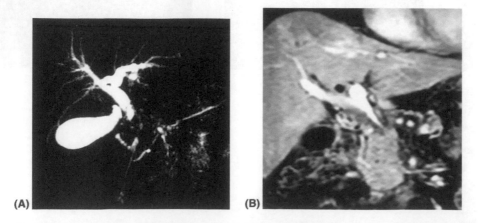

Figure 4. *Extrahepatic cholangiocarcinoma*: Thick slab MRCP (**A**) showed dilatation of the biliary tree above a stricture of the CBD. Pancreatic duct and distal CBD were not dilated. Venous phase images from post-Gd T1w series (**B**) showed the main portal vein to be strictured by a circumferential plaque of tumor (arrow) which was also obstructing the CBD (**C**). Arterial MIP from the post-Gd T1w series (**D**) showed encasement of the gastroduodenal artery. (*Continued*)

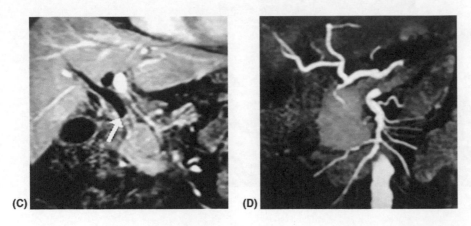

(C)

(D)

Figure 4. (*Continued*)

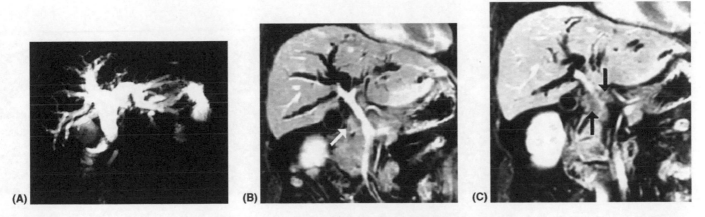

(A)

(B)

(C)

Figure 5. *Extrahepatic cholangiocarcinoma:* Thick slab MRCP (**A**) showed diffuse dilatation of the biliary tree above a stricture in CBD—note distal end of CBD was not dilated. RAO coronal post-Gd T1w venous phase images (**B, C**) showed abnormal enhancement in the tumor surrounding CBD (arrows). The right side of the lower end of portal vein showed minor irregularity suggesting local invasion here.

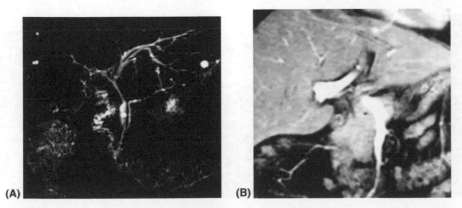

(A)

(B)

Figure 6. *Extrahepatic cholangiocarcinoma:* Thick slab MRCP (**A**) showed only mild dilatation of the left lobe ducts—the right lobe ducts were decompressed by the presence of a stent. RAO coronal post-Gd T1w images in early and late venous phase (**B, C**) showed low-signal tumor mass surrounding the duct between the hilum of the liver and the head of the pancreas. Delayed 10-minute post-Gd T1w image (**D**) showed enhancement in the tumor (arrows). (*Continued*)

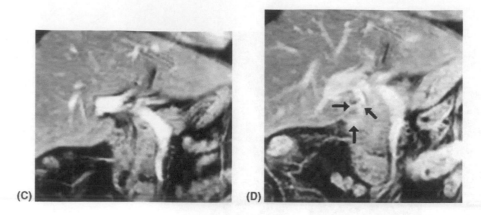

(C)　　(D)

Figure 6. (*Continued*)

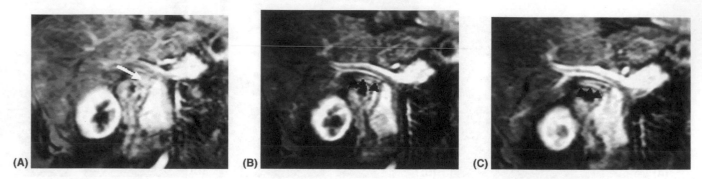

(A)　　(B)　　(C)

Figure 7. *Extrahepatic cholangiocarcinoma:* RAO coronal post-Gd T1 image in late arterial phase (**A**) showed a tumor nodule (arrow) adjacent to the intensely enhancing head of pancreas. Slightly more anterior slices (**B**, **C**) showed localized thickening of the common duct (arrowheads) immediately superior to head of pancreas.

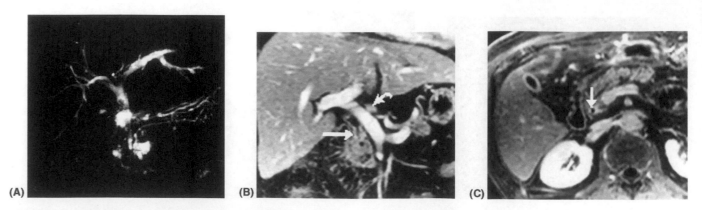

(A)　　(B)　　(C)

Figure 8. *Extrahepatic cholangiocarcinoma:* Thick slab MRCP (**A**) showed dilatation of the biliary tree above strictured CBD. The pancreatic duct was not dilated. RAO coronal post-Gd T1w image in portal venous phase (**B**) showed a tumor nodule stricturing the CBD at the margin of the pancreatic head (arrow). Note the enlarged porto-caval lymph node (curved arrow). Axial delayed phase post-Gd T1w image (**C**) showed irregular enhancement around the CBD at the site of the tumor (arrow).

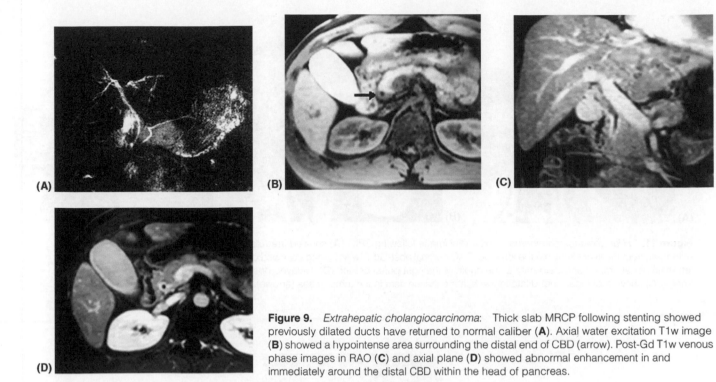

Figure 9. *Extrahepatic cholangiocarcinoma:* Thick slab MRCP following stenting showed previously dilated ducts have returned to normal caliber (**A**). Axial water excitation T1w image (**B**) showed a hypointense area surrounding the distal end of CBD (arrow). Post-Gd T1w venous phase images in RAO (**C**) and axial plane (**D**) showed abnormal enhancement in and immediately around the distal CBD within the head of pancreas.

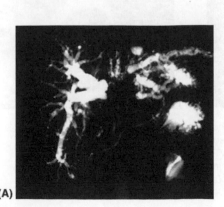

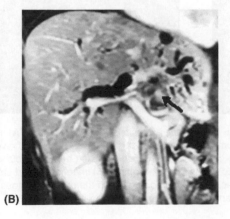

Figure 10. *Hilar cholangiocarcinoma:* Thick slab MRCP (**A**) showed bi-lobar obstruction at the liver hilum, normal pancreatic duct and distal CBD. RAO coronal post-Gd T1w image in venous phase (**B**) showed a heterogeneous tumor mass (arrow) centered to the left of the portal vein bifurcation, but obstructing both left and right hepatic ducts.

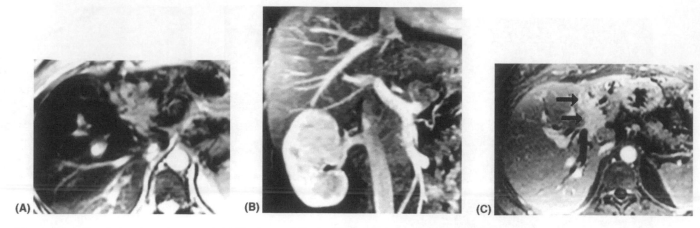

Figure 11. *Hilar cholangiocarcinoma*:   Axial T2w image following SPIO (**A**) showed irregular tumor extending from the liver hilum into the left lobe. RAO coronal post-Gd T1w MIP image showed occlusion of the left main portal branch and deformity at the origin of the right portal branch (**B**). Delayed post-Gd T1w axial image (**C**) showed bi-lobar duct dilatation with late enhancement in the tumor mass (arrows).

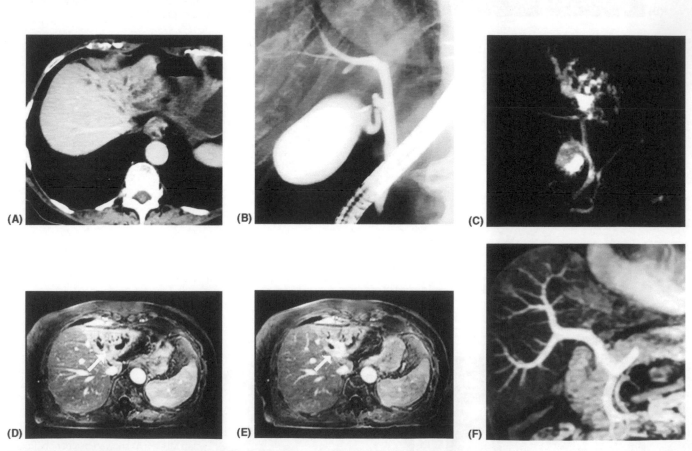

Figure 12. *Hilar cholangiocarcinoma with intrahepatic extension*:   Post-contrast CT (**A**) showed dillated ducts within an atrophic left lobe but the tumor mass could not be defined. ERCP (**B**) showed obstruction of the left hepatic duct. Thick slab MRCP (**C**) confirmed obstruction of the left hepatic ducts with upstream dilatation. Axial post-Gd T1w venous phase (**D**) and delayed phase (**E**) images showed an irregular tumor which was hypointense on the early images, but enhanced brightly on the delayed images (arrows). RAO coronal MIP in venous phase (**F**) showed amputation of the left main portal branch.

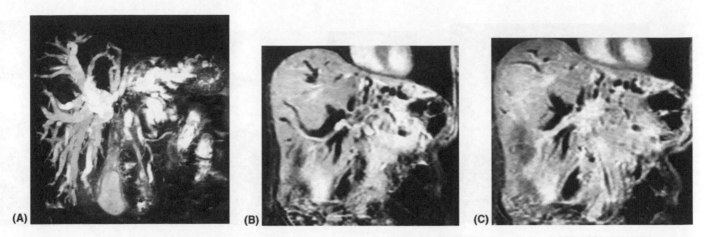

Figure 13. *Hilar cholangiocarcinoma with intrahepatic extension*: Thick slab MRCP (**A**) showed gross dilatation of all the intrahepatic ducts. RAO coronal post-Gd T1w images in venous phase (**B**) and delayed phase (**C**) showed an ill-defined tumor mass at the liver hilum with delayed enhancement.

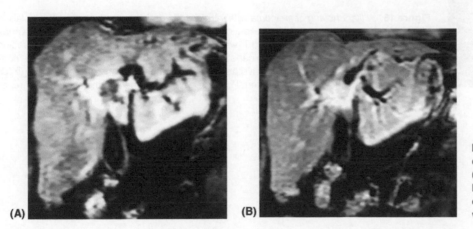

Figure 14. *Hilar cholangiocarcinoma*: RAO coronal post-Gd T1w images in arterial phase (**A**) and delayed phase (**B**) showed an initially hypovascular mass at the hilum which enhanced brightly on delayed images and was obstructing the left intrahepatic ducts.

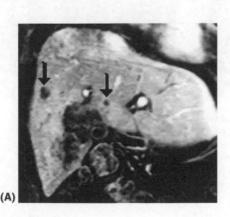
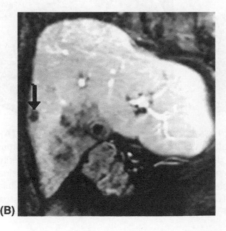

Figure 15. *Hilar cholangiocarcinoma with intrahepatic extension and metastases*: RAO coronal venous phase post-Gd T1w images (**A**, **B**) showed an irregular heterogeneous tumor at the hilum with small hypointense lesions in the adjacent parenchyma (arrows).

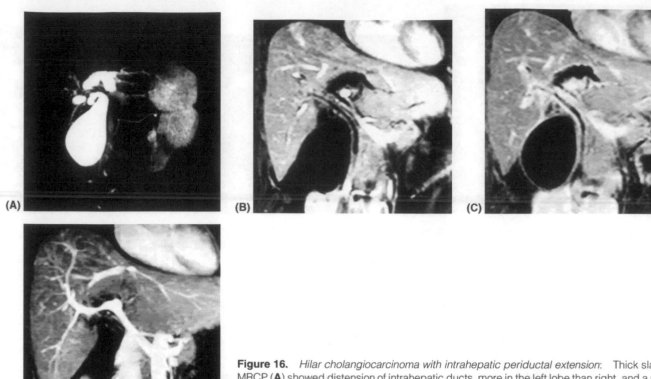

Figure 16. *Hilar cholangiocarcinoma with intrahepatic periductal extension*: Thick slab MRCP (**A**) showed distension of intrahepatic ducts, more in the left lobe than right, and a normal pancreatic duct. RAO coronal post-Gd T1w images showed abnormal soft tissue surrounding a stent in the right hepatic and common hepatic ducts (**B**) which showed marked enhancement in delayed images (**C**) indicating extensive periductal infiltration. Venous phase MIP image (**D**) showed amputation of the left main portal branch and encasement of the right portal branch.

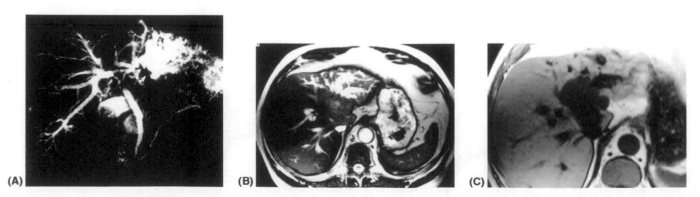

Figure 17. *Hilar cholangiocarcinoma with intrahepatic extension*: Thick slab MRCP (**A**) showed ductal obstruction at the hilum with particular dilatation of the left lobe ducts. Axial true FISP image (**B**) showed typical appearance of converging dilated ducts in the left lobe but the outline of the perihilar mass was not clear. Unenhanced axial in-phase (**C**) and opposed-phase (**D**) T1w images showed a clear-cut area of fatty change affecting segment 8. Axial T2w post-SPIO image (**E**) showed the edge of the perihilar tumor extending into the right lobe. RAO coronal post-Gd T1w image showed the hypovascular tumor encroaching on the main portal vein and occluding its left branch (**F**). (*Continued*)

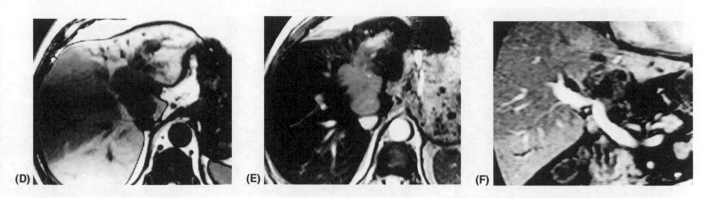

Figure 17. (*Continued*)

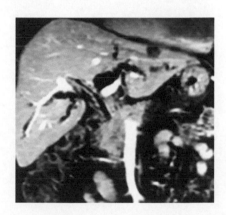

Figure 18. *Hilar cholangiocarcinoma with left lobe metastasis*: RAO coronal post-Gd T1w image showed bi-lobar duct dilatation with abnormal soft tissue surrounding the CHD and right main hepatic duct, which had been previously stented. Note also a hypointense nodule (metastasis) in the superior aspect of the left lobe.

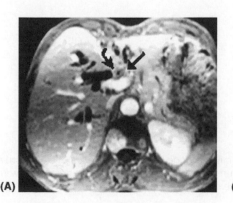
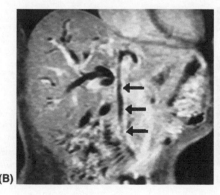

Figure 19. *Effects of stenting*: Periductal extension of tumor was present in both left and right lobes, but the left lobe had been previously stented. In axial (**A**) and RAO coronal (**B**) post-Gd T1w images, local enhancement was seen around the stented duct (arrows), while the non-stented right hepatic duct, which was also involved with tumor, showed much less enhancement [curved arrow in (**A**)]. Diagnosis—hilar cholangiocarcinoma with intrahepatic periductal extension.

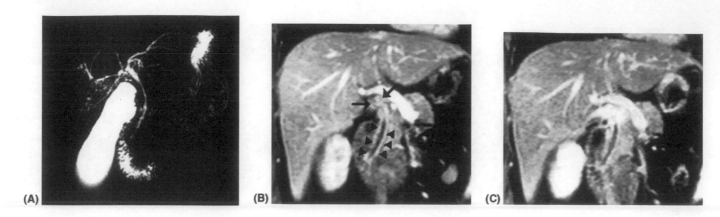

Figure 20.   *Effects of stenting:*   Following placement of a stent, thick slab MRCP (**A**) showed only minimal dilatation of the intrahepatic ducts. RAO coronal post-Gd T1w image in venous phase (**B**) showed increased enhancement of the wall of the CBD surrounding the stent (arrowheads), with an isointense irregular tumor at CHD level (arrows). Delayed imaging (**C**) showed brightly enhancing tumor infiltration around the CHD, but the early enhancement in the wall of CBD had faded. Diagnosis—cholangiocarcinoma confined to hilar region, with periductal inflammatory reaction induced by presence of stent.

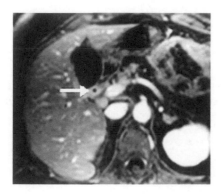

Figure 21.   *Extrahepatic cholangiocarcinoma with lymph node metastasis:*   Axial post-Gd T1w image showed localized thickening of the CBD (arrow) with no tumor mass. Note the enlarged lymph node lying between the CBD and the IVC.

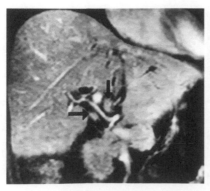

Figure 22.   *Cholangiocarcinoma in PSC with lymph node metastasis:*   Typical site of lymph node spread from cholangiocarcinoma was shown in this RAO coronal arterial phase post-Gd T1w image with enlarged nodes medial and lateral to the common hepatic artery (arrows).

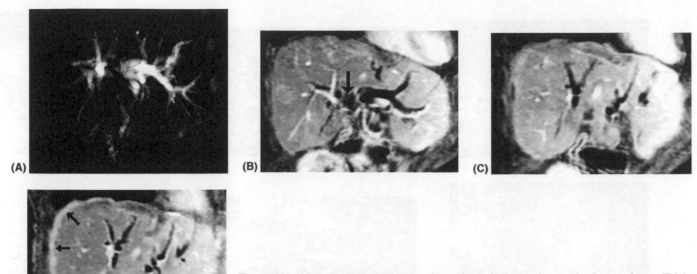

Figure 23. *Hilar cholangiocarcinoma with peritoneal metastasis over the liver surface*: Thick slab MRCP (**A**) showed bi-lobar obstruction by a hilar mass. RAO coronal post-Gd T1w image in venous phase (**B**) showed the hypointense tumor at the hilum (arrow). More anterior slices in the portal venous phase (**C**) showed enhancement over the liver surface which became more intense on delayed imaging [arrows in (**D**)].

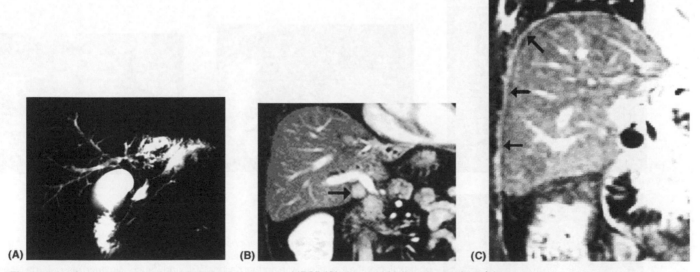

Figure 24. *Cholangiocarcinoma with peritoneal spread*: MRCP (**A**) showed bi-lobar obstruction of the intrahepatic ducts with atrophy of the left lobe. Post-Gd T1w venous phase coronal image (**B**) showed obstruction of the left portal vein branch and a prominent enlarged node at the porta hepatis (arrow). Delayed post-Gd T1w image (**C**) showed patchy enhancement of the diaphragmatic and parietal peritoneum (arrows) indicating peritoneal metastasis, confirmed at laparoscopic biopsy.

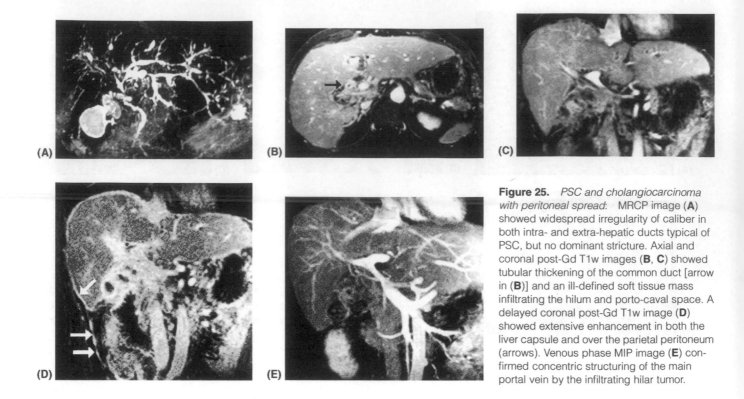

Figure 25. *PSC and cholangiocarcinoma with peritoneal spread*: MRCP image (**A**) showed widespread irregularity of caliber in both intra- and extra-hepatic ducts typical of PSC, but no dominant stricture. Axial and coronal post-Gd T1w images (**B**, **C**) showed tubular thickening of the common duct [arrow in (**B**)] and an ill-defined soft tissue mass infiltrating the hilum and porto-caval space. A delayed coronal post-Gd T1w image (**D**) showed extensive enhancement in both the liver capsule and over the parietal peritoneum (arrows). Venous phase MIP image (**E**) confirmed concentric structuring of the main portal vein by the infiltrating hilar tumor.

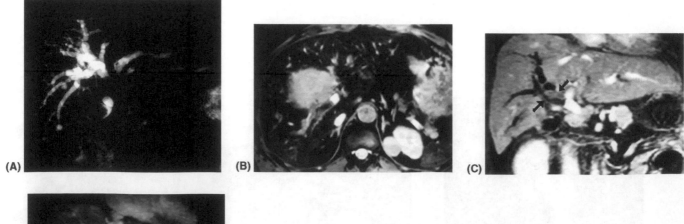

Figure 26. *Differential diagnosis: hilar cholangiocarcinoma or colorectal metastasis?*: In a patient with a history of previous colonic carcinoma, thick slab MRCP (**A**) showed bi-lobar obstruction at the liver hilum with normal caliber CBD and pancreatic duct, also a large stone in the gallbladder. Post-SPIO T2w images (**B**) showed a perihilar tumor extending into the right lobe. RAO coronal post-Gd T1w image (**C**) showed a hilar mass obstructing the right-sided ducts and invading the right portal vein (arrows). Venous phase MIP (**D**) confirmed occlusion of the right main portal branch by tumor. Histology—colorectal metastasis.

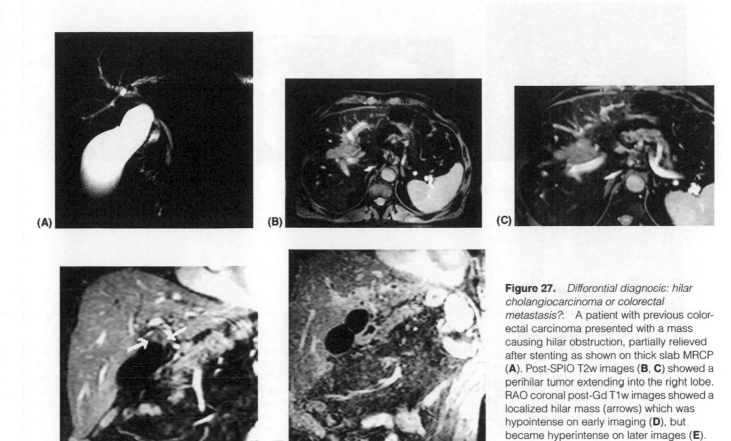

Figure 27. *Differential diagnosis: hilar cholangiocarcinoma or colorectal metastasis?:* A patient with previous colorectal carcinoma presented with a mass causing hilar obstruction, partially relieved after stenting as shown on thick slab MRCP (**A**). Post-SPIO T2w images (**B**, **C**) showed a perihilar tumor extending into the right lobe. RAO coronal post-Gd T1w images showed a localized hilar mass (arrows) which was hypointense on early imaging (**D**), but became hyperintense on later images (**E**). Biopsy—cholangiocarcinoma.

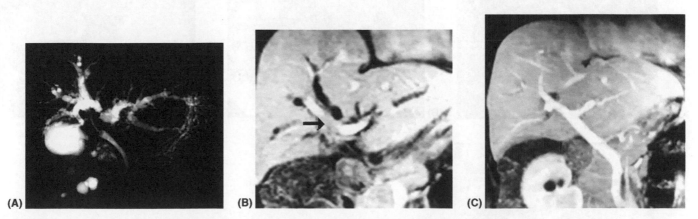

Figure 28. *Differential diagnosis: cholangiocarcinoma or NHL ?:* A patient with previous non-Hodgkin's lymphoma, but no other evidence of active disease, presented with a first episode of jaundice. Thick slab MRCP (**A**) showed a stricture involving the left and right hepatic ducts and CHD. RAO coronal post-Gd T1w image in venous phase (**B**) showed an isointense hilar mass (arrow), closely related to the portal vein bifurcation. Venous phase MIP (**C**) showed no evidence of vascular invasion. Histology—NHL.

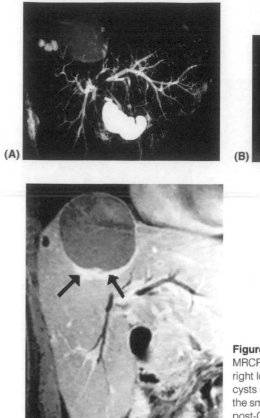

(A)

(B)

(C)

(D)

Figure 29. *Differential diagnosis: cystadenocarcinoma or cholangiocarcinoma?.* Thick slab MRCP (**A**) showed a hilar stricture with bi-lobar obstruction, also a cluster of small cysts in the right lobe and a large right lobe mass only faintly visible. Axial T2w image (**B**) showed the small cysts and the large mass to be equally hyperintense. Axial unenhanced T1w image (**C**) showed the small cysts to be hypointense, while the large mass was hyperintense. RAO coronal delayed post-Gd T1w imaging (**D**) showed a large cystic mass with a late-enhancing plaque of tumor in its inferior aspect (arrows). Histology—cholangiocarcinoma invading a simple cyst.

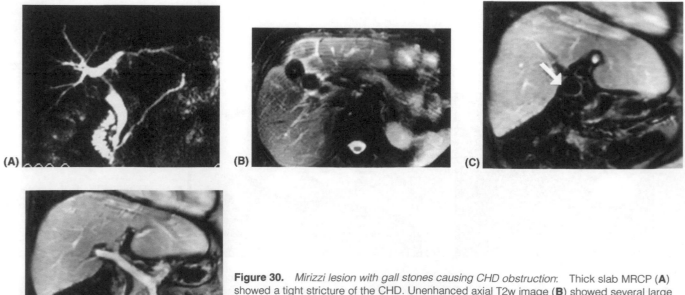

(A)

(B)

(C)

(D)

Figure 30. *Mirizzi lesion with gall stones causing CHD obstruction:* Thick slab MRCP (**A**) showed a tight stricture of the CHD. Unenhanced axial T2w image (**B**) showed several large stones in the gallbladder encroaching on the liver hilum. RAO coronal post-Gd T1w image in venous phase (**C**) showed the CHD stretched over the surface of an adjacent stone (arrowed). Portal venous phase MIP (**D**) showed no sign of vascular involvement.

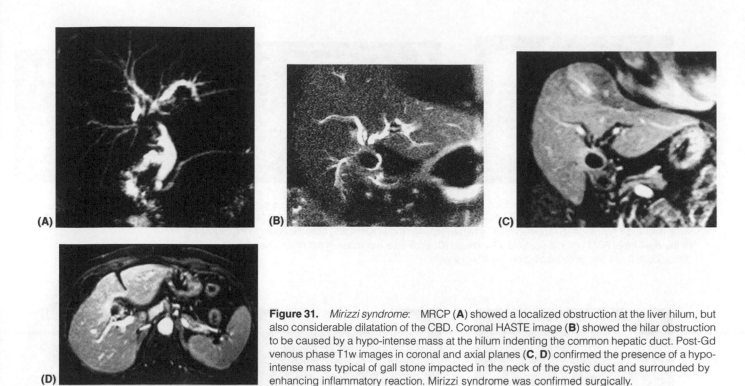

Figure 31. *Mirizzi syndrome*: MRCP (**A**) showed a localized obstruction at the liver hilum, but also considerable dilatation of the CBD. Coronal HASTE image (**B**) showed the hilar obstruction to be caused by a hypo-intense mass at the hilum indenting the common hepatic duct. Post-Gd venous phase T1w images in coronal and axial planes (**C**, **D**) confirmed the presence of a hypo-intense mass typical of gall stone impacted in the neck of the cystic duct and surrounded by enhancing inflammatory reaction. Mirizzi syndrome was confirmed surgically.

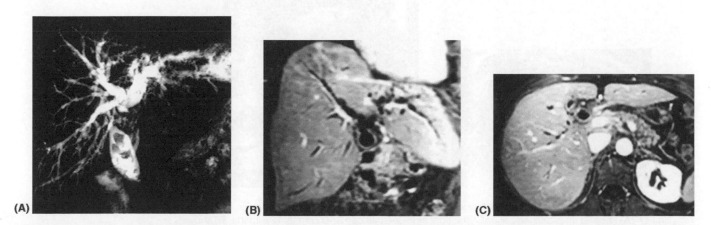

Figure 32. *Mirizzi syndrome*: MRCP (**A**) showed obstruction at the liver hilum with dilated ducts in both left and right lobes and normal caliber CBD, with numerous angular stones in the gallbladder. Coronal and axial post-Gd T1w images (**B**, **C**) showed no evidence of a mass or vascular involvement but a circumscribed hypointense lesion representing an impacted stone in the neck of the gallbladder, which was obstructing the hepatic duct at the porta hepatis.

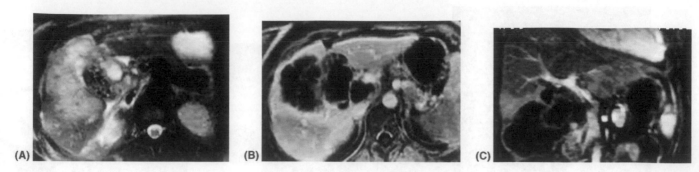

Figure 33. *Carcinoma of the gallbladder.*   Axial unenhanced T2w image (**A**) showed a heterogeneous mass involving much of the right lobe and extending into the hilum, and involving the stone-filled gallbladder. Axial post-Gd T1w image (**B**) showed a large heterogeneous tumor extending from the hilum to the periphery of the right lobe. RAO coronal post-Gd T1w image (**C**) showed the position of the mass arising in the gallbladder fossa and encroaching on the hilar vessels.

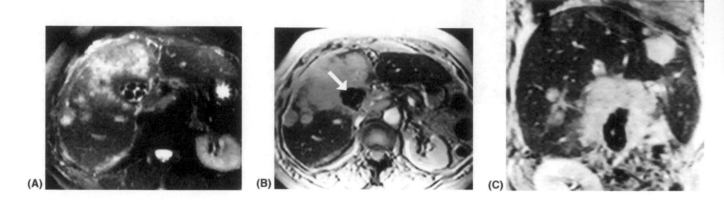

Figure 34. *Carcinoma of the gallbladder with metastases:*   Unenhanced axial T2w image (**A**) showed a large heterogeneous tumor with satellite lesions involving both left and right lobes, and enclosing a stone-filled gallbladder centrally. Axial post-SPIO T2w image (**B**) showed the tumor margins more clearly and highlighted the enclosed gall stones (arrow), which were again visible on the RAO coronal post-SPIO T2w image (**C**) which also showed metastases in both left and right lobes.

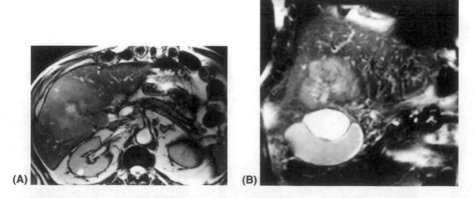

Figure 35. *Carcinoma of the gallbladder with intrahepatic extension and local metastases:*   Axial true FISP image (**A**) showed an ill-defined centrally placed tumor. Unenhanced RAO coronal T2w image (**B**) showed an ill-defined tumor mass in the right lobe associated with cystic elements inferiorly, with fluid components of differing characteristics. RAO coronal post-Gd T1w images showed a heterogenous tumor with satellite lesions and gallbladder involvement with more marked enhancement in the early phase (**C**) than in the portal venous phase (**D**). (*Continued*)

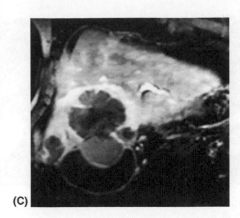

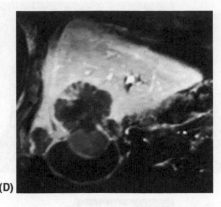

(C)   (D)   **Figure 35.** (*Continued*)

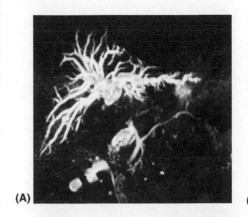

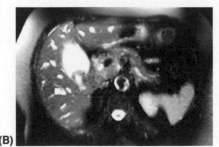

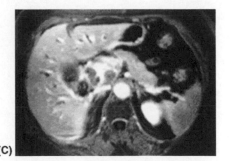

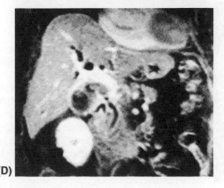

(A)   (B)   (C)

(D)

Figure 36. *Carcinoma of the gallbladder producing hilar obstruction*: MRCP (**A**) showed generalised dilatation of the intrahepatic ducts with CBD and pancreatic duct of normal caliber. Axial HASTE image (**B**) showed a polypoid filling defect in the neck of the gallbladder, contiguous with an ill-defined iso-intense hilar mass. Axial and coronal post-Gd T1w images (**C**, **D**) both showed a lobulated tumor mass extending from the position of the gallbladder neck to encase the portal vein and common hepatic duct.

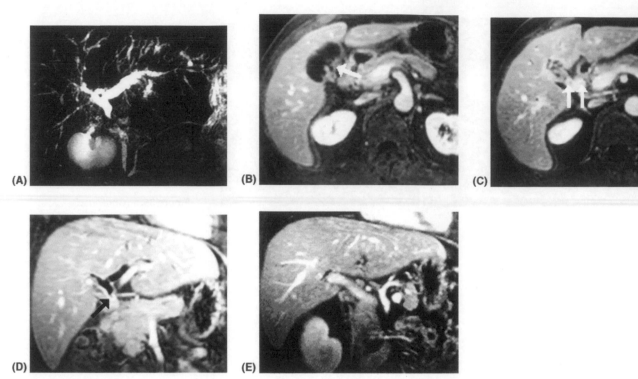

Figure 37. *Gallbladder carcinoma in PSC:* MRCP (**A**) showed widespread intrahepatic duct changes typical of PSC, with a dominant stricture at the level of insertion of cystic duct into common hepatic duct. Note also the deformity of the superior wall of the gallbladder. Axial post-Gd T1w images in venous phase (**B, C**) showed nodular thickening of the supero-medial wall of the gallbladder [arrow in (**B**)] with intense enhancement of the thickened cystic duct and common hepatic duct [arrows in (**C**)]. Coronal post-Gd T1w images in venous phase (**D**) showed a concentric mass around the brightly enhancing hepatic duct [arrow in (**D**)] and a slightly more posterior coronal oblique image (**E**) showed enlarged lymph nodes on both sides of the portal vein.

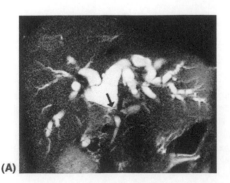

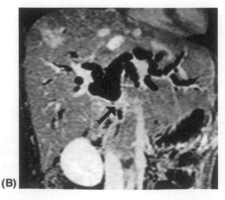

Figure 38. *Differential diagnosis: cholangio-carcinoma or benign stricture?:* In a patient with no previous history of PSC, a hilar stricture with suspicion of an intraluminal mass (arrow) was shown on thick slab MRCP (**A**). Delayed RAO post-Gd T1 imaging (**B**) confirmed an enhancing nodule within the CHD (arrow). The pre-operative diagnosis was of intraductal cholangiocarcinoma; the histology of resected specimen showed only inflammatory fibrosis, no tumor.

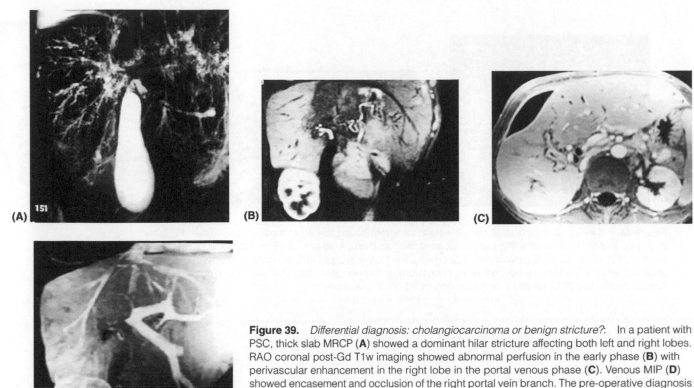

Figure 39. *Differential diagnosis: cholangiocarcinoma or benign stricture?.* In a patient with PSC, thick slab MRCP (**A**) showed a dominant hilar stricture affecting both left and right lobes. RAO coronal post-Gd T1w imaging showed abnormal perfusion in the early phase (**B**) with perivascular enhancement in the right lobe in the portal venous phase (**C**). Venous MIP (**D**) showed encasement and occlusion of the right portal vein branch. The pre-operative diagnosis was of cholangiocarcinoma complicating PSC; resection histology showed fibrosis only, no tumor.

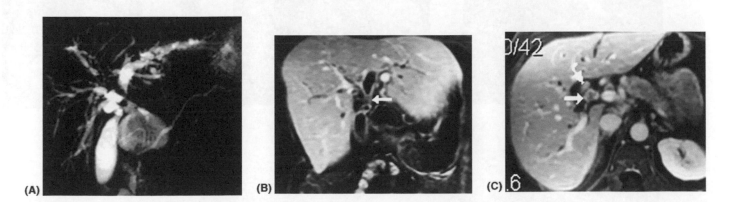

Figure 40. *Differential diagnosis: cholangiocarcinoma or benign stricture?.* In a patient with known PSC, thick slab MRCP (**A**) showed a dominant hilar stricture. RAO coronal post-Gd T1w image (**B**) showed a soft tissue nodule lying in the CHD and obstructing both left and right hepatic ducts (arrow). Axial post-Gd T1w imaging (**C**) also showed irregular thickening and enlargement of the CHD in the hepatic hilum (arrow) with an enlarged node lying anteriorly (curved arrow). Pre-operative diagnosis was of cholangiocarcinoma complicating PSC; resection histology showed fibrosis, no tumor.

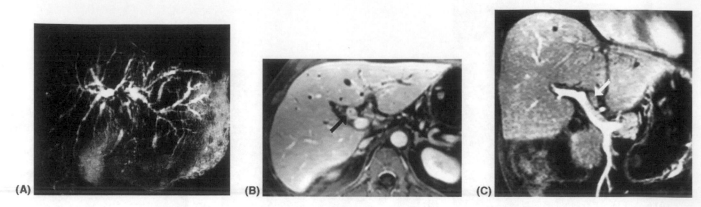

Figure 41. *Differential diagnosis: cholangiocarcinoma or benign stricture?.* In a patient with known PSC, thick slab MRCP (**A**) showed a dominant stricture at the liver hilum. Axial post-Gd T1w image (**B**) showed localized but eccentric thickening of the CHD (arrow). RAO coronal post-Gd T1w image (**C**) showed an enlarged lymph node (arrow), but no vascular compromise. Pre-operative diagnosis was of cholangiocarcinoma complicating PSC; resection histology confirmed cholangiocarcinoma.

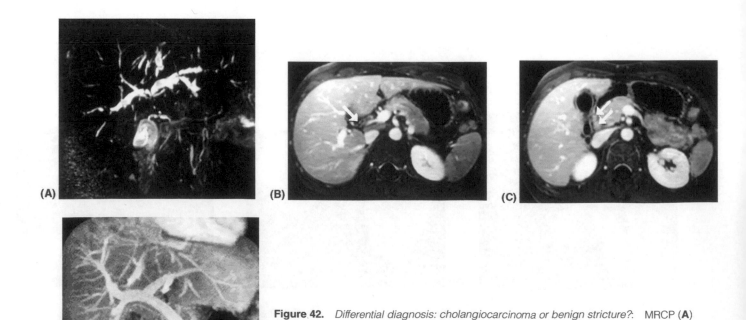

Figure 42. *Differential diagnosis: cholangiocarcinoma or benign stricture?.* MRCP (**A**) showed a hilar obstruction with intrahepatic duct abnormalities typical of PSC. Venous phase post-Gd T1w axial image (**B**) showed no mass, but tubular thickening of the CBD (arrow). Enlarged nodes (arrows) were shown on a more caudal slice (**C**). Venous phase MIP image (**D**) showed no venous involvement. Histology at transplantation showed no evidence of malignancy.

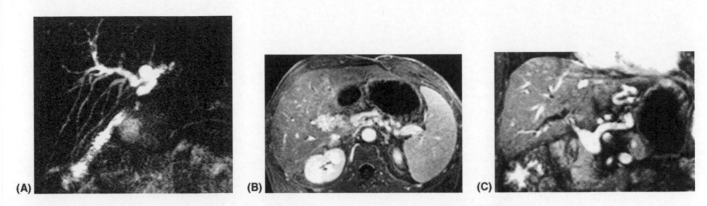

Figure 43. *Recurrent hilar cholangiocarcinoma or fibrotic stricture?:*   A patient underwent transplantation for PSC, and a small cholangiocarcinoma was discovered at pathology of the explanted liver. The patient developed jaundice 3 years later, and MRCP (**A**) showed obstruction of left and right hepatic ducts by a stricture at the site of choledochojejunostomy. Axial post-Gd T1w image (**B**) showed cavernous transformation of the transplant portal vein while the coronal post-Gd T1w image (**C**) showed stenosis of the portal vein at the liver neo-hilum, with large varices arising from the gastric coronary vein. No malignancy was found on biopsy, and after stenting the patient was well 18 months later.

CHAPTER 14

Some Unsolved Problems in Liver Imaging

387

LIMITATIONS IN DETECTING SMALL VOLUME DISEASE

Assessments of the sensitivity of imaging techniques for detecting metastases are heavily dependent on the method used to establish the absence of disease—how "true" are the "true negative" cases. Direct examination of the liver by an experienced surgeon assisted by intra-operative ultrasound will reveal additional metastases in a small proportion of patients (about 6% in our experience) compared with optimum pre-operative imaging. Pathological examination of the excised liver specimen, particularly if sliced at 3–4 mm intervals, occasionally detects further very small lesions.

Currently, with SPIO-enhanced MRI, we are detecting about 90% of metastases in these surgical cases, including 65–75% of sub-cm sized lesions. The existence of undetected disease in the residual liver segments after resections is confirmed by the significant incidence of recurrent metastases at new sites in the post-operative population. For further improvements in the treatment of liver metastases, we need to improve our imaging to detect smaller lesions with greater certainty.

Liver metastases all start out as microscopic deposits, and it has been estimated that the average age of colorectal metastases at the time of diagnosis is 2–3 years. Pathologic observations have consistently confirmed the presence of micro-metastases in terminal portal venules, and recent studies using optical microscopy in mice have demonstrated how tumor emboli become established as metastatic deposits in the liver parenchyma. All this circumstantial evidence confirms the view that livers which appear macroscopically normal in some patients with primary colorectal cancer (and other tumors) often harbour microscopic metastases. With this background, it would appear that attempts to clear the liver of metastatic disease by surgical resection or thermal ablation—macroscopic methods—are unlikely to succeed. In practice however, the five year survival of patients undergoing hepatic resection for colorectal metastases has improved from about 20–25% 15 years ago to 45–50% in the current decade. Concurrently, the proportion of patients in whom surgical resection is deemed worthwhile has increased. The net effect is that more extensive disease is being treated more aggressively and more often. This major increase in surgical treatment has been facilitated not only be improvements in surgical techniques, anaesthesia, and peri-operative care, but also by more consistently effective pre-operative imaging. With current techniques, we should now detect virtually all metastases larger than 1 cm, and also a significant proportion of lesions in the 5–9 mm range. Still, with non-invasive imaging we fail to find some lesions which are macroscopically detectable by other means, and all sub-mm foci of tumor remain occult.

How to Do Better with MRI

In order to detect smaller lesions we need to improve two aspects of imaging—spatial resolution, and contrast between tumor, and normal tissue. Improving the spatial resolution of MRI, given the large field of view needed to encompass the liver, could be achieved by increasing the field strength to give better signal to noise ratio (SNR), or by increasing gradient strength. Although early results using 3T show some promise, at the time of writing the degree of improvement available with this approach remains uncertain. Parallel imaging improves temporal resolution and so may help to eliminate or minimize motion artifacts which is a significant limitation of image quality in some patients, but at the expense of some reduction in SNR.

Improving Contrast Resolution

To detect tiny mass lesions, we need to maximize the contrast between tumor and liver. Currently available liver-specific contrast media allow us to do this either by eliminating the signal from normal liver on T2*w imaging while leaving the tumor signal unaffected (SPIO) or by maximizing liver signal while leaving tumor tissue unaffected (T1 agents in hepatocyte phase). Each of these approaches has specific limitations, but both offer the potential to improve on current results.

Attributes of SPIO-Enhanced Imaging

Metastases have no Kupffer cells so they take up no SPIO. Current acquisition techniques are limited by SNR—we need thinner slices with better SNR to detect smaller lesions. A second limitation of T2*w post-SPIO imaging is that small lesions may be confused with vessels. This distinction should be feasible by obtaining dynamic T1W images after initial SPIO injection. Distinction of metastases from small benign lesions can usually be achieved by comparing the post-SPIO T2w images with pre-contrast FSE or HASTE images.

Finally, it is not yet clear at what microscopic level the field distortion produced by iron particles would obliterate the signal from adjacent tumor—how big is the field inhomogeneity effect produced by SPIO particles within a single Kupffer cell?

Attributes of Tissue-Specific T1 Agents

Compared with T2*w imaging, T1w imaging has the advantage of better SNR, so existing 3D sequences already offer spatial resolution in the 2–3 mm range. With most lesions, tumor-to-liver contrast is maximal in the hepatocyte phase, so high-resolution delayed T1w images offer the promise of increased sensitivity for small lesions. The problem of differentiating on delayed images small metastases from vessels seen in cross-section should be solved by comparing the same sections on the post-injection dynamic phase imaging. However, unlike SPIO, a significant proportion of the T1 agents remains in the extracellular fluid space, allowing diffusion of the contrast agent into tumors. Even on delayed images, when the enhancement effect in liver parenchyma mostly arises from intracellular retention of the contrast agent by hepatocytes, the tumor to liver signal difference is diminished by the presence of extracellular contrast within tumors.

The Problem of Specificity

Recent improvements in imaging resolution have allowed us to detect smaller liver lesions more effectively. Unfortunately, this improvement does not translate directly to an equal improvement in the early diagnosis of metastases, because of the relative high incidence of small benign malformations which were previously undiscovered and inconsequential. With better imaging, we may find many more small lesions, but differentiating early metastasis from incidental benign lesions has become problematic.

The question of the optimum slice thickness for liver examination using contrast-enhanced, multi-detector, multi-slice CT has recently been explored. The consistent finding of several different studies is that thinner slices allow more small lesions to be detected, not surprisingly. It is also clear that the majority of the additional lesions detected are benign malformations, even in patients with established malignant disease. Although thinner slices do allow us to find more small metastases, this advantage may be offset by the increased number of false positive findings.

In general, the smaller lesions are at the time of detection, the greater is our difficulty in distinguishing benign from malignant.

Although simple cysts are usually unmistakeable on heavily T2w images down to 2–3 mm size, the same is not true of other benign lesions. Tiny malformations which are probably hemangiomas, von Meyenburg complexes or biliary adenomas are being found more often on imaging, but can be very difficult to see or feel at surgery and may even escape the attention of the pathologist. We need a better understanding of the structure and natural history of these lesions and we need to explore in more detail their enhancement and signal characteristics, and correlate these with histology.

In conclusion, we need to continue seeking new approaches to improve the effective detection and recognition of small malignancies.

SMALL HYPERVASCULAR NODULES IN THE CIRRHOTIC LIVER

In order to understand our current difficulties in characterizing small hypervascular lesions in cirrhosis, we first need to look back at the recent evolution of our current state of knowledge. For many years it has been recognized that HCC is a fairly frequent complication of advanced cirrhosis. About 15 years ago, it became clear that the usual pathogenesis of HCC in cirrhosis was via stepwise de-differentiation of benign regenerative nodules through several stages to frank malignancy. The overlapping and somewhat confusing terminology (macroregenerative nodules, borderline nodules, adenomatous hyperplasia, adenomous hyperplasia with atypia, early HCC, early advanced HCC) that was used to describe these stages was effectively replaced about 10 years ago by a simple classification proposed by an international working party. We now have benign regenerative nodules, malignant HCC, and dysplastic or borderline nodules. Dysplastic nodules are sometimes sub-divided into high grade and low grade histology, and some authors separate early HCC on grounds of size and some histological features. In parallel with the improved understanding of pathology, imaging began to characterize the vascularity of these nodules. Because HCCs are characteristically hypervascular during the arterial phase of enhancement while regenerative and dysplastic nodules enhance most in the portal phase, it was argued that all hypervascular nodules in cirrhosis were likely to be HCCs. However, more recent evidence has shown that a small minority (about 5%) of HCCs remain hypovascular during the arterial phase, while a similar small proportion of histologically dysplastic nodules show arterial hypervascularity. Size remains an important discriminating feature—the larger a nodule is, the more likely it is to be malignant. Purely dysplastic nodules are rarely larger than 3–4 cm and in our experience of larger nodules which show the imaging features of dysplasia, foci of HCC have always been present at explant histology, even when not detected on imaging.

In the last 5 years, the use of thin slice CT and MRI with multiple phases of enhancement has allowed the more frequent detection of hypervascular nodules of sub-cm size. Although many of these small lesions are still confirmed as HCC in explant histology, there is now a substantial body of evidence from biopsy studies, resection specimens, and sequential imaging studies to show that a significant proportion of these nodules are non-malignant. Details of the histology vary between different reports, but the common features are that the hepatocytes appear normal, portal tracts are present, patchy or scar-like fibrosis is common, and there is an increase in unpaired arteries (which explains the hypervascularity). The histologic appearances described are similar to those of focal nodular hyperplasia, they overlap with the features of hyperplastic nodules found in chronic Budd-Chiari syndrome, and they show many similarities to nodular regenerative hyperplasia. Such nodules have been described in patients with autoimmune hepatitis and post-viral cirrhosis, but are most commonly found in patients with alcoholic liver disease.

So far there are few pointers from imaging studies to discriminate between benign and malignant hypervascular nodules of sub-cm size. There is evidence from multi-arterial phase MRI studies and also from studies using sonographic contrast agents that rapid washout of contrast is a common feature of small HCCs, whereas the enhancement of benign nodules persists into the portal phase. Another pointer is that nodules which are hyperintense on T2w imaging are very likely indeed to be malignant. However, possibly the most useful feature is one which has not yet been thoroughly explored—the use of liver-specific contrast agents, particularly SPIO. Our own experience suggests that nodules which fail to take up SPIO may be regarded as malignant and in the series from our own institution, explant histology has not shown HCC in small nodules which take up SPIO normally, even if they showed arterial hypervascularity with gadolinium. Further work in this area is continuing, meanwhile a practical approach to radiological decision-making is suggested in chapter 9.

REFERENCES

Detecting Small lesions

1. Ward J, Guthrie JA, Wilson D, et al. Colorectal hepatic metastases: detection with SPIO-enhanced breath-hold MR imaging—comparison of optimized sequences. Radiology 2003; 228:709–718.
2. Ward J, Robinson PJ, Guthrie JA, et al. Liver metastases in candidates for hepatic resection: comparison of helical CT and gadolinium- and SPIO-enhanced MR imaging. Radiology 2005; 237:170–180.
3. Finlay IG, Meek D, Brunton F, McArdle CS. Growth rate of hepatic metastases in colorectal carcinoma. Br J Surg 1988; 75:641–644.
4. Ishii S, Mizoi T, Kawano K, et al. Implantation of human colorectal cancer cells in the liver studiesd by in vivo fluorescence videomicroscopy. Clin Exp Metastasis 1996; 14:153–164.

Small Hypervascular Nodules in Cirrhosis

5. Kondo F, Koshima Y, Ebara M. Nodular lesions associated with abnormal liver circulation. Intervirology 2004; 47:277–287.
6. Nakashima O, Kurogi M, Yamaguchi R, et al. Unique hypervascular nodules in alcoholic liver cirrhosis: identical to focal nodular hyperplasia-like nodules? J Hepatol 2004; 31:992–998.
7. Sobue S, Nomura T, Nakao H, et al. Clinicopathological study of hepatic nodular lesions in patientes with alcoholic liver cirrhosis. Alcohol Clin Exp Res 2004; 28:186S–190S.

Index

Note: Italics indicate illustrative figures.